THIRD (ACADEMIC) EDITION
(Updated January 2022)

ARTIFICIAL INTELLIGENCE IN HEALTHCARE

AI, Machine Learning, and Deep and Intelligent Medicine
Simplified for Everyone

PARAG MAHAJAN, MD

MedMantra, LLC
New Mexico

Third Edition of "ARTIFICIAL INTELLIGENCE IN HEALTHCARE: AI, Machine Learning, and Deep and Intelligent Medicine Simplified for Everyone" by Parag Mahajan, MD

Published by MedMantra, LLC

1330 San Pedro Drive NE STE 205A, Albuquerque, NM 87110

MedMantra.com

ISBN: 978-1-954612-02-0 (Paperback)

ISBN: 978-1-954612-03-7 (eBook)

Library of Congress Control Number: 2021930824 | Permalink: https://lccn.loc.gov/2021930824

Register your copy:

First edition: July 2018 | Second edition: April 2019 | Third edition: February 2021

The 2nd edition was first updated and renamed as "General Edition" in April 2021 and further updated in January 2022

The 3rd edition was first updated and renamed as "Academic Edition" in April 2021 and further updated in January 2022

Register your copy of this book by following the instructions mentioned at MedMantra.com/aih

Registration entitles you to a completely free eBook of the next edition/update.

Speaker invitations and business consultation requests:

Contact the author by email (DrParag@MedMantra.com) for speaker invitations or business consultation requests.

DEDICATION

Nobody has been more important to me in the pursuit of writing this book than the members of my family. I would like to thank my parents, whose love and encouragement are with me in whatever I pursue. I would especially like to mention the forever cheerful attitude of my father, who maintained it even while recently being treated for stomach cancer. Most importantly, I wish to thank my loving and supportive wife, Anuradha, and my two wonderful daughters, Anoushka and Paavni, who provide unending inspiration. I would also like to thank my role models, Elon Musk and Stephen Hawking, who inspired me to delve into the quest of the unknown.

Artificial Intelligence (AI) in Healthcare - Professional Certification Courses - 100% Online

Learn at your own pace from the comfort of your home

Pioneered by MedMantra Academy

- **Level 1 (Basic) Course** (12 Modules) - **2-24 Weeks**

- **Level 2 (Executive) Course** (20 Modules) - **4-24 Weeks**

- **Level 3 (Expert) Course / Healthcare AI Application Programing Course** (10+ Projects & 3+ Tutorials) - **2-24 Weeks**

- **Courses starting from US$ 99**

ENROLL NOW!

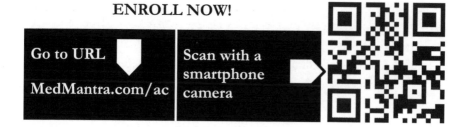

| Go to URL | Scan with a |
| MedMantra.com/ac | smartphone camera |

Claim Your Surprise Gift

Thank you for checking out my book. To show my appreciation, I've prepared a special gift for all my readers that will help you master all aspects of artificial intelligence in healthcare. The gift is in the form of regularly updated & free bonus articles, videos, training courses, and lots more...

Access it by visiting: MedMantra.com/aih

TABLE OF CONTENTS

"The question of whether a computer can think is no more interesting than the question of whether a submarine can swim."

- Edsger W. Dijkstra

SECTION 1
ARTIFICIAL INTELLIGENCE IN HEALTHCARE

CHAPTER ONE

A BRIEF INTRODUCTION TO AI
IN HEALTHCARE

Artificial intelligence (AI) is a young discipline [see Figure 1-1] that is here to bring a paradigm shift to healthcare. While it cannot replace doctors or healthcare workers in the foreseeable future, it is certainly poised to bring about a foundational shift in medical systems worldwide.

Artificial intelligence is a broad term that encompasses any code, algorithm, or combined technology designed to mimic human intelligence or behavior. Various subdomains make up this entity we commonly refer to as AI. Each AI-enabled technology can be applied to a different aspect of human ability.

Think of artificial intelligence as the "man-made" form of all human processes. *In simple terms, AI is a machine, device, robot, or tool that is powered by software programmed to display the characteristic reasoning and thinking patterns of humans.* To date, these machines have achieved specific purposes by reacting to specific actions according to how they have been programmed, that is, the data sets that they have used as learning material.

Most of us use AI in our daily lives without realizing it. The most prevalent way is its reach into social media to develop marketing strategies by evaluating consumer behavior through AI-powered algorithms. From browsing history to shopping history to movie choices, our internet actions give companies like Netflix, Amazon, and Facebook a detailed database for market analysis. Companies like *Ayzenberg*[1] developed proprietary intelligent algorithms that capture user-generated data to analyze and predict market trends. Boeing introduced its AI-powered autopilot feature years ago. However, car manufacturer *Tesla*[2] stepped up its game by providing recent models with Autopilot features as well. Tesla's self-driving technology is based on an AI-backed system to detect a car's surroundings and navigate the vehicle accordingly. Facial recognition software used at passport control in airport security, as well as virtual assistants like Siri, Alexa, and Google Home, use responsive AI technology to function.

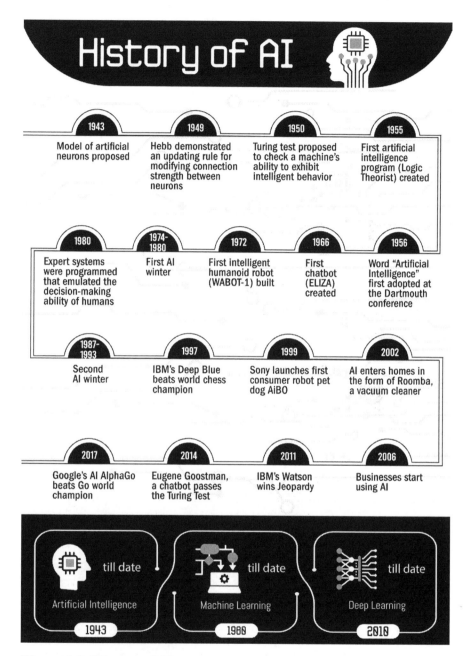

Figure 1-1. History of AI

With AI permeating every aspect of daily life, is it really a surprise that AI has found its way into the healthcare sector as well?

AI and Its Foray into Healthcare

While there are practical applications of AI in all human facets, the use of these tools in the field of healthcare shows remarkable potential for growth. Research has shown that the AI in healthcare market is expected to reach $120 billion by 2028, with an annual compounded growth rate of over 40%. It is also predicted to reduce annual healthcare costs by $150 billion by 2026.[3]

The adoption of AI-backed medical devices has only recently improved, with the United States Food and Drug Administration (FDA) approving the technology for patient use in 2017 and the Ministry of Food and Drug Safety in Korea approving it in 2018.[4]

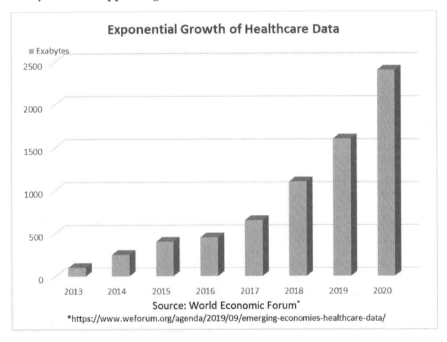

Figure 1-2. Exponential growth of healthcare data

The medical industry generates a tremendous amount of information every day [see Figure 1-2]. The use of technology to stratify and centralize this data to ensure easy accessibility has been the need of healthcare professionals for a very long time. The data available in the form of electronic health records (EHRs), X-rays, ECGs, and lab reports can be entered into algorithms for the training of AI models. AI can then develop its own "logic," which will empower medical personnel in an integrated system that translates useful information into functional tools. The ability of AI-enabled systems to work flawlessly in mimicking human cognition has dominated the rhetoric. The AI has helped healthcare in integrating statistical analysis, fast and accurate diagnosis, and the development of life-critical applications.[4]

Let us now understand the terms and acronyms commonly used with AI:

1. *Machine Learning* (ML) is a subdomain of AI involving the techniques and processes that help the machine to develop its own logic through self-learning. This knowledge can then be used to analyze patterns in large volumes of images, like making an image-based diagnosis in the fields of radiology and pathology. It can also be applied to discover anomalies in genomic structures, which can help diagnose congenital or gene-mediated diseases.

2. *Deep Learning* (DL) is a specific type of machine learning described as the modern revival of artificial neural networks (ANNs). ANNs are algorithms that mimic the biological structure of the brain. Deep learning can train AI algorithms to statistically analyze large amounts of data to accurately predict patient treatment results as well as provide personalized recommendations to patients regarding their treatment plans.

3. *Robotics* incorporates technological precision with an AI-enabled accurate diagnosis to enhance surgical procedures and can be used extensively in the medical device industry.

4. *Natural Language Processing (NLP)* **and** *Voice Recognition* can convert long-form, unstructured patient information commonly found in transcribed physician notes or electronic medical records into classified and formatted data that then becomes easy to analyze and interpret.

5. *Predictive Modeling* applies mathematical methods and tools to large data sets to forecast patient conditions or prognoses by using retrospective information for prospective action.

Bringing AI to the Patient

The dawn of the Internet of Things gave way to *the Internet of Medical Things (IoMT)*, which brought a whole new dimension to the application of AI-enabled software directly into the patient's hands. Access to technology is no longer limited to healthcare providers or medical device and pharmaceutical companies. With wearable technology in the form of fitness bands, smartwatches, smart oximeters, and glucometers connected to smartphone applications and analytical software, patients and users have direct access to health information. They can analyze, interpret, and act on their own health data, approaching physicians for consultations earlier for interventions. This focus on preventive health has gained predominance in recent years, with tech giants like Apple, Google, Samsung, and IBM competing to commercialize services, applications, and devices that integrate AI tools to improve diagnostic and prognostic accuracy.

A recent study done by *Hannun and colleagues*[5] used a deep learning algorithm to analyze 91,232 single-lead ECGs. The AI was able to diagnose abnormal readings with ECG pattern recognition as well as trained cardiologists.

In 2017, Apple[6] and Samsung[7] applied deep learning algorithms to their smartwatches, which were able to detect atrial fibrillation through an inbuilt ECG monitor and heart rate readings. This received FDA approval and is widely used by consumers to date.

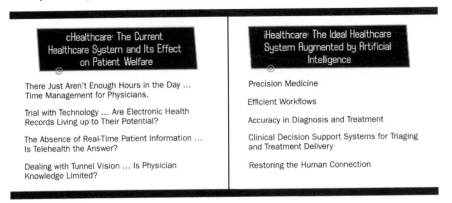

cHealthcare: The Current Healthcare System and Its Effect on Patient Welfare	iHealthcare: The Ideal Healthcare System Augmented by Artificial Intelligence
There Just Aren't Enough Hours in the Day ... Time Management for Physicians.	Precision Medicine
	Efficient Workflows
Trial with Technology ... Are Electronic Health Records Living up to Their Potential?	Accuracy in Diagnosis and Treatment
The Absence of Real-Time Patient Information ... Is Telehealth the Answer?	Clinical Decision Support Systems for Triaging and Treatment Delivery
Dealing with Tunnel Vision ... Is Physician Knowledge Limited?	Restoring the Human Connection

Figure 1-3. cHealthcare and iHealthcare

cHealthcare: The Current Healthcare System and Its Effect on Patient Welfare

While the rapid application of AI principles to healthcare is undoubtedly exciting, with its boundless potential to improve global health and wellness efforts, it is important to understand WHY its application was required and what factors in the current system inspired its widespread adoption. It is human nature to learn and evolve from situations that are detrimental to the longevity and quality of life, so it is but natural to infer that there were gaps in the existing healthcare facilities that facilitated the innovation required for AI-based technology. If we consider the current healthcare system (referred to *as cHealthcare*, from this point) with an objective eye, its flaws are apparent.

1. *There Just Aren't Enough Hours in the Day ... Time Management for Physicians.*

When it comes to creating a relationship between doctor and patient, a series of issues come into play. One of the main things that isn't always considered is the fact that doctors must spend adequate time with patients to make sure they understand what the patient is going through. Unfortunately, there is a serious dearth of this valuable time, and physician visits always seem rushed and haphazard. Research has demonstrated that patient satisfaction is directly dependent on the quality of communication with healthcare providers.

Ludmerer noted, "For over a century, the goal of medical education has been to produce thinking physicians, scientifically competent, who are sensitive to the emotional as well as the medical condition of the patient".[8]

Ninety-three percent of all human communication is based on body language, while only 7% is dependent on the exchange of words. Physicians struggling with increased workloads will find themselves running out of time and rushing through patient interactions. These distracted visits are noted by patients, who tend to lose trust in their providers as a result.[9,10]

Contrary to popular belief, this overload is rarely due to an increase in patient load. However, systems worldwide are so dependent on recording and documentation of patient interactions that most physicians and other medical experts are busy trying to keep up with the data that is constantly being provided to them. There is a continual need to fill in patient notes, transcribe patient information, and input patient data into paper files or electronic systems, which may be handled by scribes or physician assistants in some cases, but which is still dependent largely on skilled manual labor. This situation is similar in both outpatient clinics and inpatient care.

A study in 2018, conducted in an intensive care unit of a hospital, used a sensor network to analyze how long healthcare workers spent in direct patient contact. The study aimed to be more accurate than traditional surveys, which were subject to participants' memories or human observers, which themselves were prone to observational bias. The results of the study demonstrated that physicians spent 14.7% of their shift time in patient rooms or at bedsides, while they spent 40% of their time in the physician workroom, tied to their desks, busy with electronic medical record review and documentation. This limited interaction with patients further fuels patient dissatisfaction and distrust, as patients perceive it as indicative of substandard care delivery.[11]

There was also a concern regarding the lack of real-time information about patients, apart from time spent at the clinic. The rationale was that patients are not diagnosed based on data from their daily lives. With limited face-to-face interactions during physical consultations, the doctors can offer insight only into obvious findings without a holistic view of the patient's health status.

2. *The Absence of Real-Time Patient Information ... Is Telehealth the Answer?*

Before the COVID-19 pandemic in 2020, doctors generally did not have time to follow up with patient information after patient visits, considering their ongoing workload. While an accurate diagnosis is dependent on the patient's ability to recall their symptoms or experiences with medication for their next in-person visit with their doctor, it is natural for this information to be unreliable or incomplete. 2020 provided a turning point for this physician-patient interaction with the introduction of remote patient monitoring devices linked to smartphone applications that could easily be shared with one's healthcare provider. This was a demonstration of necessity being the mother of invention, as social distancing mandates pushed for greater adoption of telehealth facilities, with more patients opting for wearable digital health technology to monitor and evaluate their health matrices. This included smartwatches, fitness bands, blood pressure and heart rate monitors, pulse oximeters, and glucometers, which captured real-time patient information for rapid analysis. Many of these applications were backed by AI software, resulting in rapid, real-time physiological monitoring and greater compliance. The constant monitoring and generation of large data volumes proved to be another hurdle to conquer ... because now that we had a way to automatically capture this data, how would we analyze it and then act on it?[12]

3. *Trial with Technology ... Are Electronic Health Records Living up to Their Potential?*

The introduction of electronic health records (EHRs) undoubtedly has created an advantage over paper-based systems that were prone to errors and lapses in communication and continuity of care. With enhanced patient data security and the ease with which reports and patient information can be transferred from one physician to another, patients are protected from unnecessary testing, duplication of diagnostic testing, and medication errors. With better electronic medical records, it will also be easier to correlate genomic data with phenotypic data for patients.

However, the accuracy of this data is largely dependent on physicians, who enter the data themselves through charting, round notes, or handoff notes. It seems that once again, a solution to one problem opened Pandora's box and let loose another set of issues to overcome. There is a difference between being active and being productive. Electronic health records have been linked to cognitive overload and user burnout. According to the National Physician Burnout and Suicide Report 2020, which evaluated 15,000 physicians in over 29 specialties, 42% of participants reported being burnt out, while 55% of the respondents cited bureaucratic tasks like data entry, charting, and administrative work as the primary cause for burnout.

large amount of data present in electronic medical records must be properly analyzed and interpreted for it to be used to its full potential. The application of artificial intelligence algorithms is necessary to wade through the overwhelming data sets and arrive at actionable conclusions to improve care delivery. Otherwise, it is very easy to lose sight of the objective and drown in data.

Dr. Erica Shenoy, MD, PhD, Associate Chief of the Infection Control Unit at Massachusetts General Hospital, Boston, USA, noted, "AI tools can live up to the expectation for infection control and antibiotic resistance. If they don't, then that's really a failure on all of our parts. For the hospitals sitting on mountains of EHR data and not using them to the fullest potential, to industry that's not creating smarter, faster clinical trial design, and for EHRs that are creating this data not to use them ... that would be a failure".[13]

4. Dealing with Tunnel Vision ... Is Physician Knowledge Limited?

Physicians have been known to concentrate on the patient at hand, limited by the knowledge they have already attained, simply because they may not have the time to research or compare their patient status with those in large databases, with the unlimited case studies or references available in the medical literature. The research takes too long, and the interpretation of study findings is often inconclusive and may not apply to their patient demographics, which in turn makes them fall back on comfortable and repetitive models of diagnosis and treatment. This raises a pertinent question about the practical utilization of medical studies that are published.

Despite the obvious value of medical literature, it is extremely challenging for physicians to keep up with the latest advances in their fields. A report in the Journal of the American Medical Library Association found that over 7,000 articles are published monthly in primary care journals alone.[14]

Medical practice has a "TL;DR (Too Long; Didn't Read)" problem. Most physicians may not have the time to keep themselves updated with the latest advancements in their specialties. In recognition of this problem, a research project used artificial intelligence programs to comb through vast medical literature databases to derive results for focused themed research. The AI scored 49 out of 60 points, outperforming the human researchers, who scored 46 points using the same matrices for research accuracy. This shows the potential that AI has to analyze and filter required information to facilitate improved medical education.[15]

The varied factors responsible for the lacunae in *cHealthcare* are also the factors that lead to ***misdiagnosis***, which further fragments an already-fragile doctor-patient relationship.

When patients are diagnosed with the wrong illness and offered treatments that are not suitable to their needs, the result will generally be worsened patient care delivery, increased mortality and morbidity rates associated with inflated medical malpractice premiums, and the risk of legal repercussions for healthcare providers.

Reports on the economics of medical errors have revealed that medical errors cost the United States $19.5 billion per annum. In addition, the annual costs of "defensive medicine," which constitutes unnecessary investigations ordered solely to protect physicians from malpractice suits, are valued at $45-60 billion US per annum. This shines a light on the wastage of resources, time, and energy on treatment modalities that do not have a robust evidence base or clinical decision support.[16,17]

With all that can potentially go wrong in cHealthcare, does artificial intelligence have what it takes to improve the current scenario and bring much-needed reforms and support to clinical care?

iHealthcare: The Ideal Healthcare System Augmented by Artificial Intelligence

While AI doesn't aim to replace human doctors in the current healthcare system, it does have a goal to make the system more effective.

What was considered science fiction is now within our grasp. This thought brings excitement and apprehension in equal parts to the minds of healthcare providers worldwide. An imagined utopia—a healthcare system powered by AI-enabled tools and software—seems to be right around the corner. The extent to which algorithms and machine learning will penetrate the medical industry remains to be seen. If we consider this AI-driven healthcare industry (referred to as *iHealthcare* from this point), we can evaluate how making use of both human effort and advanced technology can bring us closer to efficiency and accuracy in the field of medicine.

1. Precision Medicine

Precision medicine has gained traction since the introduction of AI in healthcare, as it shows the immense possibilities in customizing care delivery or delivering solutions based on an individual patient's genetics, lifestyle, location, and environmental factors. This is opposed to the one-size-fits-all approach that traditional medicine delivers. It spans the treatment journey from diagnosis to disease detection, prognosis, and management. By taking advantage of AI algorithms, genomic and proteomic profiles of patient subgroups can be analyzed to predict risk factors for cardiovascular disease and cancer as well as prognostic factors for neurodegenerative conditions.

In the last few years, the digitization of medical records added large amounts of patient data with initiatives from the NIH (USA) called the EMERGE network and the "All of Us" program, databases from the Canadian Institutes of Health Research, and the National Health Service, UK. The application of AI algorithms to these data sets can help to derive genotype-phenotype relationships for specific genetic diseases, with the ability to deliver holistic care to patients. AI algorithms aided in the mapping of the human genome, which, along with the addition of MRI images, helped to establish the Allen Developmental Brain Atlas in 2011 and the Human Cell Atlas in 2017. This can lead to personalized treatments with FDA-approved targeted gene therapy.[18] The Tempus group[19] has developed its AI software to provide a large library of clinical and molecular data that enables doctors to make real-time decisions for data-driven, personalized therapeutics.

2. Efficient Workflows

AI in healthcare will build on systems with automation and robotics to deliver better care outcomes through a lean management strategy that reduces wastage of resources for healthcare providers while delivering value-based care to patients. The **McKinsey Group** has estimated that

AI will help in the automation of 15% of current working hours in the healthcare industry.[20]

US-based company **Olive**[21] has a machine learning algorithm that automates repetitive tasks in healthcare management, thereby freeing physicians and administrators to work on more pressing issues. The platform can automate insurance checks and claims and seamlessly integrates with a healthcare network to track down deficiencies and highlight areas for improvement. **CloudMedX**[22] uses deep learning to generate analysis that showcases areas of improvement in the patient's journey through the healthcare system. Its coding analyzer was used with existing coding and billing software to efficiently manage, analyze, and communicate structured and unstructured data to improve patient care.

3. *Accuracy in Diagnosis and Treatment*

Machine and deep learning algorithms are experts at pattern recognition and image analysis, which greatly improves the accuracy of radiological and pathological diagnoses.

Digital pathology platforms like **Proscia**[23] improve the speed and accuracy of cancer diagnostics, while **Zebra Medical Vision**[24] arms radiologists with an AI-powered assistant that analyzes and filters routine scans from those with positive clinical findings to help lighten the workload for practitioners.

4. *Clinical Decision Support Systems for Triaging and Treatment Delivery*

Clinical decision support tools have existed for years but are attracting attention now due to the application of AI algorithms to existing electronic data through health records or imaging reports.

A study conducted by *Pickhardt and colleagues*[25] used body composition markers from abdominal CT scans to develop a deep learning algorithm focused on imaging features, as compared to clinical parameters like Framingham Risk Scores and Body Mass Index (BMI), to predict major cardiovascular disease as well as survival rates for adult patient populations. The algorithm outperformed established clinical indicators.

5. Restoring the Human Connection

AI-enabled systems have the potential to reduce the cognitive load that overwhelms physicians and leads to increased incidents of burnout. The World Health Organization (WHO) states, "Although the global economy could create 40 million new health-sector jobs by 2030, there is still a projected shortfall of 9.9 million physicians, nurses and midwives globally over the same period." The automation of repetitive, time-consuming processes through AI-enabled systems also addresses the issue of shortage in manpower while aiding in the provision of care services to underserved or developing areas.[26] It is ironic that many believe the application of AI will, or the adoption of technology in diagnosis and treatment may cause, further detachment between physicians and patients by establishing additional barriers. However, it may result in just the opposite effect because it has the potential to free physicians from routine and mundane tasks so that they can provide empathy and re-establish a human connection in the doctor-patient dynamic—a skill that cannot be replaced even with the most advanced AI. In other words, AI will allow doctors to be more ... human.

Potential Liabilities with the Application of AI in Healthcare

As with most things in life, all that glitters is not gold. While AI is often touted as a concept that will revolutionize medicine and care delivery, evaluating it with a critical eye is bound to reveal inconsistencies and lacunae in its development and implementation that may make us accept the claims of its potential with a pinch of salt.

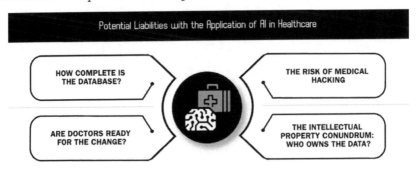

Figure 1-4. Potential liabilities with application of AI in healthcare

1. How Complete is the Database?

We must evaluate whether the raw data used to derive a conclusion is equally representative of all ethnicities and patient populations or whether it is biased toward a certain population. Precision medicine could be at risk of bias if the data did not include minority groups. In situations like this, how accurate would the analysis be if the data set provided at the source is flawed? AI may be objective, but it is not perfect. This is because of the methodology used in developing these algorithms. They not only need an abundance of information to perform analysis but also require developers to make such processes objective. Human developers are often influenced by their personal biases and may unintentionally manipulate data. This is a limitation in the development of AI in the medical world.

2. Are Doctors Ready for the Change?

The strongest resistance to the incorporation of AI into routine healthcare workflows has been from physicians who believe that the technology will eventually replace them. While the adoption of AI in healthcare is still in its nascent phase, most experts agree that its success in healthcare is due to the adjuvant efforts from healthcare professionals and that it is always the combination of technological intelligence and human intervention that brings about the best results.

Recht and colleagues[27] provide a nuanced opinion that AI may become a part of the radiology workflow by performing routine tasks like segmentation or counting, thereby enabling radiologists to perform value-added tasks like integrating clinical features with imaging reports for diagnosis while playing a critical role in integrated physician teams within healthcare systems. *Karches*[28] also maintains, "Human physician judgment will remain better suited to the practice of primary care despite anticipated advances in AI technology."

3. The Risk of Medical Hacking

Do we have the infrastructure to effectively protect and store data while maintaining patient privacy through robust encryption of medical data?

AI may be considered a double-edged sword that may be used for defense or offense, depending on the hands manning the controls. **The Future of Humanity Institute published a report on the Malicious Use of Artificial Intelligence**[29], explaining that AI-enabled tools are similar to drones that can be used to drop both medicines and bombs, leading to dynamically opposing results.

4. The Intellectual Property Conundrum: Who Owns the Data?

Healthcare is a business, and the economic gains that can be made through the correct application of AI-enabled tools in the industry could prove to be significant. It is therefore important to determine who owns this valuable data set on which AI software is applied—the data set that serves as a base for training of the algorithm, that serves to set the AI's definitions of normal so that it can then diagnose what is abnormal. Does it belong to the individual patient? To the public as a whole? To the government healthcare body that utilizes the software? Or to the private technology companies that develop the software?

Conclusion

At present, we are witnessing a meteoric rise in AI-based applications within the healthcare industry that encompasses every aspect of the patient's journey through a complex healthcare system worldwide, including consultations, symptom checking, investigations, diagnostics, and management with targeted therapeutics. The reason for the rapid adoption is the simplicity that it brings to patients, doctors, and hospital administrators. Its mimicry of human cognitive functions has enabled it to seamlessly duplicate human interventions in a field that is notorious for its intricacies and person-driven processes.

As with most novel technologies, artificial intelligence also brings its own challenges to the forefront. It raises the question of patient privacy, data security, and transparency as well as accountability if diagnosis or treatment modalities go wrong and result in poor patient outcomes. The next step in the AI journey in the healthcare industry is standardization. To ensure that technical quality and diagnostic accuracy are maintained with the applications that are actively used in patient care, a rigorous approval process is recommended. This must be delicately balanced, as too much red tape would invariably stifle the creativity with which AI designs are applied in a versatile and ever-changing field like healthcare. The US FDA has recently begun work on a new regulatory framework that aims to promote the cautious, safe, and effective development of AI-backed medical devices.[30]

There is no doubt that AI can be the defining technology of the near future. It requires clinicians with vision working alongside technical experts to set up the organizational design and the processes needed to establish an integrated and cohesive AI-enabled healthcare network. Only when the end-users work actively with the developers of the technology will AI be widely implemented to get teams out of their silos and working together.

In the words of Dr. Paul Weber[31], Associate Dean of Medical Education at Rutgers Medical School, New Jersey, USA, "We're able to train machines to exhibit human-like intelligence and apply that in a clinical setting. We haven't achieved human intelligence, but we're getting close to it."

References/Further Reading

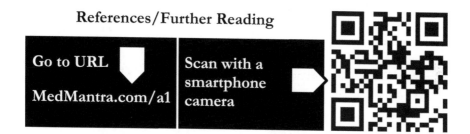

Go to URL

MedMantra.com/a1

Scan with a smartphone camera

CHAPTER TWO

AI-AUGMENTED HEALTHCARE – CURRENT STATE AND FUTURE APPLICATIONS

There's a new doctor in the exam room, one without a face, a name, or an identity. Artificial intelligence made a whirlwind entry into healthcare, taking many by surprise. While there is a new generation of healthcare workers who see AI as a natural progression of the rapid evolution of technology, there are industry stalwarts who believe that patient care and the human touch may be replaced by machines and robots. This mixed reception has led to the belief that it's man versus machine, prompting an in-depth look into both sides of the theory. Is AI the positive disruptor it has been proclaimed to be ... or is mankind putting too much faith in a machine? Do the rewards actually outweigh the risks?

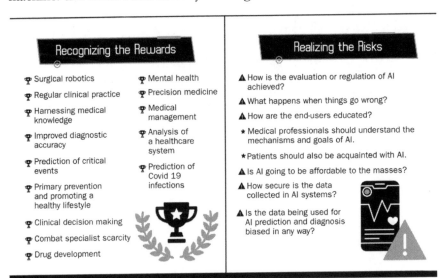

Recognizing the Rewards

🏆 Surgical robotics
🏆 Regular clinical practice
🏆 Harnessing medical knowledge
🏆 Improved diagnostic accuracy
🏆 Prediction of critical events
🏆 Primary prevention and promoting a healthy lifestyle
🏆 Clinical decision making
🏆 Combat specialist scarcity
🏆 Drug development
🏆 Mental health
🏆 Precision medicine
🏆 Medical management
🏆 Analysis of a healthcare system
🏆 Prediction of Covid 19 infections

Realizing the Risks

⚠ How is the evaluation or regulation of AI achieved?
⚠ What happens when things go wrong?
⚠ How are the end-users educated?
★ Medical professionals should understand the mechanisms and goals of AI.
★ Patients should also be acquainted with AI.
⚠ Is AI going to be affordable to the masses?
⚠ How secure is the data collected in AI systems?
⚠ Is the data being used for AI prediction and diagnosis biased in any way?

Figure 2-1. Recognizing the rewards and realizing the risks

Recognizing the Rewards

Deep learning, or machine learning, can significantly impact the fields where enormous data is available. The large volume of healthcare data has made the implementation of AI in this field a dream come true. The industry generates a large amount of information daily. The use of technological advancements to categorize, centralize, and stratify this data to ensure that it is both easy to access and easy to understand and interpret has been a long-standing requirement. AI can develop its own "logic" and can be used to empower healthcare personnel in an integrated medical system.

AI-enabled systems have the ability to flawlessly mimic human cognition, and the triumphs have dominated the rhetoric, both in the scientific community and the patient audience in general. AI has also helped in the integration of statistical analysis, rapid and accurate diagnosis even when applied to critical health conditions. Known as the "stethoscope of the 21st century," artificial intelligence has become the center of attraction for many specialists. In many hospitals, physicians are overburdened with a multitude of tasks, both administrative and clinical, and they find it difficult to concentrate on other procedures. That is why the technological stethoscope is making all the difference in the medical world.

Beyond administrative drudge work, the applications of AI are numerous and diverse. Nowadays, finely tuned technological robots and robust algorithms for diagnosis are making their way through the branches of medicine.

A. Surgical Robotics

In the field of surgical robotics, AI has allowed some semi-automated repetitive tasks to be undertaken by specific robots, thus increasing the efficiency of the process. An inability to exactly mimic body motion and human intelligence seems to be the drawback of robotics, which is being tackled by introducing applications like natural language processing, neural networking, speech recognition, and image recognition.

In recent times, *the Da Vinci robot* has demonstrated its success as a surgical robot, an extension of a human surgeon, who, with the aid of a console, controls the device/robot.[1,2]

Microsure is a spin-off company of the Eindhoven University of Technology and the Maastricht University Medical Center, which designed a robot to perform microsurgeries with precision.[3] The robot is controlled by a surgeon, whose hand movements are sensed and converted into tiny, accurate, and more precise movements executed by a set of "robot hands." The robotic system is augmented by AI, which is used to eliminate any tremors in the surgeon's hands, ensuring that the surgery takes place correctly.

B. Regular Clinical Practice

In regular clinical practice, basic AI systems or computer algorithms available today can be successfully employed for automating routine functions such as:

Alerts and reminders: This spans from the basic scanning of laboratory results to drug orders and the updating of the patient with scheduled reminders. Nonetheless, more advanced AI can interface with a patient monitor and detect changes in the condition of illness.[4]

Therapy pre-planning: This is specifically for conditions that require elaborate treatment plans. The patients get the advantage of receiving formulated plans that can improve their medical condition. Physicians can benefit from this as well.

Retrieval of information: Complex medical applications can be fitted with software search agents. These agents are more efficient than several web-crawling agents of the present day. To a large extent, the retrieval of information and upgrading of data is made easy.

C. Harnessing Medical Knowledge

The medical field has an ocean of knowledge that no doctor can churn up, and that, too, is growing at a more incredible pace. The doubling time of medical knowledge was fifty years in 1950, seven years in 1980, and only 3.5 years in 2010. In 2020, it was estimated to double in just seventy-three days, while training a doctor requires an arduous five-year course and a decade more for specialist training. An AI system can assist physicians by providing up-to-date medical knowledge from research journals, textbooks, and years of clinical practices across the globe to augment proper patient care. Furthermore, an AI system can extract information from an extensive patient database to make real-time reasoning for medical risk alerts and health outcome prediction.

D. Improved Diagnostic Accuracy

Diagnosis in Radiology

In the AI world, "complex" is just another word for "simple." AI has successfully eliminated issues occurring during certain angiograms and MRI scans. They can be instantaneously detected by image recognition and interpretation methods. This has attracted a significant amount of usage in many radiology clinics across the world.

Seattle-based ATL Ultrasound, Inc., made the imaging and monitoring of cardiac tissue structures simpler by developing different diagnostic ultrasound systems. The mechanism aims to eliminate irrelevant frequencies in returned signals. An adaptive intelligence algorithm is utilized to optimize many parameters when a patient is examined.[5] *Agilent Technologies in Andover, Massachusetts,* has successfully developed a smart ECG that can estimate the probability of acute cardiac ischemia (ACI).

In *John Radcliffe Hospital in Oxford,* a system was built to diagnose several heart diseases.[6] This AI diagnostic system was discovered to give about 80% accuracy compared to that of human doctors.

By using *InferVision*[7], diagnosis of illnesses and the reading of CT and X-ray scans have been made easier.

Medical Sieve is an algorithm launched by IBM to act as a cognitive assistant.[8] With its wide range of clinical know-how, it can offer analytical and reasoning solutions for the team. This technology can make sound clinical judgments in cardiology and radiology. In radiology, it can analyze images to detect problems with more efficiency and reliability.

Diagnosis in Pathology

Implementation of deep learning algorithms to whole-slide histopathology images can drastically improve diagnostic accuracy and efficiency. With AI augmentation, not only did pathologists' cancer diagnostic accuracy improve from a mere 73% to greater than 95%, but the time required to reach diagnosis decreased, too.[9] *IBM's intelligent system, Watson,* took ten minutes to interpret data of tumor cells.[10] When human doctors carried out the procedure, they spent about six days and ten hours making reasonable contributions from the genetic data. This also included the process of providing treatments and recommendations from their inferences.

A *smart microscope* developed at Harvard University[11] detects harmful infections of the blood. This AI-assisted tool was trained by treating about 25,000 slides with dye to increase the bacteria's visibility, after which about 100,000 images were pooled together. This system's total accuracy was measured at 95% – a figure surpassing that of resident doctors.

Neuromedical Systems, Inc., in New Jersey, came up with a method that is useful in screening cancer by scanning Pap smears and applying neural networks to review cells during the screening process.[12] *SkinVision* may be used for the detection of skin cancer[13] by recognizing moles and skin lesions.

E. Clinical Decision Making

Symptom checkers can track the progression or regression of chronic illnesses. Users can input their electronic health record (EHR) forms and attach additional reports such as ECGs or radiographs and get an online consultation within minutes. The benefit offered goes both ways. Physicians also get ample time to attend to more critical and emergent cases and let the app manage the rest of them.[14]

An example of such an app is Akira. In Toronto, a health tech company developed this "doctor-in-your-pocket" app to help users engage in virtual chats with their assigned healthcare providers. In this app, a patient can obtain a sick note that helps save the time required to travel to a doctor. Also, professionals can refer their patients to specialists via the app.[15]

F. Prediction of Critical Events

Using predictive analytics, artificial intelligence models can look at a patient's past medical records and find specific patterns to anticipate the patient developing a particular illness like cancer. Medical practitioners can analyze this information and get back on track, preventing their patients from developing heart attacks, diabetes, and other life-threatening ailments.

Diabetic retinopathy is the leading cause of blindness in the 21st century and can be diagnosed earlier with deep learning algorithms. Also, AI could do more with the help of the same retinal images taken for retinopathy. There are things that humans didn't quite know to look for in retinal scans, but the deep learning algorithms offered more insight into those. AI can extract information from the same eye scan, which predicts a five-year risk of having a life-threatening cardiovascular event, i.e., a heart attack or stroke.[16] This could be the basis of a newer, non-invasive way to detect cardiovascular diseases.

At the University of Nottingham, a study was published to back up this possibility.[17] A self-taught AI system was able to predict cardiovascular occurrences in some patients. Leading by a margin of accuracy of about 7.6%, the AI system had been trained on extensive data from nearly 380,000 patients. The degree of accuracy was revealed to be better than that of standard healthcare centers. The "Human Diagnosis Project" is an AI system that combines doctors' real-life experiences with machine learning.[18] Also called "Human Dx," the system's makers compile data from different healthcare centers in more than 80 countries. This covers a total of 500 institutions and 7,500 doctors. It has been said that the system will be capable of making highly accurate medical decisions and deliberations.

G. Primary Prevention and Promoting a Healthy Lifestyle

The increasing number of consumer wearables, such as the *Apple Watch* that can do quick ECG, and other medical devices combined with AI, are also being used to oversee early-stage heart diseases, enabling physicians and other caregivers to better monitor the health of patients and detect potentially life-threatening episodes at more treatable stages.[19] Another application, *Morpheo,* can be used for the detection of sleep disorders[20] by providing rich tracking data about sleep patterns.

H. Combat Specialist Scarcity

A worldwide shortage of radiologists is causing increased morbidity and mortality due to delays in diagnosis, mostly among cancer patients.[21] Researchers at the Artificial Intelligence Research Centre for Neurological Disorders, Beijing Tiantan Hospital, Beijing, developed BioMind, a Chinese AI that beat a team of top Chinese radiologists in rapidly and accurately diagnosing brain tumors.[22]

The combined skills of AI and radiologists can create a hybrid intelligence that could lead to better diagnostic accuracy and higher safety standards. AI systems could also serve as effective decision support backups, facilitating diagnoses and reducing physician burnout.

Babylon has developed an app that scans your symptoms for possible differential diagnoses, asks interactive questions to narrow down the searches, and refers you to a specialist or starts a video conference with a general practitioner right inside the app. This is literally a "Pocket Doctor" accessible to far-flung areas of the world – a step forward in bringing expert diagnosis to places where trained doctors are scarce.[14]

I. Drug Development

According to the California Biomedical Research Association, it takes an average of twelve years for a drug to reach patients who are in dire need of treatment. Only five out of 5,000 drugs that begin preclinical testing ever make it to human testing and only one of these five drugs is approved for human usage. Furthermore, it costs a company a minimum of US $359 million for research to develop a new drug.[23]

AI frameworks are helping researchers to streamline the drug discovery and repurposing processes. AI reduces the time taken to market new drugs and significantly cuts the money invested in the development of drugs.

The creation or discovery of new drugs using AI technology requires more research and funds. If both factors were constant, AI would make a significant impact in the healthcare industry. More so, the limit of medical innovations would be infinite. Atomwise uses a database of molecular structures with supercomputers and programmed algorithms to uncover therapies. They launched a search online to virtually discover safe and existing medications that had the potential to be re-engineered for the treatment of the Ebola virus.

The company's AI technology found two drugs that were predicted to be capable of reducing the infectivity of Ebola. The best part of this is that the analysis took less than 24 hours to complete, whereas human intervention would probably take months, if not years.[24]

J. Mental Health

Cogito Corp. is a company that has improved its customer service interactions by integrating AI-powered voice recognition and analysis. *Cogito Companion*[25], the company's venture into the mental healthcare space, is an app that helps track behavioral patterns. By turning on location, the app can determine whether a patient is in their home. Communication logs make it possible to know if the patient is in touch with people. The company has said that the app does not reveal the identity of the caller. The patient's active and passive behavioral signals are monitored. If the patient has a care team, this team can monitor reports that indicate a change in the patient's overall mental health.

"Audio check-ins" are analyzed by an ML (machine learning) algorithm. Simply called voice recordings, the check-ins are akin to an audio diary. The algorithm picks up emotional cues from the audio. Characteristic voice properties that distinguish one human from another are intonation, energy, and dynamism in a conversation. Humans train this algorithm to differentiate between a "competent" and "trustworthy" sound.

They may also train the algorithm to identify a depressed patient's tone and differentiate it from that of a manic bipolar patient who is depressed. Patients can sufficiently track their moods with such real-time information, whereas healthcare practitioners can track patients' health progress. It can be seen that AI can understand human conversation facets and the mental health aspect of humans.

K. Medical Management

The first virtual nurse is known as *Molly*. A medical start-up called Sensely developed this AI nurse. With a friendly face and a pleasant voice, she monitors the health conditions and treatment of subscribers. The machine learning module offers support to patients with chronic conditions while they are getting regular treatments from doctors. *Molly* has a strong focus on chronic diseases, and it provides customized monitoring and follow-up care.[26]

Like Molly, there is *AiCure,* which monitors the frequency with which patients take their medications. Patients who find it challenging to follow medical prescriptions and advice have found the best use for this app. Endorsed by the National Institutes of Health, *AiCure* uses a webcam (on a smartphone) coupled with AI to confirm if a patient adheres to prescriptions and thereby supports patients in managing their health conditions.[27]

L. Precision Medicine

Genetics and genomics tend to be positively impacted by artificial intelligence. This is why *Deep Genomics* was created. This app finds mutations and linkages to diseases by identifying similar patterns in a database of genetic information. In due time, some systems will inform doctors about the consequences of the alteration in genetic variation – be it therapeutic or natural.

M. Analysis of a Healthcare System

In the Netherlands, over 90% of healthcare invoices are digitized. The hospital, healthcare provider, and treatment can be contained in the data. To mine this data, *Zorgprisma Publiek* Company uses IBM's Watson in the cloud to analyze invoices.[28] This company helps hospitals improve their healthcare practices. Also, patients who are unnecessarily hospitalized are well-taken care of. However, primarily, the company detects repetitive mistakes made in a clinic when treatments are administered.

N. Prediction of COVID-19 Infections

To tackle the COVID-19 global pandemic, The COVID Symptom Study, a smartphone application that was previously named the COVID Symptom Tracker, was launched in the US and the UK. Considering the large number of COVID patients who complained of loss of smell and taste, researchers wanted to use the app to determine if this symptom was specific to COVID-19. Data donated by 2,618,862 individuals were analyzed using an AI algorithm, which analyzed combinations of presenting symptoms to predict the probability of infection, which narrowed down the possibilities to 805,753. They then predicted that 140,312 out of the total participants, or 17.42% of them, were likely to be infected with COVID-19. The analysis also identified four major symptoms, which included loss of smell or taste, a cough that was dry, persistent, and severe, muscular fatigue or body pain, and loss of appetite. A total of 18,401 participants underwent a SARS-CoV-2 test, and it was revealed that 65% of those who tested positive for COVID-19 had experienced the loss of smell and taste, as opposed to only 21.7% of those who had a negative test. Considering the strong correlation between the symptoms and the disease, researchers think that this may help to provide rapid screening and diagnosis in populations who don't have access to widespread testing, although a major limiting factor is that the data is mainly self-reported and could be open to bias.[29]

Realizing the Risks

The rising global burden of disease, mismanagement of prescriptions, absence of collaborative treatment, diagnosis of rare diseases, increasing patient traffic, and growing patient data load are vital challenges in the healthcare sector. While one must acknowledge the need for faster and better healthcare resources, mankind cannot throw caution to the wind, embracing AI without being aware of possible drawbacks. AI should not be integrated haphazardly – logical reasoning is for humans, not robots.

To demonstrate the potential pitfalls in machine-based learning, its effects in systems outside healthcare can be evaluated. An "AI lawyer" was launched in September 2015 by a teenage British programmer.[30] This bot successfully helped people appeal their parking tickets. When the parking tickets are received, this bot sorts out what to do with them by asking relevant questions. Ten months after the launch, about 250,000 parking tickets had been appealed in New York and London. The success rate was penned only as 64%. In a field as sensitive as healthcare, is that success rate good enough?

Another potential area for improvement is the fact that AI researchers sometimes design the systems without keeping the end-user's comfort in mind. When evaluating the retail industry, for example, people who use eBay do not call it "AI for shopping"; it is called eBay for a reason: to appeal to the needs of the consumer so seamlessly that they don't even realize that they are using an AI-based software.

Just as every complex machine carries a description for use, the pooled information reduces the complexities of AI and the logical patterns obtained from data interpretation. Another machine cannot do this. Because AI is human-made, the operational understanding is transferred from humans to machines. This gives rise to questions that need to be asked, like:

A. How is the Evaluation or Regulation of AI Achieved?

The evaluation process is the only way the technologies' real potential can be determined for future purposes. Before an AI system is certified for diverse applications, it is subjected to a thorough analysis, one in which all processes are well documented and identified.[31]

This opens up Pandora's box of questions. How do we plan to evaluate and attach credibility to the AI software that works? Should all AI be approved? What is the vetting process? Who decides what can be used clinically? What are the benchmarking norms?

Published and released by the United States Food and Drug Administration (FDA) in January 2021, the "Artificial Intelligence/ Machine Learning (AI/ML)-Based Software as a Medical Device (SaMD) Action Plan" attempts to provide a holistic and well-rounded approach to AI-based systems by providing oversight based on lifecycle regulation. The plan aims to outline ways to support the development of "Good Machine Learning Practices" to evaluate, standardize, and improve algorithms that are based on AI. This is similar to the good practices currently existing in software engineering and quality systems. Advocating transparency to end-users fosters a patient-centered approach while boosting confidence in the idea of AI-enabled services through the advancement of real-world performance monitoring pilots.

The establishment of a total product lifecycle (TPLC) to provide oversight of AI/ML-based applications will have to be supported by the collection and monitoring of real-world data. This will allow manufacturers to figure out how their products are being used, identify the scope for improvements, and react proactively to make their products safer or more user-friendly.

This again raises a plethora of concerns for uniformity in data collection, like what type of reference data would be considered appropriate in measuring the performance of AI/ML in the field or what kind of oversight should be performed by the stakeholders. How much data is enough, and how often should the information be shared with the governing agency? What are the steps to standardize, validate and test algorithms, models, and claims by AI-supported device companies, and how should user feedback be collected and incorporated into the end design?

These standards introduced by the FDA have not been combined into a single document or provided with a robust legal framework. This gives rise to another challenge because "AI regulation" involves ethical, technical, and security-based issues, which are otherwise tackled through many different legal avenues and may differ from country to country.[32]

Validating healthcare systems that use AI is still an issue that is largely unresolved and therefore raises many questions. The goal of these regulations or standards is to ensure that the systems are safe, accurate, and precise enough for both physicians and their patients to use them with confidence.

A surprising discovery made by researchers led by the University of Cambridge revealed that out of around 300 COVID-19 machine learning AI-based models described in 2020, none have proven to be suitable for the detection or diagnosis of COVID-19 from medical imaging like chest X Rays or CT scans. This is due to flaws in methodology, biases, lack of reproducibility, and "Frankenstein datasets." These were considered to be a major weakness, considering the urgency with which COVID-19 models are needed.

"However, any machine learning algorithm is only as good as the data it's trained on," said first author Dr. Michael Roberts from Cambridge's Department of Applied Mathematics and Theoretical Physics. "Especially for a brand-new disease like COVID-19, it's vital that the training data is as diverse as possible because, as we've seen throughout this pandemic, there are many different factors that affect what the disease looks like and how it behaves."[33]

B. What Happens when Things Go Wrong?

In Montreal in 2010, a surgical operation took place by robots. The robot anesthesiologist (called McSleepy) teamed up with the surgical robot to conduct the first in-tandem performance. "The DaVinci allows us to work from a workstation operating surgical instruments with delicate movements of our fingers with a precision that cannot be provided by humans alone," said Dr. A. Aprikian, MUHC urologist in chief and Director of the MUHC Cancer Care Mission. Both doctors were widely commended for their stellar performance throughout the procedure.[34]

Five years later, a retrospective analysis of FDA data was performed by the Massachusetts Institute of Technology (MIT).[35] The objective of this research was to ascertain the safety of robotic surgery. Due to technical malfunctions, 144 patients died, while 1,391 patients sustained injuries during the study period. However, it was said that many procedures yielded results and were without problems. At the same time, complex surgical procedures such as gynecology recorded a high number of events. This incident does question the ability of surgical robots to replace human physician conducted procedures, presently.

It also highlights the missing piece of the puzzle- accountability. Who or what is responsible if things go sideways? This technology is recent, and litigation against robots hasn't been considered extensively. Thus, this is still a gray area. When a physician neglects some procedures or violates standards of care, it is regarded as medical malpractice. Theoretically, AI lacks awareness of the concept of negligence. For the robot to be held responsible for some performance standards, the existence of this standard is fundamental.

Thus, who takes the blame when the robot is unsuitable? Will the surgeon in charge of the robot be held responsible? Maybe the manufacturer of the robot? Or is it the design engineer who should be charged?

C. How are the End-users Educated?

AI will not become a reality if the fears and doubts surrounding its development are not addressed. The world needs to know the benefits and risks of this technology. Some people believe that AI can be so sophisticated that the human race will become extinct. Others fear that AI may overtake the control of our lives. Both Stephen Hawking and Elon Musk, stellar scientists, have predicted that full AI may spell doom for the human race. There must be a concerted effort to reach out and educate people about the real-life benefits of AI in healthcare in order to allay these fears.

Medical professionals should understand the mechanisms and goals of AI.

Without the support of physicians on the field, large-scale implementation of AI will be difficult in the years to come. Like with all things, the fear and apprehension of the unknown are more than likely the causes of the reluctance to embrace the benefits of AI.

An international study surveyed 1,041 radiologists and radiology residents and found that "fear of replacement and lack of adequate knowledge about the applications of AI significantly affected the perception and therefore the adoption of AI in medical professionals. 48% of radiologists and residents have an open and proactive attitude towards AI, while 38% fear replacement by AI." The authors have suggested that AI be incorporated into the training curriculum so that medical professionals are aware of it as they enter practice, and it could lead to more proactive clinical adoption.[36]

Patients should also be acquainted with AI.

Research conducted by the Harvard Business Review indicates that patients are hesitant to use health care services provided by medical artificial intelligence even when it has proven to outperform human physicians. Patients believe that their medical needs are unique and cannot possibly be addressed successfully by algorithms. Manufacturers of these AIs, such as IBM, Google, Facebook, and Baidu, should communicate effectively and transparently with the general public about AI's advancement – including the benefits and risks, to overcome the public's misgivings.[37]

D. Is AI Going to be Affordable to the Masses?

Data must be readily available for AI technologies to correctly train models, but extracting patient data from charts, reports, radiographs, and handwritten notes is cumbersome and showcases technical infrastructural deficits. The significant initial capital expenditure required to purchase the expensive clinical robotic surgical systems is a big drawback in its early adoption by the medical community. Most of the systems require the construction of new infrastructure. Also, the cost necessary to acquire the highly paid and highly skilled surgeons proficient in robotics seems to be a considerable hindrance. In order to effectively revolutionize healthcare, AI should be made available to everyone – ordinary people and not just the scientific community or those who can afford it.

E. How Secure is the Data Collected in AI Systems?

User-generated data and medical data are the bedrock of AI algorithms. However, studies have shown that the younger generation of patient populations are reluctant to share their data with large corporations.

According to the recently published FDA guidelines[32], the responsibility of data security issues while using AI algorithms would lie with the AI systems administrator (AI Officer). If these regulations are applied, it may go a long way in assuring the end-users about the security of their information, knowing that they can hold a human being accountable.

F. Is the Data Being Used for AI Prediction and Diagnosis Biased in any Way?

AI solutions have brought into the forefront a completely new criterion in the evaluation of intelligent technology: non-discrimination and equality in treatment provided. Because most medical data is recovered from electronic health records, fed and imported by human minds, it may introduce evaluation criteria that are discriminatory, even though it may be unintentional on the part of the data provider. This bias may be based on traits like ethnicity, race, or gender. The recent FDA guidelines[32] state that the data used to train the AI-based systems needs to be examined and evaluated in detail to ensure that it does not have filters that feed into this bias and adequately represent the patient population it is meant to help.

Conclusion

While it is incredibly tempting to dive headfirst into AI as a potential replacement for physicians in healthcare, as the old saying goes, we have miles to go before we sleep! AI has demonstrated its efficacy in augmenting healthcare services to a large extent; however, there are obstacles that need to be overcome, fine lines that need to be ironed out before complete implementation. Does AI actually excel on the basis of accuracy? If it were to replace doctors, what would be the unique or specific contributions it would make that could outweigh the potentially harmful effects that it could render in the medical world?

References/Further Reading

Go to URL	Scan with a
MedMantra.com/a2	smartphone camera

CHAPTER THREE

FDA-APPROVED AI APPLICATIONS IN MEDICINE

The Food and Drug Administration (FDA) is a United States federal agency established in 1906. Its sole purpose is to protect public health, guaranteeing the safety, effectiveness, and protection of drugs, biological products, and medical devices for both humans and animals. It also includes the scrutiny of the food supply, cosmetic products, and products that release radiation.

The FDA aims to advance public health by approving and promoting innovative technologies that help make medical products more efficacious and affordable.[1] The organization functions to provide the public with correct, evidence-based information necessary for using medical products for adequate health maintenance.

Why is FDA approval important? The answer is that it authenticates research on how certain drugs and medical devices work and what effects they have on both children and adults. It lets people know that a product is safe for use and also enables companies to design devices that meet their standards nationwide.[2]

After a company designs a new device or product, it must be approved by the FDA. Prior to being tested on people, the device must be tested on animals to identify whether it can cause any serious harm. After animal testing, the company must submit an Investigational New Drug (IND) application to the Food and Drug Administration.

The results submitted with the application should include the manufacturing process of the product along with the company's plan to test it in public. After approval of the IND application, the FDA directs the beginning of clinical trials to test the product on people. This takes place in four phases. At first, small-scale trials are done, followed by large-scale ones. The results of the trials are then submitted to the FDA.

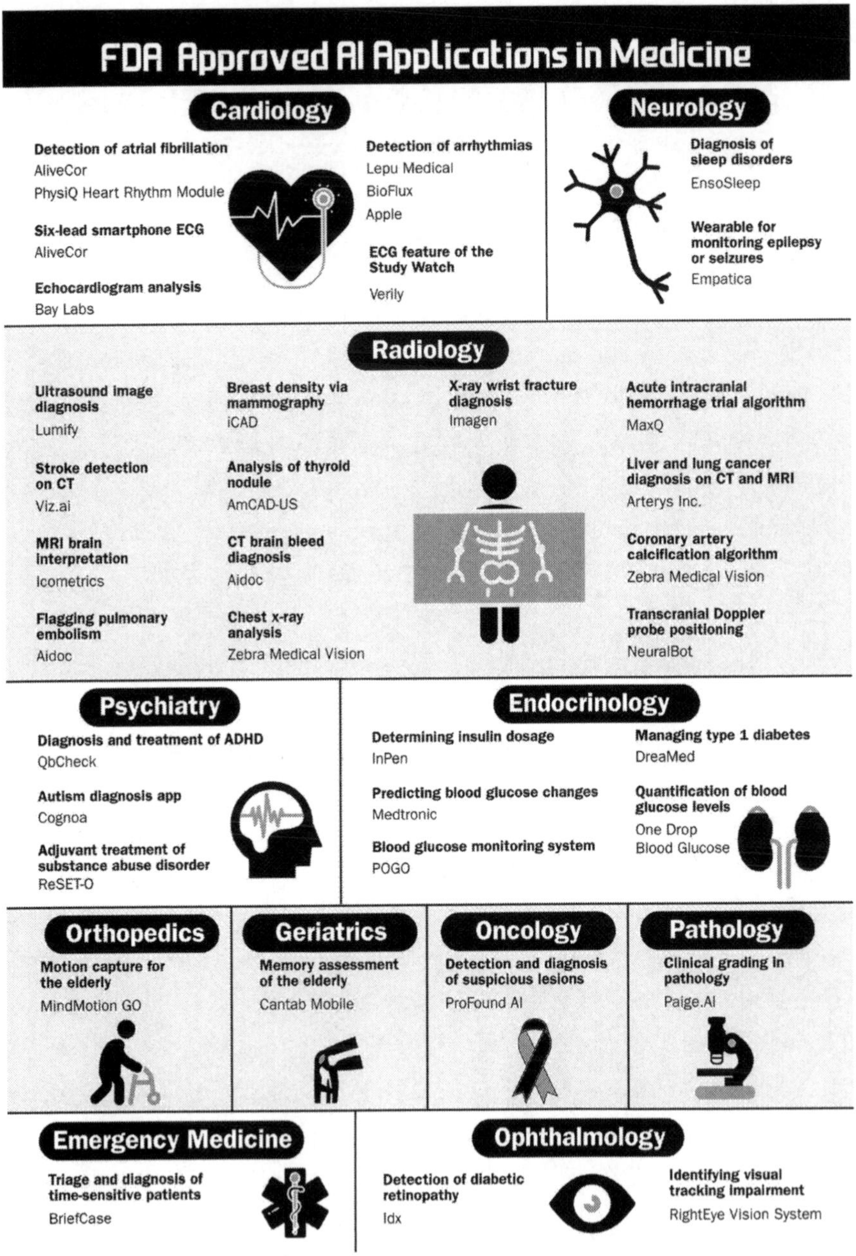

FDA Approved AI Applications in Medicine

Cardiology

Detection of atrial fibrillation
AliveCor
PhysiQ Heart Rhythm Module

Six-lead smartphone ECG
AliveCor

Echocardiogram analysis
Bay Labs

Detection of arrhythmias
Lepu Medical
BioFlux
Apple

ECG feature of the Study Watch
Verily

Neurology

Diagnosis of sleep disorders
EnsoSleep

Wearable for monitoring epilepsy or seizures
Empatica

Radiology

Ultrasound image diagnosis
Lumify

Stroke detection on CT
Viz.ai

MRI brain interpretation
Icometrics

Flagging pulmonary embolism
Aidoc

Breast density via mammography
iCAD

Analysis of thyroid nodule
AmCAD-US

CT brain bleed diagnosis
Aidoc

Chest x-ray analysis
Zebra Medical Vision

X-ray wrist fracture diagnosis
Imagen

Acute intracranial hemorrhage trial algorithm
MaxQ

Liver and lung cancer diagnosis on CT and MRI
Arterys Inc.

Coronary artery calcification algorithm
Zebra Medical Vision

Transcranial Doppler probe positioning
NeuralBot

Psychiatry

Diagnosis and treatment of ADHD
QbCheck

Autism diagnosis app
Cognoa

Adjuvant treatment of substance abuse disorder
ReSET-O

Endocrinology

Determining insulin dosage
InPen

Predicting blood glucose changes
Medtronic

Blood glucose monitoring system
POGO

Managing type 1 diabetes
DreaMed

Quantification of blood glucose levels
One Drop
Blood Glucose

Orthopedics

Motion capture for the elderly
MindMotion GO

Geriatrics

Memory assessment of the elderly
Cantab Mobile

Oncology

Detection and diagnosis of suspicious lesions
ProFound AI

Pathology

Clinical grading in pathology
Paige.AI

Emergency Medicine

Triage and diagnosis of time-sensitive patients
BriefCase

Ophthalmology

Detection of diabetic retinopathy
Idx

Identifying visual tracking impairment
RightEye Vision System

Figure 3-1. FDA-approved AI applications in medicine

Thereafter, the FDA decides whether to approve the product. The product's packaging is then reviewed to ensure the communication of correct information to healthcare professionals as well as users. The company's manufacturing sites are then inspected by the FDA, after which an approval or a response letter is issued. After approval of the product, the company is responsible for submitting post-marketing monitoring for safety updates to the FDA.

The approval of various AI-powered algorithms by the FDA has paved the way for their implementation in the healthcare field.[3] FDA's AI medical device database is available at: https://www.fda.gov/medical-devices/software-medical-device-samd/artificial-intelligence-and-machine-learning-aiml-enabled-medical-devices (https://bit.ly/3BGRsUA)

List of FDA-approved AI applications in medicine

1. Cardiology

Detection of atrial fibrillation

AliveCor

The AliveCor Kardia system was approved by the FDA in 2014 for the company's cellular phone application Kardia.[4] This allowed ECG monitoring and detection of atrial fibrillation through a smartphone. A published article in 2017 showed that remote interpretation of ambulatory patients using a single-lead iECG demonstrates a greater likelihood of identifying asymptomatic atrial fibrillation than routine care. In addition, patients reported general satisfaction with the ease of use and security of data with AliveCor.

PhysiQ Heart Rhythm Module

Approved in August 2018, the PhysiQ Heart Rhythm Module[5] is intended for use by healthcare professionals to calculate heart rate and its associated variability and detect atrial fibrillation using itinerant ECG via single-lead. The PhysiQ Heart Rhythm Module is aimed for use in sub-acute clinical settings as well as non-clinical sites for ambulatory patient monitoring. It is not intended for use in patients who require life support, life-sustaining systems, or ECG alarm devices.

Detection of arrhythmias

Lepu Medical

It's considered to be a complete solution for patients with cardiac diseases. The company specializes in the development of high-tech medical devices for most cardiovascular disorders. Beijing's artificial intelligence ECG tracker software gained FDA approval in 2017.[6] It aims to provide the most dynamic monitoring to patients by improving the detection efficacy of non-persistent arrhythmias that are otherwise difficult to identify in standard ECG assessments. The device is eligible for use in clinics and hospitals as well as community healthcare centers. It not only helps physicians with prompt and accurate data interpretation but can also be used in centers lacking professional doctors.

BioFlux

This modern cardiac monitoring software is aimed at facilitating the diagnosis of cardiac disorders, improving patient outcomes, reducing costs, and enhancing revenue generation. BioFlux is a highly accurate Mobile Cardiac Telemetry (MCT) that allows for the transmission of ECG details of ambulatory patients in real-time.[7] It received FDA approval in December 2017.

Apple

The AI-powered Apple watch application has demonstrated the detection of cardiac arrhythmias with a precision value of 97%, according to the mRhythm study.[8] The Apple watch uses deep learning algorithms for the accumulation of relevant heart rate data. Apple worked with the FDA and, in September 2018, was successful in achieving the administration's approval of an ECG app for the detection of arrhythmias. Its arrhythmia notification feature helps people identify irregular heart rhythms, thereby helping to prevent stroke.

Echocardiogram analysis

Bay Labs

Cleared by the FDA in January 2018, Bay Labs makes it possible to perform echocardiogram analysis using its AI software.[9] The AI algorithm automatically selects the appropriate clip while also calculating the ejection fraction of the left ventricle of the heart. Thus, it removes the need for manual selection of visuals, reducing the variability as well as the time required. The technology enables physicians to interpret echocardiograms with a higher accuracy rate, resulting in augmented patient care.

ECG feature of the Study Watch

Verily

Verily intends to assemble information as an element of research, as opposed to the Apple Watch, which works as a consumer device.[10] It was approved by the FDA in 2019 and is available by prescription only. It functions to document, store, transfer, and present single-channel ECG rhythms. It is aimed for use by physicians as well as patients with diagnosed or suspected heart disorders. Verily allows for real-time use of algorithms on the device with encrypted record compression.

Six-lead smartphone ECG

AliveCor

FDA gave its first-ever approval in 2019 to AliveCor for a six-lead ECG device, making the KardiaMobile 6L the pioneer in personal ECG service.[11] This opens the doors for both clinicians and patients to have a more in-depth view of the patient's heart, thereby improving clarity for arrhythmias that are indicative of various heart conditions. According to AliveCor CEO Ira Bahr, AliveCor has made cardiovascular care more convenient, more obtainable, and less costly than ever before. 6L means that the technology enables the physician to visualize the heart from six perspectives, allowing them to better examine the heart than if a single-lead ECG were used.

2. Radiology

Ultrasound image diagnosis

Lumify

An initiative of Philips, the Lumify ultrasound device, has made ultrasound examinations more accessible and less expensive.[12] Having earned FDA approval in October 2016, the latest ultrasound technology is available for purchase by healthcare institutions across the United States. The system eliminates the need for purchasing imaging equipment and includes the transducer and online portal accessibility along with the app. The Lumify application is available for use in acute care, internal medicine, musculoskeletal and emergency settings, and general clinical practice.

Analysis of thyroid nodule

AmCAD-US

This is a computer-based application that obtained its FDA approval in May 2017.[13] It is an ultrasound image analysis system that carries out the risk scoring for thyroid nodules. It is the first computer-assisted ultrasound device approved by the FDA. The software helps physicians analyze thyroid ultrasound images obtained from FDA-cleared sonographic systems. It is aimed at visualizing ultrasound images of thyroid nodules larger than 1cm. In addition, the software device presents detailed data with the help of ultrasonic visuals and quantification of the nodules of the thyroid gland. It allows healthcare professionals to make effective and precise diagnoses. Combined with physicians' expertise, this technology provides the best solution for fast-paced medical needs.

Stroke detection on CT

Viz.ai

This AI-powered stroke identifying software provides timely detection and triage of large vessel obstruction strokes and alerts specialists by sending radiological images to their smartphones.[14] This allows them to provide prompt care. As a result, there is a dramatic reduction in time delays before life-saving treatment is administered. Viz.ai is an innovative technology approved by the FDA in February 2018 and has transformed care for stroke patients.

Liver and lung cancer diagnosis on CT and MRI

Arterys Inc.

This AI-powered software earned FDA clearance in February 2018. It uses CT and MRI scans for the assessment of the lungs and to look for lesions. The cloud-based tool utilizes AI to segment lesions and nodules. Furthermore, its evaluation is as good as a board-certified radiologist. The software is intended to allow radiologists to detect and measure suspected tumors and track the progress of established cases. This technology enables radiologists to validate, assess, enumerate, and report lung and liver nodules. Albert Hsiao, MD, co-founder of Arterys, states that the software is aimed at maximizing radiologists' precision and efficiency in the interpretation of suspected cases for prompt care provision.

MRI brain interpretation

Icometrics

This is an important tool to provide enhanced monitoring and improved patient outcomes.[15] It speeds up the radiology workflow by more than 50%. It enables early diagnosis and quantification of brain conditions and lesions like multiple sclerosis, dementia, etc. Also, it enhances patient care through a quick treatment response. With Icometrics, which the FDA approved in April 2018, patients' data security and privacy are given high importance.

X-ray wrist fracture diagnosis

Imagen

After receiving FDA clearance in May 2018, Imagen has acted as an adjunct to the clinician's assessment.[16] It is the latest computer-aided detection technology based on artificial intelligence. It is aimed for use by healthcare professionals to quickly detect and diagnose wrist fractures. Its OsteoDetect software employs AI not only to detect but also to mark the location of the fracture. It can be used in primary care and emergency settings, as well as in specialist areas such as orthopedics.

Transcranial Doppler probe positioning

NeuralBot

This software guides the operator in correctly positioning transducers, one on each side on the temporal region of the head, with the help of robotic actuators using certain algorithms.[17] It obtained the FDA seal in May 2018. When used with the Lucid M1 System, NeuralBot acts as an ultrasound device guiding the user in setting up and acquiring the velocity of cerebral blood flow. It is aimed for use by trained professionals and is used as an adjunct to conventional practice.

Coronary artery calcification algorithm

Zebra Medical Vision

The Israeli deep learning startup got FDA approval in July 2018.[18] Zebra Medical envisions formulating artificial intelligence gear for medical imaging and radiology. It is intended to enable clinicians to quantify coronary artery calcifications. It is a software that uses specific algorithms to carry out automated scoring of coronary calcification. It can identify patients at risk of a cardiovascular event. Also, it potentially offers more effective treatment, a reduced incidence of adverse outcomes, and decreased healthcare costs.

CT brain bleed diagnosis

Aidoc

The AI-powered software offers workflow optimization to assist radiologists in triage. It obtained FDA approval in August 2018 for the detection of acute intracranial hemorrhage. This technology provides a comprehensive solution to detect acute pathologies. It is not limited to the brain; rather, it can potentially be used for the whole body. By studying a variety of radiology images, Aidoc notifies radiologists of suspected cases to prioritize more serious cases for prompt diagnosis and treatment. Thereby, it dramatically reduces report turnaround time and enhances the confidence of radiologists in improving patient care.

Breast density via mammography

iCAD

This automated software based on machine learning delivers quick and reproducible breast density analyses.[19,20] The AI-based system obtained FDA approval in August 2018. It potentially identifies patients with diminished sensitivity to digital mammography due to an increased density of breast tissue. It not only identifies but also calibrates dense breast tissue according to the reporting system of the American College of Radiology (BIRADS). This helps healthcare providers better detect cases of suspected breast cancer and provide greater patient satisfaction for enhanced care.

Acute intracranial hemorrhage trial algorithm

MaxQ

The CEO and chairman of MaxQ AI, Gene Saragnese, stated that their software could improve the detection of suspected bleeding in patients and reduce the time to identify such cases.[21] This intelligent tool helps to prioritize and grade patients who need a prompt diagnosis with the help of clinicians' judgments. The software is the workflow tool formulated to help physicians triage patients suspected of having an acute intracranial hemorrhage. The system earned its FDA approval in late October 2018. It is a game-changing tool that does not eliminate the need for clinicians but, rather, works as an adjunct to enhance patient care. Like other sibling tools, it assists in quick diagnosis and eases specialists' workload. The company's compatibility with other healthcare firms, like Neurologica, makes the implementation of its tool easier, thereby allowing it to make a massive contribution to the well-being of patients around the world.

Chest x-ray analysis

Zebra Medical Vision

This software is a complete triage solution aimed at prioritizing and flagging acute cases.[22] It is a remarkable innovation that facilitates healthcare settings and unleashes the power of AI with the help of algorithms. This tool was approved by the FDA in May 2019 and helped to reduce radiologists' workload, as it enables radiologists to view only the flagged cases. It detects pneumothorax and other acute pathologies on chest x-rays and aims to further add algorithms to augment the potential for finding other acute pathologies.

Flagging pulmonary embolism

Aidoc

Alongside intracranial hemorrhage detection, Aidoc specializes in marking acute pathologies of the lungs.[23] This product gained FDA approval in May 2019. It reduces the time required for detecting pulmonary embolism, thus decreasing the number of deaths caused by it. The AI-based software provides triage for the workflow that facilitates the challenging diagnosis of pulmonary embolism. This makes it a life-saving tool, producing unprecedented results. It can be utilized by professional healthcare providers in emergency care as well as by fellows and residents.

3. Psychiatry

Diagnosis and treatment of attention deficit hyperactivity disorder (ADHD)

QbCheck

This AI-driven software works on algorithms to assist doctors in ruling out or diagnosing ADHD.[24] The tool optimizes treatment as well as augments communication with patients. QbCheck does not work independently for diagnoses. Instead, it is formulated to work in conjunction with patient assessment and interview. It received its FDA clearance in March 2016, is portable, and ensures patient data safety and security. QbCheck allows physicians to interpret reports easily and also offers online training.

Autism diagnosis

Cognoa

The pediatric behavioral health company Cognoa has developed a diagnostic app for the detection of autism spectrum disorder (ASD).[25] At present, autism diagnosis occurs at an average of four years of age, which is beyond the primary brain development phase. Cognoa, however, aims to facilitate pediatricians in the primary care of autistic children as young as 18 months to provide them with the earliest possible diagnosis and treatment. This is a significant breakthrough that can have a lifelong impact on autistic children. The application was approved by the FDA in February 2018 and provided a breakthrough in the diagnosis and management of autism. It is intended for physicians, employers, and parents to learn about the importance of early detection and treatment and understand how to impact behavioral health in children.

Adjuvant treatment of substance abuse disorder

ReSET-O

This application provides a complete solution for people with substance abuse disorder, including opioid abuse disorder.[26] It enhances outpatient therapy and provides patients with access to lessons and motivational reinforcements for assisted recovery. Further, it enables physicians to bridge the gaps in patient care. Approved by the FDA in December 2018, ReSET-O is a prescription digital therapy used in conjunction with other medicines. The AI-based software is easy to use and is available on smartphones.

4. Endocrinology

Determining insulin dosage

InPen

InPen is an application intended for use by diabetic patients aged 12 and above to self-inject insulin.[27] This app can be used at home, and one pen is reusable for a single patient. It obtained its FDA approval in July 2016. The insulin dose calculator of the InPen application calculates the insulin dose and the amount of carbohydrate intake according to data entered by the user. However, some specifications must be registered in the app under a doctor's supervision before use, and meal sizes must be predetermined.

Quantification of blood glucose levels

One Drop Blood Glucose

This application, based on AI algorithms, calculates blood glucose levels and is automated to send the information to another application. The FDA approved this application in November 2016, giving some autonomy to patients in terms of monitoring their blood glucose levels, thereby making care accessible to many and reducing healthcare costs. It also includes lifestyle recommendations to motivate patients to monitor their behavior and diet.

Predicting blood glucose changes

Medtronic

Based on machine learning, the Medtronic app is the pioneer in innovations that predict future blood glucose levels in the body. It predicts patients' low blood glucose levels for the next one to four hours. The app was approved by the FDA in March 2018 and is available in the App Store for download free of cost. It enables users to determine the pattern of changes in their blood glucose levels. Thus, it prevents the occurrence of hypoglycemic events in patients with chronic diabetes, as well as in new cases.

Managing type 1 diabetes

DreaMed

The data science-based revolutionary app provides insulin treatment plans specific to each patient. It works by transforming patients' real-time data into insulin management insights.[28] It helps with self-management, providing easy access to functional expertise. It was approved by the FDA in June 2018. The AI-driven software aims to improve the lives of diabetic patients by providing them with decision support technology. DreaMed is widely accessible, providing optimal glycemic control to patients, improving the quality of life for the masses, and reducing overall costs.

Blood glucose monitoring system

POGO

Pogo is an automatic blood glucose testing system that eliminates the need for test strips and lancets. It consists of a 10-test cartridge that does the work for you. Pogo received its FDA approval in June 2018. It is easy to use, time-saving, and effective. Patients can use their personal Pogo device without the limitation of place and time, as well as without the hassle of handling the lancet and strips. This AI technology produces fast results with a one-step procedure. It can also be synchronized with other compatible apps like patterns for patients to track their blood glucose levels from their smartphones or desktop computers.

5. Geriatrics

Memory assessment of the elderly

Cantab Mobile

This is a tablet-based tool approved by the FDA in January 2017. The application was designed by Cambridge Cognition, a UK-based company that deals with memory issues in the elderly. The app includes three different exercises that take ten minutes to perform in order to test applicants' memory. It functions by marking suspected cases of Alzheimer's and dementia. Early detection means an improvement in the quality of life of older adults who have suffered without this tool. It helps clinicians figure out the earliest signs of memory impairment so that further treatment can be optimized in a timely fashion. It also tests for depression and differentiates between memory disorders and mood impairment. This app acts as an adjunct to clinical care. Its simplicity of implementation and handling allows it to be used by support staff as well.

6. Neurology

Diagnosis of sleep disorders

EnsoSleep

This cloud-based technology helps physicians with diagnoses. It enables them to assess the quality of sleep. The software was approved by the FDA in March 2017 and is intended for use under a physician's supervision for the analysis of sleep disorders in order to score sleep study outcomes, leg movement, sleep staging, arousal detection, and obstructive apnea.

Wearable for monitoring epilepsy or seizures

Empatica

This AI-based wearable device is a health tool for patients with epilepsy. It can be worn on the wrist and constantly monitors physiological signals. In the case of a risk of seizure, it immediately alerts patients' healthcare providers, family, and friends. The tool obtained FDA approval in February 2018 for use in adults and children above six years of age.[29] It allows medical care to be given outside of hospitals and in the homes of patients. The cloud-based app is synchronized with the Alert app in a patient's smartphone, which immediately calls or sends a text message to caregivers in an emergency, along with the patient's GPS location. This allows the caregiver to reach out for help immediately.

7. Emergency medicine

Triage and diagnosis of time-sensitive patients

BriefCase

This computer-based radiological device was approved by the FDA in August 2018. It is used to analyze CT images of the cervical spine. The software is aimed at assisting hospitals and radiologists in triage by flagging high-risk cases and communicating suspected findings in the cervical spine. It uses artificial intelligence to analyze visuals. The device works alongside the conventional clinical care provided by physicians as a tool for transmitting information rather than as a diagnostic device.

8. Ophthalmology

Detection of diabetic retinopathy

Idx

The artificial intelligence-based device Idx is used to identify eye diseases that are greater than mild-level in diabetic patients. Early detection of diabetic retinopathy is essential before permanent damage to the eyes occurs. In April 2018, the FDA approved the device for use by doctors in the primary care setting. With the help of AI algorithms, Idx can analyze images taken from a retinal camera. The quality images screen the patient for diabetic retinopathy and provide doctors with direction for further management. Cases lesser than the mild level are flagged and recommended for reference to the eye specialist, or they are shown as negative, and re-screening is advised after 12 months.

Identifying visual tracking impairment

RightEye Vision System

The system was approved by the FDA in September 2018. It is used for tracking eye movements to associate them with various oculomotor and neurological health conditions.[30,31] The system performs analysis of eye movements to detect visual tracking impairment. It measures the objective eye movement, which assists physicians in the diagnosis of conditions like Parkinson's disease by reducing the likelihood of misdiagnosis. It is a tool that not only directs clinicians to a correct diagnosis but also empowers them to detect the disorder at an earlier stage.

9. Orthopedics

Motion capture for the elderly

MindMotion GO

This home neurological rehabilitation software from a Switzerland-based company received its FDA clearance in May 2018. It is a remarkable software therapy that can be used in patients' homes for those who have mild to moderate degrees of neurological impairment. The motion capture technology uses a set of activities displayed in 3D to enhance patients' care and task capabilities. It promotes patient recovery by safely acquiring patient data through their formulations, which will have beneficial outcomes beyond healthcare.

10. Pathology

Clinical grading in pathology

Paige.AI

The AI-based system Paige.AI has been successful in achieving clinical-level accuracy in computational pathology.[32] It is software that complements the efforts of pathologists to diagnose and manage cancers by providing decision support for improved patient care. The system was approved by the FDA in March 2019. It uses deep learning algorithms to detect various cancers, including those of the skin, breast, and prostate, with almost 100% accuracy.

11. Oncology

Detection and diagnosis of suspicious lesions

ProFound AI

The software obtained its FDA seal in December 2018. This computer-assisted software device is aimed at detecting and diagnosing abnormal lesions. It has the latest AI technology that holds immense potential for breast imaging.[33] It works concurrently with compatible digital breast tomosynthesis (DBT) systems to help clinicians interpret lesions. It detects the grade of soft tissue densities, including their mass, asymmetries, and tissue distortions, as well as the possibility of calcifications in the three-dimensional DBT. By spotting the densities and calcifications, the tool assists physicians in identifying true lesions. In addition, the software algorithm scores the probability of malignancy in a case on a percent scale. Thus, it is a remarkable time-saving tool that provides diagnostic confidence to radiologists.

References/Further Reading

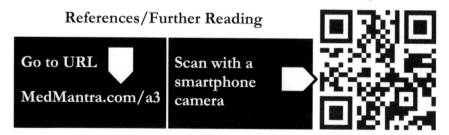

Go to URL
MedMantra.com/a3

Scan with a smartphone camera

"Whether we are based on carbon or on silicon makes no fundamental difference; we should each be treated with appropriate respect."

- Arthur C. Clarke

Section 2

Artificial Intelligence and Machine Learning Simplified

CHAPTER FOUR

ARTIFICIAL INTELLIGENCE AND MACHINE LEARNING SIMPLIFIED

Thousands of real-world problems are getting solved by the new powerful artificial intelligence (AI) based techniques, which are machine learning (ML), deep learning (DL), artificial neural networks (ANNs), etc. The application of associated algorithms and AI techniques has gained remarkable popularity. The terms associated with AI may be somewhat complex and technical due to the combination of computing, electronic signal processing, mathematics, machine learning, linguistics, psychology, and most importantly, neuroscience.

In as much as this concept seems very technical, this chapter aims to break it down to such a level that rookies in the world of technology can understand it. Even non-practitioners can relate to a certain level. The main objective of this chapter is to ensure that certain complicated areas in this field of study are better understood by a good number of the masses.

Artificial Intelligence (AI) means the ability of machines to perform tasks like those performed by human intelligence. AI is a branch of computer science which deals with stimulating intelligent behavior in computers. It consists of two different types, general and narrow. General AI can perform like human intelligence and can do all tasks in all areas like a human being. Narrow AI has the ability similar to or better than human intelligence but limited to one particular area or task (like recognizing images and nothing else).

ML is a field of study that gives computers the ability to learn without being explicitly programmed (Arthur Samuel, 1959).[1] ML is a subset of AI [see Figure 4-1]. ML involves "training" a computer software algorithm (collection of commands/rules/codes) by giving it large amounts of data and then allowing it to adjust itself so that it can learn and improve its accuracy and efficiency.

ML can be divided into two main fields: Conventional (or sometimes called shallow) and deep ML. So, DL is a subset of machine learning. As of today, there is no clear definition of the term "shallow learning" in ML, as opposed to DL, which refers to automatic learning from data using artificial neural networks. Practically, DL and ANNs are interrelated, DL would not exist without ANNs, and DL and ANNs have revolutionized the field of AI. That's the reason DL and ANNs are given significant importance when it comes to the topic of AI. DL mimics the working of the human brain in processing data for a variety of use cases.

Generally, AI is referred to as the whole system which can do a specific task. ML usually works with numerical data arranged in rows and columns. DL is more flexible with data; it can work with images, text, numerical data, voice, etc.

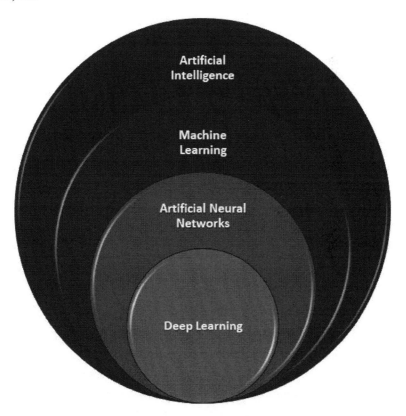

Figure 4-1. Relationship between artificial intelligence, machine learning, artificial neural networks, and deep learning

Machine Learning Algorithms

Introduction

Machine learning is based on the idea that algorithms can learn from data, identify the underlying patterns, and make decisions based on it with minimum human help. ML algorithms help recognize patterns in existing databases to predict or classify data.[2] New insights into these patterns can be made using mathematical models. It's not a new concept, but it's the one that has gained fresh momentum. With technological advancements in computational power, the rise of the internet, and smartphones, machine learning researchers got everything they dreamt of. These advancements led to the development of technologies that are applicable in almost every field.

All we need is data

The essential prerequisite for learning systems and corresponding algorithms are sufficient computing capacity and access to vast amounts of data. They are indispensable for the training of algorithms and modeling. Data can be images, words, clicks, speech, numbers, etc., whatever we can store digitally. "Big Data" has helped solve a lot of problems regarding data storage, transfer, and handling, and leveraging cloud services. We can use machine learning models on devices like smartphones, IoT (internet of things) devices with very little computational power when compared to the big servers with powerful hardware.

Despite not being recent technologies, ML and AI have significant practical importance. We use AI and ML technologies every day in our lives, knowingly or unknowingly. This applies to many areas of life and business. Internet users have benefited from this technology for long without even thinking about algorithms that work in the background. The areas of application are diverse. Consider spam detection, content personalization, document classification, sentiment analysis, customer churn forecast, email classification, upselling opportunities analysis, traffic jam prediction, genome analysis, medical diagnostics, chatbots, and much more.

The spectrum of applications spans from film and music recommendations within private environments to enhancing marketing campaigns, customer services, and logistics pathways within the business arena. A wide range of ML methods is available, including linear regression, instance-based learning, decision tree algorithms, Bayesian statistics, cluster analysis, neural networks, deep learning, and dimensionality reduction. There is a multitude of opportunities for different industries.

Making it work

For machine learning to learn from data, it must be trained by a human. This learning process begins with a prepared data set (called training data set), which is searched for patterns and correlations by a machine learning algorithm. After completing the learning process, the trained model is evaluated on unknown data. If it performs well, it is used to make predictions; otherwise, we use different parameters (settings) and algorithms to find the best results for our task.

The development of an ML model is an iterative process often run through several times until the result has reached a certain quality. There are always development loops in practice where a person must evaluate the results from the machine learning algorithm.

Machine Learning Approaches [see Figure 4-2]:

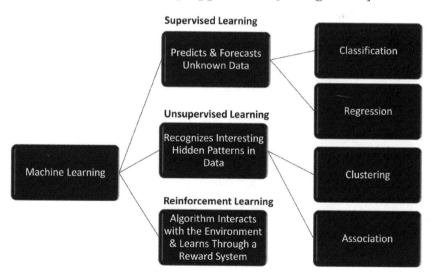

Figure 4-2. Classification of different machine learning approaches

Supervised Machine Learning

Supervised machine learning means working with labeled data. It is like telling the algorithm what pattern to look for. Like, when we watch something on YouTube, you're telling the algorithm to find similar content for you. So, it shows similar content on your home page. The model learns the mapping based on training data. In supervised learning, the relationship to a target variable is always learned, and the model tries to predict it correctly. The target variable can be a class (e.g., termination yes/no) or a numerical value (e.g., sales for the next month). The algorithm trains based on given pairs of inputs and outputs (labels). The algorithm compares the original output with the accurate output, recognizes its mistakes, and learns in this way. After that, it modifies the model accordingly. Using the model, prediction of the labels for further data that do not yet have a label can be made [see Figure 4-3].

Supervised learning is mostly used when it is possible to derive probable future events from historical data.[3] A successful learning process is used to make reliable predictions for future or unknown data. In marketing, supervised learning is often used to classify customer data. Supervised learning is very popular. Examples of supervised learning are:

- Predicting power consumption for a period of time based on past consumption

- Risk assessment in a healthcare scenario

- Prediction of failure of industrial machinery

- Forecasting customer behavior

- and many other use cases.

Unsupervised Machine Learning

The algorithm does not receive labeled data in unsupervised machine learning. It receives data from which it must independently recognize interesting and hidden groups and patterns. The fundamental difference to supervised machine learning is that unsupervised machine learning is not designed to calculate a prediction for a known target variable (e.g., classification or forecast).[4]

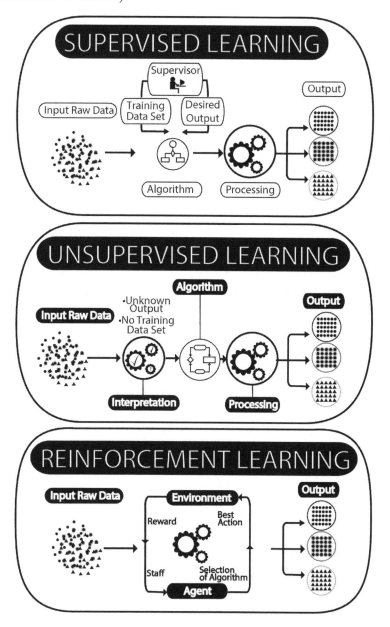

Figure 4-3. Flowcharts showing how supervised, unsupervised, and reinforcement learning works

Unsupervised ML is put into use for data without historical labels. Therefore, the system is not provided with a "correct answer." The algorithm is supposed to decode the existing data. For this purpose, the data must be examined by the algorithm for a pattern to be identified in it [see Figure 4-3 depicting unsupervised learning cycle].

Unsupervised ML can be divided into two types of problems:

Clustering: Clustering is a method of grouping objects into clusters such that objects with the most similarities remain in a group and have fewer or no similarities with objects in another group [see Figure 4-4]. Cluster analysis finds similar features amongst the data objects and groups them as per the presence or absence of these similar features.

Association: Association is a method used for finding relationships between variables in a large dataset. It determines a set of items that occurs together in the dataset. Association rule makes marketing strategy more effective. For example, people who buy X product (e.g., bread) also tend to purchase Y (butter/jam) product.

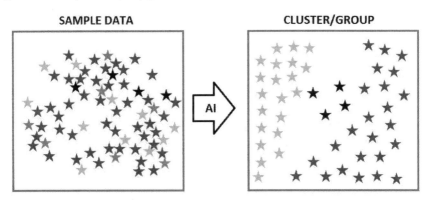

Figure 4-4. Clustering

Unsupervised learning is known to work especially well with transaction data. For example, identifying different customer groups around which to build marketing campaigns or other business strategies. Movie or YouTube video recommender systems involve grouping together users with similar viewing patterns to recommend similar content. Another real-world use case is in genetics - clustering DNA patterns to analyze evolutionary biology. Commonly used unsupervised ML algorithms include k-means clustering, k-NN (k-nearest neighbors), principle component analysis, and singular value decomposition.[5]

Partially Supervised Machine Learning

Partially supervised ML (semi-supervised ML) uses both sample data with specific target variables and unknown data and is, therefore, a mixture of supervised and unsupervised learning. The areas of application for partially supervised learning are basically the same as for supervised learning. The difference is that only a small amount of data with a known target variable is used for the learning process and a large amount where this target variable does not yet exist.[4] This has the advantage that training can be carried out with a smaller amount of labeled data. Procurement of labeled data is often extremely complex and cost-intensive. Since people often must create this data through manual processes (e.g., manual labeling of images), especially in the image or object recognition. Here a small data set of known (labeled) images is created. This is usually done by people. Then rest of the data is labeled using this model. Subsequently, for example, an artificial neural network is trained for classification and then applied to the rest of the data. This way, the sample data for the unknown data can be created correctly and quickly.

Reinforcement Learning

Reinforcement learning (RL) algorithms learn using trial and error to achieve an objective. RL consists of three parts, the agent (learner), the environment (everything the agent interacts with), and actions (what the agent does). Agent receives a reward or a penalty for its action based on the objective or the policy. The goal is to maximize rewards. The algorithm is not shown which action is the right one in which situation but instead receives positive or negative feedback from the cost function (a mechanism that returns the error between predicted outcomes and the actual outcomes). The cost function is then used to estimate which action is the right one at which point in time. Thus, the system learns "to reinforce" through praise or punishment to maximize the reward function.

The main difference from unsupervised and supervised learning is that reinforcement learning does not require sample data in advance. The algorithm can develop its own strategy in many iterative steps in a simulation environment [see Figure 4-4].

Reinforcement learning is used in robotics, computer games, and navigation. Through trial and error, the algorithm recognizes the actions that bring the greatest reward in reinforcement learning. The target of the agent is to select actions that maximize the expected reward within a specific time. The target can be achieved relatively rapidly if an appropriate strategy is employed. Learning the best strategy is the aim of reinforcement learning. Reinforcement learning is the great hope of many AI researchers for solving complex problems, such as autonomous driving, autonomous robotics, and the development of general artificial intelligence.

Autonomous vehicles use reinforcement learning to learn to drive, keeping safety first, and obeying traffic rules. The reinforcement learning agent (algorithm) learns from the system of rewards and penalties to achieve specific goals like keeping the vehicle in lane, avoiding collision, overtaking correctly, and more. The agent interacts with (but cannot change) the environment (roads, traffic, etc.) around it.

Commonly Used Machine Learning Algorithms:

ML algorithms can be broadly classified into conventional and deep ML algorithms. All ML algorithms that are not deep are called conventional (or occasionally shallow). Examples of conventional ML algorithms include linear regression, decision tree, K-nearest neighbor, Naïve-Bayes, support vector machines, etc.

Regression

Regression is a statistical method that helps us understand the relationship between two or more variables. It helps to understand which factors are important and should be considered and which can be ignored.

Regression finds the relationship between the dependent and independent variables. The dependent variable is the factor/value which we are trying to calculate; as it depends on other factors, it is named so. Independent variables are the values/factors which influence the prediction values. Regression is of two types, linear and polynomial regression.

1. *Linear Regression*

It is one of the most versatile statistical methods. Simple linear regression is a linear regression analysis that allows for only one predictor to be considered. Here we use only one variable to predict the output. In linear regression, the regression model predicts the values for the dependent variable based on the independent variables. For example, increasing sales are observed with increasing purchasing power of the customers. Usually, increasing the dosage of an antihypertensive drug leads to decreasing blood pressure in patients, which is a linear correlation.

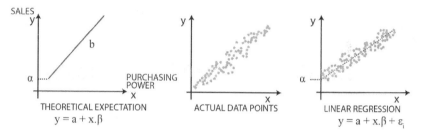

Figure 4-5. Straight-line through the data points showing linear regression

Linear regression is represented as a straight line that, at its best, determines the relationship between the input variable 'x' and the output variable 'y'.[6] This is done by determining certain weights for the input variables that are also referred to as coefficients β, and the 'y' is predicted based on the input 'x.' The linear regression learning algorithm is aimed at the determination of the value for the coefficients. Our goal is to best fit a line that can describe the properties of data [see Figure 4-5]. We are therefore looking for a function in regression that describes our point cloud - with which we are confident that we can make predictions about the dependent variable. Here, the target value (dependent variable) is 'y, and the input value is 'x.' So, we work in a two-dimensional world. It should also be noted that a point cloud can never be perfectly described by a straight line. In a two-dimensional system (one input and one output), we speak of simple regression.

Variables that mathematically define the function are often represented as Greek letters (β, α, ε, etc.). The model describes how a series of input values (n = number of x-dimensions) and a series of weights (n + 1) results in a function that calculates a y-value. Here we use n + 1 weights as n + 1th weight is the intercept of the line. This calculation is also known as forward propagation. How do we make the forward propagation spit out the correct values? We employ backpropagation.

Backpropagation is an optimization method that uses the gradient method to calculate the error of forward propagation and adapt the weights in the opposite direction of the error. It is optimized in such a way that the error is minimized. It is an iterative process in which a forward propagation is carried out repeatedly based on training data, and with each iteration step, the prediction results are compared with the specified results (the marked training data), and the errors are thus calculated. The resulting error function is convex (U-shaped), derivable, and has a central global minimum. We find this minimum through this iterative approach. For more than 200 years, science has known linear regression, and it has been thoroughly researched. A few good rules of thumb during the usage of these methods include the removal of very similar variables (correlated) and the removal of noise from the data, if feasible. Therefore, linear regression is both a quick and easy method and an excellent first algorithm to try out.

2. *Polynomial Regression*

Polynomial regression (PR) is used to fit nonlinear relationships in data. In many cases, the relationship between the dependent and independent variables cannot be expressed appropriately through a straight line. In such cases, we use different curves to fit our data and predict better results [see Figure 4-6]. PR helps us develop flexible ML models that calculate the potential death rate by analyzing many dependent factors or variables. In COVID-19 pandemic, these variables can be pre-existing chronic diseases, living or working in crowded places, access to face masks, etc. PR is often used to monitor the spread of tumors in cancer patients, as the tumor spread often has a non-linear character. We need to use this algorithm carefully, as a wrong approach could lead to overfitting (the algorithm performs well on the given data, but in practical application, it struggles to provide proper predictions).

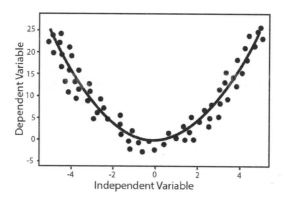

Figure 4-6. Graph of polynomial regression - a curve representing data properties

Logistic Regression

Logistic regression works where the dependent variable is categorical, i.e., data containing the only integral value to represent its class. It is used to predict whether an event or person passes or fails, wins or loses, healthy or sick, etc. It can also be extended to multi-class classification or multinomial logistic regression, where instead of two categories, dependent variables can be classified into more than two categories. It mostly deals with problems related to binary classifications (i.e., problems with two class values).

This is an alternative method that has been adopted from the field of statistics by machine learning. As with linear regression, the goal of logistic regression is the determination of the values for the coefficients that weight each of the output variables. A nonlinear function called the logistic function is used to convert the prediction for the output.[7] The logistic function resembles 'S' [see Figure 4-7]. Its task is to convert the given value into a range that is from 0 to 1. This is essential because the rule may be applied to the logistic function's output to bind the values to 0 and 1 (e.g., if the output is less than 0.5, the output is 0) and for the prediction of a class value.[4]

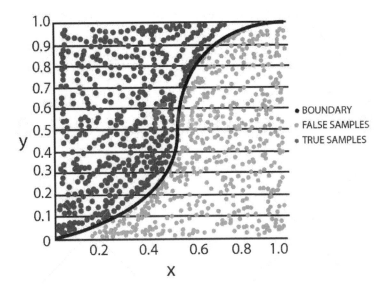

Figure 4-7. Logistic regression - 'S' shaped logistic function acting as a boundary between two classes

As the model learns, there is an option to use the logistic regression predictions as a probability for the instance of the given data assigned to either class 0 or class 1. This is particularly helpful in solving the problems where a prediction needs to be better justified. As with linear regression, logistic regression works better if both the attributes that are not related to the output variable and the attributes that are relatively very similar are eliminated. Logistic regression is, therefore, a quick model to learn. It can also solve the problems of binary classification very effectively.

When formulating the regression model, it must be decided which variables are included in the model as dependent and as independent variables. Theoretical considerations play a central role in this. The model should be kept as simple as possible. It is therefore advisable not to include too many independent variables. The ordering of independent variables also plays a significant role in logistic regression. If all independent variables are completely unrelated, then the order in which they are introduced into the model is irrelevant. However, the variables are rarely completely unrelated. The method of variable inclusion is, therefore, relevant.

With the help of logistic regression, we can make statements about the probability with which a certain form of an independent variable will be found in a condition of the dependent variable. Imagine the example of caffeine consumption and the ability to concentrate. Instead of measuring the concentration on a continuous scale from 1 to 100, you could simply ask the test subjects whether they are feeling focused or not.

Discriminant Analysis

Discriminant analysis (DA) is used to analyze problems to differentiate or discriminate data into discrete/distinct classes. For example, a physician could perform a discriminant analysis to identify patients at high or low risk for heart attack. DA can also be used in real life to differentiate between the price sensitive and non price sensitive buyers of groceries in terms of their psychological attributes or characteristics. DA contains the statistical properties of the data that are calculated for each class. It includes the following for a single variable input:

- the mean for each class

- the variance calculated for all the classes.

The predictions are made via the calculation of a discriminant value for each of the classes and making a prediction for the class that has the highest value. This method assumes that the data has a Gaussian distribution or normal distribution (bell curve) and different classes have class-specific means and equal variance/covariance. If these assumptions are violated, logistic regression will outperform Linear Discriminant Analysis (LDA). Therefore, it is recommended to eliminate the outliers from the data in advance. Discriminant analysis is best suited for tackling predictive modeling problems.

Decision Trees

A decision tree is drawn upside down with its root at the top and leaf nodes at the bottom. The tree is split into branches and edges. Trees cover both classification as well as regression-related problems. It is a flowchart-like structure, and its internal nodes denote different test conditions, the branch denotes the outcome of the test, and the last nodes (leaf nodes) hold class labels or output [see Figure 4-8].

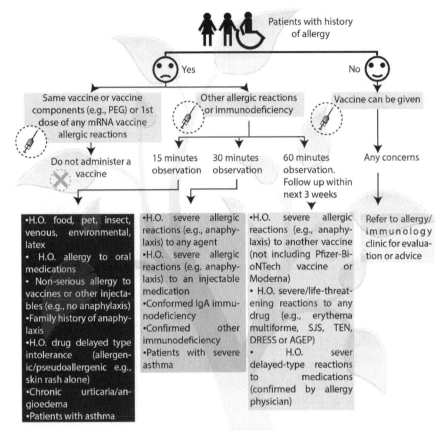

Algorithm for COVID-19 vaccination and physician response for patients with suspected allergy

Abbreviations: Erythema multiforme (EM), Stevens-Johnson syndrome (SJS), toxic epidermal necrolysis (TEN), Drug reaction with -eosinophilia and systemic symptoms (DRESS), Acute generalized - exanthematous pustulosis (AGEP). polyethylene glycol (PEG)

Figure 4-8. A decision tree contains root at the top and leaves at the bottom

A decision tree is a robust algorithm used for the predictive modeling of ML. The model of a decision tree is represented as a binary tree. A binary tree has a straightforward structure because it consists of algorithms and data structures. Each node is used to represent an individual input ('x') and a division point of this variable (provided that the variable is a numeric one). The end nodes of the tree consist of an output variable ('y') that is used in making a prediction: the tree divisions run through to the end node, and the class value is the output at the same end node. Trees are quick to learn and very quick in determining predictions. Additionally, they are often precise in solving diverse problems and do not need special preparation of the data.

One must descend along the tree from the root node to the leaf node to get a classification or output. A tree essentially contains the rules for answering only one question. In a problem with low complexity, a binary decision tree is used for prediction. Decision trees are less appropriate for predicting continuous values and are prone to errors due to the relatively small dataset.

Decision trees may either be manually written by experts or automatically deduced from gathered experience using ML techniques. There are many competing algorithms available for this. According to the top-down principle, the decision trees are mostly inferred recursively (from root to leaf nodes). For this purpose, the dataset needs to contain values using which decisions can be made. A split on the data is performed at each node based on one of the input features, generating two or more branches as output. More and more splits are done in the upcoming nodes, and increasing numbers of branches are generated to partition the original data. This continues until a node is generated where all or almost all of the data belong to the same class, and further splits or branches are no longer possible.

Ultimately, a decision tree describing the experience of the training data in formal rules is created. Now, the trees may be used for the automatic classification of other data records or for the interpretation and evaluation of the resulting set of rules.

All algorithms for the automatic induction of decision trees are based on the same recursive top-down principle. The only difference is in their criteria for the selection of the values and attributes of the rules at the nodes of the tree, in their criteria for the cancellation of the induction process, and in the likely post-processing steps that subsequently optimize a branch of a tree that has already been calculated (or entire trees) using various criteria.

A considerable benefit of the decision trees is that they are relatively easy to both understand and explain. This is especially useful when the basic properties of the data cannot be determined from the outset.

An often-mentioned drawback of the decision trees is the relatively low quality of classification when the trees are made use of for automatic classification. Because of their discrete set of rules, the trees perform somewhat worse for most real-world classification problems as compared to the other classification techniques like artificial neural networks or support vector machines. This implies that even though the trees can create easily understandable rules for people, these understandable rules often do not have the best possible quality for problem-solving in the real world. Another drawback is the possible sizes of the decision trees if no simple rule can be induced from the training data.

This can have several negative effects: on the one hand, a human viewer quickly loses the overall view of the connection between the many rules, and on the other hand, such large trees tend to lead towards over-adaptation to the training data record so that the new data records are automatically incorrectly classified. Methods were therefore developed to shorten the decision trees to a reasonable size. For instance, one may either limit the maximum depth of the trees or set in place a minimum number of objects per node.

The error rate of a decision tree is equal to the number or amount of the wrongly classified data objects relative to all the data objects in a data record. This number is determined regularly on either the training data used or, even better, on a set of data objects that are categorized as accurately as possible, disjointed from the training data, also called test data.

Depending on the area of application, it can be particularly important to keep either the false positive objects (incorrect classification of disease when no disease is present in the test subject) or the false negative objects (fails to indicate the presence of a condition when it is present) especially low. For example, in emergency medicine, it is far less harmful to treat a healthy patient than not to treat a sick patient. The effectiveness of decision trees is, therefore, always context-dependent.

Decision trees can be combined with neural networks. In this way, it is possible to replace inefficient branches of a tree with neural networks to achieve a higher classification quality that cannot be achieved with the trees alone. The advantages of both classification methods can also be used by mapping partial structures into the other methodology: The trees do not need as much training data for induction as the neural networks, and due to this, they can be quite inaccurate, especially when they're small. The neural networks, on the other hand, classify more precisely but require more training data. Therefore, one can try to use the properties of the decision trees for the generation of parts of neural networks by the so-called TBNNs (Tree-Based Neural Networks) that translate the rules of the decision trees into the neural networks.[8]

Naïve-Bayes

This is a relatively basic but astonishingly strong predictive modeling algorithm. It assumes that the presence of a particular feature in a class is unrelated to the presence of any other feature. For example, a fruit may be considered to be an apple if it is red, round, and about 3 inches in diameter. All the properties of a class contribute independently to calculating probability, and that's why it is known as 'naïve.' In other words, it means each input variable is independent. It is based on the Bayes theorem.

It calculates two kinds of probabilities:

i.   the probability of each class,

ii.   the conditional probability for each class for each specified value.

These probabilities are calculated directly from the training data. After the calculation is done, the probability model is employed for the determination of the predictions for the new data utilizing the Bayes theorem. For the data that has real value, a Gaussian distribution or normal distribution (bell-shaped) is usually assumed to make the estimation of these probabilities easier.

K-Nearest Neighbors (k-NN)

This algorithm assumes that similar things exist near or in close proximity to each other. The k-NN algorithm is another basic but effective ML algorithm. It uses the entire dataset at once to calculate similar clusters of data points. To make a prediction, it tries to fit each data point into each of the clusters and finally classifies it to the best-suited one. Generally, it uses Euclidean distance to calculate the similarity between data points, but we can use several other techniques that best suit our problem. We need to tell the algorithm how many data points need to be in a cluster. This led to its naming as k-Nearest Neighbors. It puts the 'k' number of nearest points in the same cluster. It votes for the most frequent label (in classification, i.e., integers) or averages the labels (in regression, i.e., a number with decimals) as output [see Figure 4-9].

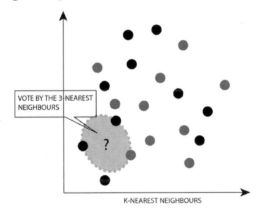

Figure 4-9. Graphical representation of k-NN showing a cluster of three nearest data points

It should also be pointed out that k-NN may require a large amount of storage space or a lot of memory to store all the data. However, this algorithm will only perform a calculation (or training) whenever there is a requirement for a prediction. If the training instances are updated and monitored over time, the predictions are kept accurate. Generally, we use the most relevant features or variables to predict the output.

For a small application, the risk is particularly great if the training data are not equally distributed or if there are only a few examples. If the training data is not evenly distributed, a weighted distance function can be used that assigns greater weight to closer points than more distant ones. A practical problem is the large storage and computing effort requirement of the algorithm with high dimensions and a lot of training data.

Genetic Algorithms (GAs)

GAs are search-based optimization techniques based on genetics and the principle of natural selection. Optimization means finding input values such that we get the best output. Generally, it refers to maximizing or minimizing a function. Genetic algorithms mimic the principle of biological evolution. To find an approximate answer to a problem of optimization, evolutionary principles such as mutation or selection are applied to the populations of solution candidates.

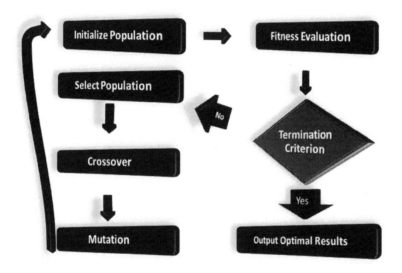

Figure 4-10. Flowchart showing a genetic algorithm

We have a pool or a population of possible solutions to the given problem. These solutions then undergo recombination and mutation (changes like in natural genetics), producing new children, and the process is repeated over various generations. Each individual (or candidate solution) is assigned a fitness value (based on its objective function value), and the fitter individuals are given a higher chance to mate and yield more "fitter" individuals. This is similar to

"Survival of the Fittest." In this way, we keep "evolving" better individuals or solutions over generations till we reach a stopping criterion. The algorithm terminates when either a maximum number of generations has been produced or a satisfactory fitness level has been reached for the population [see Figure 4-10].

Let us imagine a box with auto parts. If the box is shaken long enough, there is a chance (however small) that after a while, a roadworthy car will be assembled within the box. This random generation model makes it extremely unlikely that anything nearly complex, let alone a living organism, could arise. As we would like to further develop the population of the solution candidates, there is a requirement for a suitable representation.

The fitness function mimics the environment of biological evolution. This is often identical to the function to be optimized. A method for selecting the solution candidates according to their fitness is used for the simulation of the selection of biological evolution. A simple method is to convert fitness into a probability of selection, which is then used to decide which individuals will be transferred to the next generation without change.[9] This is repeated until we get desired results.

GAs generally perform better for real-world problems than other optimization processes like Gradient-based methods. GAs also deliver fast results that suit real-world applications.

Learning Vector Quantization (LVQ)

LVQ is a prototype-based supervised classification algorithm. It applies a winner-take-all Hebbian learning-based approach. It is a precursor to self-organizing maps (SOM) and related to the k-nearest neighbor algorithm (k-NN). It compresses data by assigning reference vectors to data points and sending only the optimum reference vectors instead of the entire data. The LVQ model is based on the similarity (or dissimilarity/distance) measure between the test object and the reference vectors, called codebook vectors or prototypes.[10] For each data point, the LVQ model, determines the prototype closest to the input. This winner prototype is then moved closer if it correctly classifies the data point or moved away if it classifies the data point incorrectly. LVQ models can be applied to multi-class classification problems, especially in classifying text documents.

Support Vector Machines (SVMs)

The function of SVMs is to find a hyperplane in N-dimensional space (N = number of features) that distinctly classifies data. A hyperplane refers to a straight line/plane that divides the input variable space. It can also be referred to as a decision boundary [see Figure 4-11]. There may exist many such hyperplanes, but our objective is to find the one with maximum margin. This may be represented in two dimensions as a straight line or as a plane in three dimensions.[11]

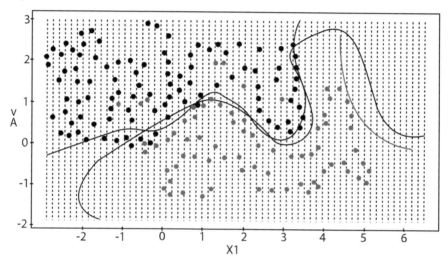

Figure 4-11. Graphical representation of a support vector machine

A vector in a vector space symbolizes each object. Support vectors are the data points that are closer to the separating hyperplane. The position of these support vectors influences the orientation of the hyperplane. We try to find the maximum separation between these support vectors and the hyperplane. The optimal or best hyperplane that can divide the two classes is a straight line that has the largest margin.

During the insertion of the hyperplane, it is not required to consider all the training vectors. The vectors that are at a greater distance from the hyperplane are 'hidden' to an extent behind the other vectors and do not affect the separation plane's position. The hyperplane is only dependent on the closest vectors, and only they are required to describe the layer precisely in a mathematical manner.

It is impossible to 'bend' a hyperplane, and so a clean separation with a hyperplane is feasible only if the objects are linearly separable. This condition is not commonly met for real sets of training objects. In most real-life datasets, data cannot be separated using a straight line. Support vector machines make use of the kernel trick to draw a nonlinear class boundary.

For such data, we apply some mathematical transformations to add more dimensions. SVMs convert non-separable problems into separable problems and are most useful in nonlinear separation problems. Now, this data can be separated using a straight line. Most of the algorithms have inbuilt features to calculate best-suited transformations, so it's not done manually. When transforming again into the lower-dimensional space, the linear hyperplane becomes a nonlinear hyperplane, possibly even a non-contiguous hyperplane that divides the training vectors cleanly into two classes—using which predictions can be made for new data points.

Bagging and Random Forest

One of the most well-known and powerful algorithms in ML is random forest. It is a type of ML ensemble algorithm that is also known as either bootstrap aggregation or bagging. An ensemble method is a technique that combines the predictions from multiple machine learning algorithms together to make more accurate predictions than any individual model.

In bootstrap, we make small groups of our original data, and then we calculate the mean of each small group and average it out. We use this average as the mean of the original data instead of calculating the mean of it directly. It can be applied to find other quantities.

Numerous samples of the training data are obtained, and models are created for each data sample. When the making of a prediction is required for new data, each of the models makes a prediction, after which each prediction is averaged to obtain a better estimate of the actual output.

A random forest is a classification procedure in which the decision trees are created in such a way that suboptimal divisions are carried out by introducing randomness instead of selecting optimal division points. The models created for each data sample, therefore, differ more than they would otherwise but are correct in their exclusive and distinctive way. Through the combination of their predictions, the true base output value is better estimated. In simple words, a large number of individual decision trees are made, and the most common answer among their predictions is selected.

Boosting

Boosting is an ensemble method for the creation of a sole good classifier from several relatively weak classifiers. For this purpose, a model is created from the training data and a second model for the improvement of the errors of the first model.[12] The peculiarity of Boosting is that the models are continually added until the ideal prediction of the training set or the addition of a maximum number of models.

It learns from the mistakes of the previous model and tries to correct them in the next model till we get good results.

Boosting is of three types:

AdaBoost (Adaptive Boosting)

It is the first successful boosting algorithm. AdaBoost uses decision trees with a single split, and these decision trees are called decision stumps. In the first decision stump, all observations are equally weighted. Incorrectly labeled decisions are weighted more than the correctly classified observations to correct errors of the previous model. It can be used for both classification and regression (predicting continuous numerical value) tasks.

The models are built one at a time and perform the task of updating the weights of the training instances, which affect the performance of the next tree in the sequence. After the creation of all the trees, the predictions for new data can be made [see Figure 4-12]. Since a lot of attention is paid to correcting errors using this algorithm, we get clean data.

Algorithm Adaboost - Example

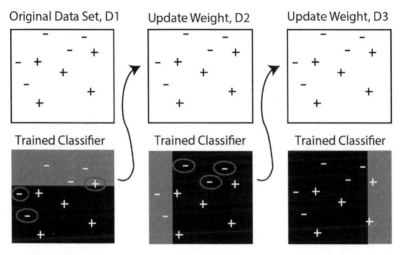

Figure 4-12: AdaBoost – the final model can classify data points more accurately

Gradient Boosting

It employs gradient descent to find the shortcomings of the previous model. Instead of changing weights for predictions, it tries to predict new values in place of erroneous values. The final model can correct a lot of errors from previous models. This leads to better results over time.

XGBoost

It stands for extreme gradient boosting. It is a library that is focused on computational speed and model performance. It supports multiple interfaces like:

- Command-line interface (CLI)

- C++

- Python

- R

- Julia

- Java and Java Virtual Machine (JVM) like Scala and Hadoop

Gradient boosting is slow due to higher computational cost. It provides Parallelization, Distributed Computing, Out-of-Core Computing, and Cache Optimization features. It is an open-source software that is available for use under the Apache-2 license.

Differences between bagging and boosting

Bagging employs parallel models, and their output is averaged according to problem type (classification or regression). Whereas in boosting, a single learner is improved over time using different approaches [see Figure 4-13].

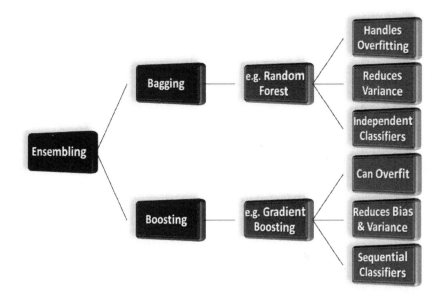

Figure 4-13. Differences between bagging and boosting

Neural Networks (NN)

Artificial neural networks are the basis of deep learning. They are inspired by the working of neurons in the human brain.

An overview of biological neural networks

To date, the most powerful computing machine ever known is the human brain. No other machine has been able to supersede its complexities. A neuron consists of a cell body from which multiple dendrites come out, along with a long tube-like axon having multiple axon terminals at its other end [see Figure

4-14]. Axon terminals are interfaces where the neurons communicate with one another, and a synapse (a gap) connects the terminals to dendrites.

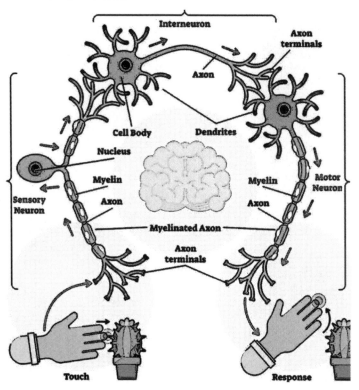

Figure 4-14. Three types of neurons, sensory neuron, interneuron, and motor neuron

A neuron, also known as a nerve cell, is an electrically excitable cell that receives, processes, and transmits information through electrical and chemical signals

© Can Stock Photo / normaals

A neuron in the brain can be considered to be equivalent to a tiny transistor in a computer, also called a node in the artificial neural network. The concept of neurons (brain cells) and network of neurons are the models upon which the inner workings of the human brain depend on. In fact, an estimated number of 100 x 10^9 neurons are contained in the human brain, with each connected through their pathways to the rest of the brain [see Figures 4-15 and 4-16].

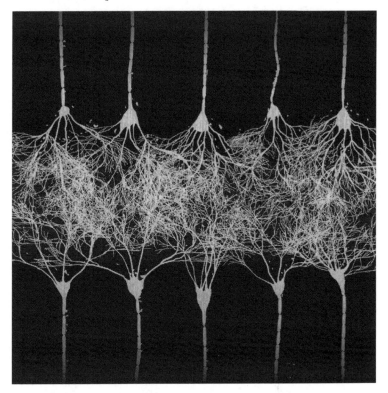

Figure 4-15. Neurons or nerve cells form a massive network

© Can Stock Photo / whitehoune

In the biological neural network, the transmission of input signals (sensory data) occurs from one layer of neurons to another through their numerous interconnections. Usually, a single neuron in the deeper layers can receive thousands of input connections, and each neuronal layer may contain a few dozen to millions of neurons.

In generating input signals, all five senses are of utmost importance. Other processes that may apply include ingestion – breathing, eating, and drinking. Before the output is delivered, multiple biochemical-physiological processes occur in the deeper neuronal layers. Then, the brain acts by instructing to act (motor signals), recollecting memory, and so on.

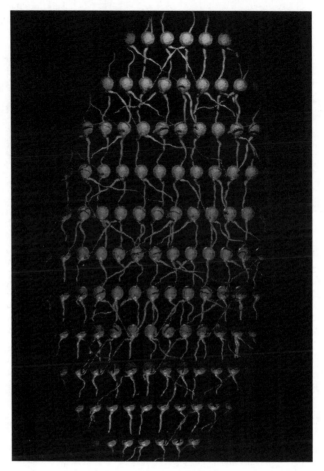

Figure 4-16. Neurons or nerve cells form a network

© Can Stock Photo / tdhster

The neural networks are the reason our brain carries out the functions of 'thinking' or 'processing' every action. As soon as our body – muscles and organs inclusive – receive the subsequent instructions from the brain, the action takes place. Nevertheless, the neural networks of the brain are capable of changing and updating by modifying their processes as a response to new learning and more experience.

If a computing machine wants to perform human-like activities, then it should replicate the functionalities and capability of the human brain. This includes intelligence. Thus, an artificial version of a network of neurons must be successfully implemented by the machine.

An overview of artificial neural networks (ANNs)

Artificial neural networks (ANNs) are algorithms that are modeled to a certain extent on the human brain. Neural networks are a very active research area and are considered the basis for artificial intelligence. They work on various data sources such as images, sound, text, tables, or time series in order to extract information and recognize patterns.

Multiple neurons in various layers of the human brain are interconnected to form massive biological neural networks. The ANNs are designed to mimic biological neural networks. The neuron or nerve cell equivalent in the ANN is called a "node." The ANNs are actually virtual or simulated networks created inside the computer software. The ANNs need not be programmed to do a particular task; they can rather be trained or learn on their own, similar to a human brain!

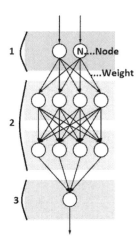

Figure 4-17: Artificial Neural Network (ANN) - an artificial network of interconnected nodes (N). Layer 1 represents the input layer, layer 2 represents the hidden layer, and layer 3 represents the output layer. Each connection between two nodes is represented by a variable number called a weight (W)

© Can Stock Photo / korolev

One or more nodes are arranged in multiple layers in a typical artificial neural network. A typical ANN has three distinct layers. These are an input layer, the hidden layers, and the output layer [see Figure 4-17]. The input layer lies at the top of the network. The hidden layers lie below the input layer, and the output layer lies at the bottom of the network. In a typical ANN, each node in the hidden and output layers is connected with each and every node in the layer above. Each connection represents a variable number called a "weight." Input layer nodes receive the data to be processed. Output layer nodes output the result(s) obtained after processing the data in the hidden layers.

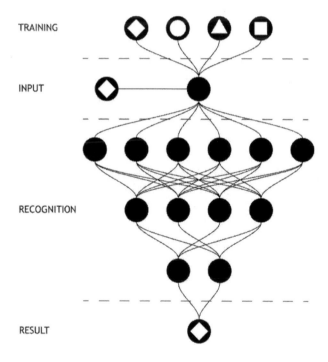

Figure 4-18. Artificial Neural Network (ANN)

© **Can Stock Photo / korolev**

When the ANN is being trained, the input layer nodes receive the data and pass it on to the nodes in the next hidden layer. The same thing happens when a trained ANN is performing a task it is trained to do. The input data is passed on from the input layer node(s), through the hidden layer nodes, and finally to the output layer node(s). The output layer node(s) give out the output data or the result [see Figure 4-18]. Since the data flows forward from the input to the output layer, this type of network is called a "feed-forward network." Data, in this case, is in the binary form - a matrix of numbers 0 and 1 in varying combinations. Any type of input data like an image, text, or audio is represented in the ANN in a binary form.

When the input layer has more than one node, each node receives the same input data. The number of output layer neurons is determined by the number of classes in the data. When the data passes through a connection between any two nodes, a mathematical function applies a weight (a small variable number that can either be positive or negative) to the data and modifies it. In simple terms, the mathematical function multiplies the input data value with the variable number of the connection weight and passes on the product to the node below it. Each node has a threshold value. The node adds all input data values, and if this summation value exceeds the threshold, then the node is activated and passes on the modified data to all the connected nodes in the next layer – a process called excitation.

Different connections may have different weights. During the training of an ANN, these weights need to be adjusted so that a correct result is obtained from the output layer. It has been proven that, given enough time to try to find the optimum weights for different connections, any artificial neural network can output the correct result! Various optimization techniques are used to expedite this process of finding optimum weights for various connections in an ANN, like gradient descent and stochastic gradient descent, to name a few. In fact, the current rapid and significant increase in the processing power of the graphics processing units (GPUs) has enabled us to reduce this optimization time from years/months to a few days/hours. This is one of the most important reasons why the ANNs have become practical and economical today.

While training an ANN for a given input data, our aim is to match the output data with the expected answer, as, answer to the input data (question) is already known. Without any training, the ANN may not give a correct answer. The difference in the actual output and the expected output (correct answer) is gradually reduced during training by changing the connection weights. This process of changing the connection weights is done in a reverse direction (bottom-up), starting from the output layer and gradually (layer by layer) moving up towards the input layer. This is the reason the process is called backpropagation. It is usually shortened to backprop.

During training, a sufficient number of pre-evaluated input data samples are used. Training is complete when the actual output exactly matches the expected output for all of the sample data. The connection weights present at this time remain fixed when the trained ANN is used in the future until it receives further training. This can be explained by a simple real-world example. Imagine as if we need to train an ANN to correctly recognize two distinct forms of oral medication - a capsule and a round flat tablet. In an ANN with one input node and one output node, we can assume that a capsule is represented by a 1 and the tablet by a 0 (binary digit). When training this ANN, our aim should always be to obtain an output of 1 when the input node sees a capsule and an output of 0 when the input node sees a tablet. When we start training the ANN to recognize a capsule, we feed the ANN with different images of capsules and use the above-described backpropagation method to gradually change the weights of different connections till we always obtain an output of 1. A similar process is repeated when training the ANN to recognize a tablet until we always obtain an output of 0. The fully trained ANN can then correctly recognize any type of capsule or tablet not seen by it before. The more and varied samples an ANN is trained with, the more accurate it becomes.

Shallow ANNs have very few hidden layers, while deep ANNs have a high number of hidden layers. Deeper ANNs are designed to carry out complex data recognition tasks, like identifying images and finding patterns in a large text database. In a deeper ANN, the superficial hidden layers learn to recognize simpler features and the deeper layers learn to recognize more complex features. The deeper the hidden layer, the more complex the feature it can recognize. For example, in a deep ANN trained to recognize human faces, the superficial hidden layers recognize simpler features like edges and overall shape of the face, and the deeper hidden layers recognize complex features like the size and shape of the nose, the color of the iris and the size and shape of the eyebrows, etc.

A complex ANN model [see Figure 4-19] with more efficient problem-solving ability and increased abstraction can be created by:

- Increasing the frequency of hidden layers

- Increasing the number of paths between neurons

- Increasing the number of neurons in a given layer

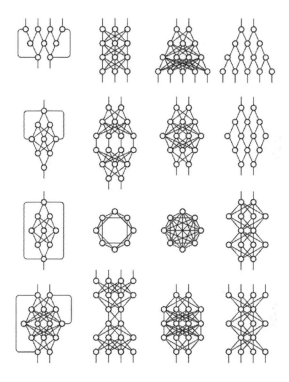

Figure 4-19. Different types of Artificial Neural Networks (ANNs)

© Can Stock Photo / korolev

However, increased model complexity is often associated with an increased chance of overfitting. Overfitting means the failure of an ANN algorithm such that it gives suboptimal results when fed unknown data but gives optimum results when fed training (previously known) data. Increased time requirements and computational resources can be consequences of complexities in model and algorithm as well.

Parallelism is the 'term' employed in modeling and processing nonlinear relationships between the input and output nodes. ANNs can be used in a lot of applications and are the important components of a broad field of machine learning.[13]

The complexity of ANNs is difficult to analyze because they are very powerful – the reason they have been termed as 'black box algorithms.' The inner workings of these algorithms have complexities that cannot be explained; finding solutions to problems by using ANN should be done, bearing this in mind.

Deep Learning (DL)

Deep learning is a subset of machine learning. It uses ANNs to learn from data. Recall that artificial neurons or processing nodes are used to transform input data throughout the different layers of an ANN. Deep learning neural networks have a greater number of hidden layers of artificial neurons and a complex architecture. The chain of transformations that occur from input to output layers is called the credit assignment path (CAP). In a deep learning model, the concept of depth is measured using the CAP value. While some scientists consider deep learning to be really deep when CAP > 10, others consider CAP > 2 as deep.[13] Shallow learning algorithms have a lesser number of hidden layers of neurons (usually a single) and are less complex as compared to deep learning algorithms.

Deep learning excels in the area of unsupervised feature extraction. Further learning, understanding, and generalization are made by using feature extraction, where meaningful data features are automatically constructed by an algorithm. Feature extraction in shallow ML is a manual process that requires domain knowledge of the data that we are learning from.

Neural networks and deep learning concepts leverage statistical techniques and signal processing techniques – which include processing and transformations which are nonlinear. Since nonlinear functions are generally not attributed by a straight line, the relationship between the dependent and independent variables (output and input, respectively) requires more than a slope for the modeling. Functions that are nonlinear include logarithmic terms, polynomial terms, and exponential terms. Nonlinear transformations are often adopted to model several phenomena in the human environment. The same applies to ML and AI solutions as it concerns transformations between the input and output layers.[13]

Large numbers of input features in the data can cause poor performance of DL algorithms. Dimensionality reduction reduces the number of input features using methods like feature selection, linear algebra methods, projection methods, and autoencoders. The benefits of dimensionality reduction are:

- Simplification
- Computational reduction
- Memory power reduction

Following are the examples of deep learning algorithms:

- Convolutional neural networks (CNN)
- Recurrent neural networks (RNN)
- Recursive neural networks (RCNN)
- Deep belief networks (DBN)
- Convolutional deep belief networks (CDBN)
- Feed-forward neural networks (FNN)
- Self-organizing maps (SOM)
- Multi-layer perceptron (MLP)
- Deep Boltzmann machines (DBM)
- Stacked de-noising auto-encoders (SDAE)
- Gated Recurrent Unit (GRU)

Before DL can be leveraged for proffering solutions to problems, some factors must be considered, including:

- Selection of algorithms
- Implementation of algorithms
- Performance assessment of algorithms

Computer Vision

It is an interdisciplinary field that deals with empowering computers to deal with images and videos. More generally, it seeks to automate visual tasks that humans can do.

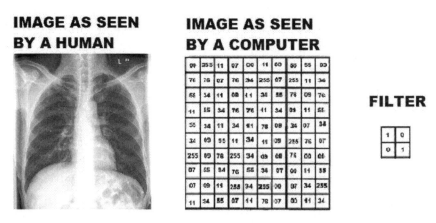

IMAGE AS SEEN BY A HUMAN

IMAGE AS SEEN BY A COMPUTER

FILTER

Figure 4-20: Chest radiograph image as seen by a human and a computer, and an example of a filter (small matrix).

The discovery of convolutional neural networks, popularly known as CNNs by Yann LeCun in 1988, revolutionized this field. CNN is a unique framework of the artificial neural network. CNN was designed to function as the human visual cortex, which is responsible for vision. Among the most popular uses of CNN is image identification or classification. For instance, Facebook makes use of CNNs for its auto-tagging feature. Amazon uses CNNs to create product recommendations, while Google uses them to search the photos of its users. Image classification will play an important role in all medical specialties, particularly in the diagnosis of medical images in radiology, pathology, dermatology, orthopedics, ophthalmology, and more.

Computers are able to detect, classify, and locate objects in images and videos using CNNs along with some additional layers of pooling and dense layers. Together they are able to understand the contents in images and videos. Let us learn more about the use of CNNs for the classification (differentiation) of images. The major function that image classification does is to accept the input image and then define the group/type it belongs to. People learn this skill from birth, and as a result, they can conveniently identify pictures of animals and daily use objects. A trained doctor can easily identify the image to be a chest X-ray. However, what the computer sees is quite different.

A computer can never see an image as a person does. Instead, it sees an array of pixels [See Figure 4-20]. For instance, if the size of an image is 300 x 300 pixels, in this situation, the array size will become 300 x 300 x 3. 300 stands for the width, the other 300 stands for the height, while 3 is the value of RGB (Red, Green, and Blue) channels. The value assigned by a computer ranges from 0 to 255 to every one of these specific numbers. This value defines the intensity of a pixel at a particular point.[14,15]

If the computer wants to find a solution to this challenge, it will, first of all, search for the low-level features. According to human understanding, such features, for instance, are either the shoulder bones, ribs, or air-filled lungs. However, for a computer, the edges, curvatures, or boundaries are low-level features. Also, with the help of groups of convolutional layers (forming the whole network), the computer can see more of the high-level features (shoulder bones, ribs, heart, or the air-filled lungs).[14,15]

To explain in detail, the image passes via a series of convolutional, nonlinear, pooling, and fully connected layers. Then it produces the output [see Figures 4-20 and 4-21].

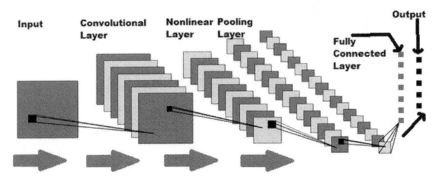

Figure 4-21. Image data passes through various layers of a neural network

The convolutional layer always comes first. The matrix of pixel values (the image) is added to it. Just imagine that the input matrix reading starts from the top left of the image. The software chooses a small matrix there, which is known as a filter (or a core or a neuron). Then this filter creates a convolution, i.e., it moves along the input image. The function of the filter is the multiplication of its values by the original values of the pixel. All of the multiplications are then added up to obtain a single number. The filter starts reading the image from its top left corner and gradually moves further right by a unit after carrying out the multiplication operation. When it reaches the right edge of the image and completes the multiplication operation there, it moves to the left side one row below and continues with the process. After moving the filter through every position on the image, it now obtains a matrix that is smaller than the input matrix [see Figure 4-22].

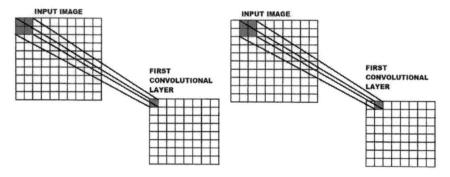

Figure 4-22. The filter starts reading the input image data from its top left corner and gradually moves further right by a unit after carrying out the multiplication operation. The filter moves through every position on the image to obtain a matrix that is smaller than the input matrix

The whole network is required to recognize top-level features in an image, and it consists of several convolutional networks (layers) mixed with nonlinear and pooling layers. When the image passes through one convolutional layer, the output of the first layer becomes the input for the second layer. And this happens with every further convolutional layer. After every convolution operation, a nonlinear layer is included. It contains activation functions that feature nonlinear properties. This property enables a network to be highly intense. After the nonlinear comes the pooling layer. It is concerned with the height and the width of the image and carries out downsampling on the image (decreased image data). This means that if some features (like edges) have already been identified in the previous convolution operation, then a detailed image is no longer needed for further processing, and it is compressed to less detailed pictures. It is vital to include a fully connected layer (dense layers) after completing a series of convolutional, nonlinear, and pooling layers. The function of this layer is to carry data from the convolutional networks.

Computer vision is used for:

- Object Classification

- Object Identification

- Object Verification

- Object Detection

- Object Landmark Detection

- Object Segmentation

- Object Recognition

Outside of just recognition, other methods of analysis include:

- Video motion analysis

- Image segmentation

- Scene reconstruction

- Image restoration

Natural Language Processing (NLP)

NLP is a technology that is aimed at enabling people and computers to communicate with each other on equal footing. It combines knowledge from linguistics with all the latest methods in AI and computer science [see Figure 4-23]. For NLP to function, first, it is important to work on language recognition, i.e., to see if the current model can recognize that language properly. Currently, there are many models available for English, French, German, etc. NLP might not work on regional languages or languages which are less spoken. NLP is viewed as a promising technology within the domain of Human Computer Interface (HCI) to control devices or web applications.[16] The work of chatbots or digital voice assistants was originally based on the principle of NLP. NLP was developed in the 1950s when the scientist Alan Turing wrote and published an article called 'Computing Machinery and Intelligence' in which he presented a method called the 'Turing Test' to measure AI, which is still being used.

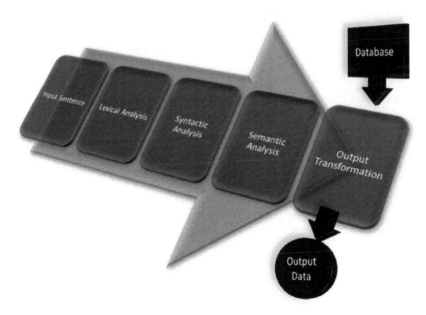

Figure 4-23. A flowchart explaining natural language processing

As early as 1954, researchers had already been able to use a machine to translate sixty sentences into the Russian language. Excited by this breakthrough, several other computer scientists believed that machine translation would soon be possible. However, it was not until the 1980s that the first systems for statistical-based machine translations were further developed. Meanwhile, some other approaches were found that translated information from the 'real' world into the language of computers.[16]

The late 1980s saw another revolutionary breakthrough as ML gained popularity. Along with the ever-increasing computing power of computers, NLP's algorithms were now functional.

Today, NLP-based computer programs can not only use datasets that have been collected manually, but they are also able to analyze text corpora like websites or spoken languages independently. The basis of NLP is the simple concept that any form of language (either spoken or written) should initially be recognized. Nonetheless, language is an incredibly complex system of characters – it is not just a word on its own that is important, but it is the connection that the word has with the other words, phrases, entire sentences, and even facts that is significant as well. While learning from birth is natural for humans, computers have to achieve this using algorithms. Humans are able to access their life experiences, but computers have to access artificially-created experiences.

NLP has various use cases; the most popular uses include:

- Content categorization.

- Topic discovery and modeling.

- Contextual extraction.

- Sentiment analysis.

- Speech-to-text and text-to-speech conversion.

- Document summarization.

- Machine translation.

Choosing the right algorithm

To choose the right algorithm, we need to try out some algorithms which fit our use case and pick the one which performs best on our dataset [see Figure 4-24]. There are no hard and fast rules regarding this, but it's more based on trial and error and experience.

To create a model, one must pass through these phases:

- Construction of the model

- Training the model

- Testing the model

- Evaluation of the model

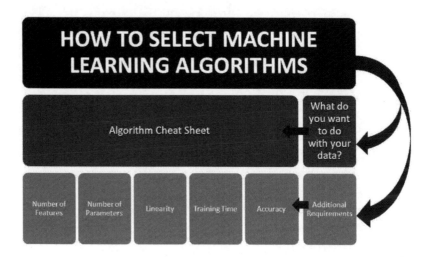

Figure 4-24. Flowchart showing machine learning algorithm selection criteria

Model Creation

Machine learning and deep learning models are usually created in the following manner:

- Selecting a specific kind of algorithm and then defining its parameters and hyperparameters.

- Training the model on labeled data.

- Evaluating the model's performance.

- Using it for prediction.

Model Evaluation

Model evaluation is an essential part of the ML workflow. There's no universal measure that is common to all. Instead, different types of measures are used to evaluate performance, which changes according to the problem being tackled. Some commonly used methods are:

- Accuracy

- Log Loss (Logarithmic Loss)

- Confusion Metrics

- Area Under Curve (AUC)

- F1 Score

- Mean Absolute Error (MAE)

- Mean Squared Error (MSE)

Model Training

Training refers to the process of feeding data to the algorithm to make it learn from the data. Training duration is the time that is taken by the algorithm to learn from the data. It depends on many factors. Simpler models can be trained in a very short duration with a small dataset. In comparison, larger datasets consume a lot of time to learn. The complexity of a model also affects the training time.

Parameters

Parameters are the knobs that can be turned to get different results from the model. The duration of the training and the algorithm's accuracy depends on these parameters. Parameters are learned from data during the training process.

Hyperparameters

Hyperparameters are the adjustable values required for the model, and these are not learned from data.

Determination of optimal hyperparameters for a machine learning model is called tuning. It creates and tests several models having different combinations of settings.[17] The metrics are then compared across all models, and best-performing settings are selected for use.

Although this is a great way to get the best hyperparameter values, the time it takes to train a model exponentially increases with the number of parameters. The benefit is that the presence of numerous parameters usually indicates that an algorithm has more flexibility. Often, it achieves excellent accuracy if one hits the correct combination of parameter settings.[4]

Python libraries for machine learning

Python is 2nd most used programming language in the world. One of the numerous reasons why Python is extremely popular with programmers is that there is a surprisingly huge collection of libraries that users can work with. The following reasons explain why Python enjoys immense popularity:

- Python is relatively easy to learn due to its clear structure and is therefore very suitable for beginners. Its programming syntax is relatively easier to learn and is at a higher level than C, C++, and Java.

- Portability is very important for Python.

- From development to deployment and maintenance, Python helps its developers be more productive.

- Python allows for relatively faster development of new applications with lesser written code.

- Due to the simplicity of Python, many developers have created new machine learning libraries. Python is immensely popular with experts because of this huge collection of libraries.[18]

TensorFlow

It is a free and open-source software library for machine learning and deep learning. It was developed by the Google Brain team, and later it was released as an open-source library. It is available for all major platforms like Windows, macOS, Linux, Android, and iOS.

- TensorFlow provides easy visualization of any part of a diagram, something that is not offered by other libraries.

- TensorFlow can train on CPU (Central Processing Unit), GPU, and TPU (Tensor Processing Unit) as well.

- TensorFlow offers pipelining using which neural networks can be trained on multiple GPUs reducing training time

- Since it was developed by Google, there is a large team of software developers who are constantly working on improvements to make the system more stable and add new features.

TensorFlow is very popular. All libraries created in TensorFlow have been written in either C or C++. Tensorflow mainly supports Python and C++. Some other languages are also being added to it.[19]

During development, first, the Python code is compiled, after which it is executed on the TensorFlow engine using C and C++.

SciKit-Learn

It is also called sklearn. SciKit-Learn is a Python library that is linked to both SciPy and NumPy. It is a free library that supports multiple machine learning algorithms, including ones like SVMs, Random Forests, k-means clustering, etc. It originally started as a Google Summer of Code project. It is written in Python and uses Numpy and SciPy for high-performance mathematical operations.

The SciKit-Learn library contains a variety of algorithms for implementing standard tasks for machine learning and data mining. These include reducing dimensionality, classification, regression, clustering, and model selection.

NumPy

NumPy is one of the most popular libraries for machine learning in Python. It supports large multi-dimensional arrays and matrices and high-level mathematical functions to operate on these arrays. It is an open-source library. It was developed to simplify array operations and increase performance. It is an abbreviated form of Numerical Python.

TensorFlow and other libraries use NumPy internally to perform various operations.

- NumPy is both very interactive and incredibly easy to use.

- NumPy helps make mathematically complex implementations easy.

- It makes it easier for one to code and grasp the concepts.

- NumPy is widely used, so there are many open-source implementations.

The NumPy interface can be used for the expression of images, sound waves, as well as other data in the form of an array of real numbers in the N dimensions.

Keras

It is also an open-source library that is written in Python. It now acts as an interface for the Tensorflow library. Its previous versions also supported various backends like Tensorflow, Theano, R, etc. Its design supports the fast development of models which is used for experimental purpose. It also supports training on GPUs as well as TPUs. Keras models can also be deployed on multiple platforms like web, android, iOS, etc.

Keras is one of the most impressive learning libraries for Python, and it offers a simple mechanism for the representation of neural networks. However, Keras is comparatively slower than other ML libraries because it creates a computational graph through the backend infrastructure and uses it to complete the processes. All the models in Keras are portable, regardless.

- Keras runs smoothly on both the GPU and the CPU.

- Keras practically supports almost all kinds of neural networks, whether they are fully connected, pooled, recurring, embedded, etc. Additionally, different types may be combined to create more complex models.

- The modular structure of Keras makes it incredibly expressive, ideal, and flexible for innovative research.

- Being a completely Python-based framework, Keras simplifies solving the problem and exploring this library.

You might be using applications that use Keras-based models on a daily basis. Apps like Netflix, Yelp, Uber, Zocdoc, Instacart, and Square, among many others, use Keras. It is a popular notion with startups that make use of deep learning technology.

Moreover, it offers a great choice of pre-trained models such as MNIST, VGG, Inception, SqueezeNet, ResNet, etc. Lastly, Keras is preferred by deep learning researchers. It is already used by researchers who work in large scientific organizations, like NASA and CERN.[11]

PyTorch

PyTorch is another popular deep learning framework. It is also a free and open-source library. It also offers a C++ interface along with the main Python interface. Caffe2 was merged into PyTorch in 2018. It feels more native to Python as compared to other frameworks.

The PyTorch library is based on Torch, which is an open-source library that is implemented in C with a wrapper in Lua. PyTorch in Python was officially introduced in 2017. From the time of its foundation, the library has become increasingly popular and has attracted more and more machine learning developers.[17]

- Research and production performance is optimized by leveraging native support for asynchronous execution of collective operations as well as peer-to-peer communications that is accessible through Python and C++.

- PyTorch is not simply an integration of Python into a monolithic C++ framework – it is designed to be deeply integrated into Python to allow for its usage with common packages and libraries like Cython or Numba.

A dynamic community of developers and researchers has created a wide range of both tools and libraries for the expansion of PyTorch, and in doing so, supports the development in the area from computer vision to reinforcement learning.

PyTorch is used mostly for applications like NLP. It was originally developed by Facebook's AI research group. TensorFlow & PyTorch are both competing frameworks. It is attracting a good amount of attention, majorly in the research community.

Light GBM

It stands for Light Gradient Boosting Machine. It was originally developed by Microsoft. It is an open-source framework that also works on distributed machines. It is also compatible with popular languages like Python, R, C++, etc. It uses decision trees. It is designed for high performance.

It aids developers in the creation of new algorithms via newly defined elementary models and, particularly, decision trees. There are special libraries designed to implement this method swiftly and effectively – LightGBM, CatBoost, and XGBoost.[16] All these libraries are 'competitors' but aid in solving a common problem and can also be used in almost similar ways.

- Faster training speed and higher efficiency.

- Lower memory usage.

- Better accuracy.

- Support of parallel and GPU learning.

- Capable of handling large-scale data.

This library offers implementation of gradient boosting that is optimized, scalable, and rapid, making it highly popular with the developers of ML.

Eli5

It is a python library that is used for debugging ML and DL code. It also explains predictions made by models. It provides support for numerous libraries like scikit-learn, Keras, XGBoost, LightGBM, etc.

It is a combination of visualization and debugging for machine learning models, tracking steps of the algorithm. Most machine learning and deep learning models are also called black boxes as we don't know what's happening inside them and how they are learning it. It helps in model interpretation for those who don't understand the terminologies related to ML and DL.

In scikit-learn, it allows explaining weights and predictions of classifiers and regressors. It can print decision trees as text and many more.

SciPy

It is also referred to as Scientific Python. SciPy is an environment containing open-source libraries that are particularly helpful in Science, Mathematics, and Engineering. Some of its core packages are (also called SciPy stack):

- NumPy

- SciPy library

- Matplotlib

- IPython

- SymPy

- Pandas

SciPy is used in scientific computing, along with NumPy. SciPy makes use of NumPy as the integral data structure, and it incorporates the modules for various commonly used tasks in scientific programming like integration (calculus), linear algebra, common solving of differential equations, and signal processing.[17]

Theano

Theano is a python-based library and optimizing compiler for matrix-related computation of multidimensional arrays. It is built on top of NumPy. It may also be used in parallel or distributed environments that are similar to TensorFlow.[17]

- It is possible to make use of whole arrays of NumPy in functions that are Theano-compiled.

- Transparent usage of GPUs.

- Data-intensive calculations can be carried out a lot faster.

- Theano performs the derivation for functions that have either one or more inputs.

- Theano is very stable even for complex calculations

- Includes tools for diagnosing bugs

Theano's actual syntax is symbolic and can be difficult for beginners. Expressions are particularly defined in an abstract manner, compiled, and used later for the actual calculation.[18]

Theano was originally designed specifically for calculations that are needed for large neural network algorithms like the ones that are used in deep learning. Developed in 2007, Theano was one of the first libraries of its kind, due to which it is seen as the industry standard for deep learning and development. Additionally, it is utilized in several neural network projects nowadays, and its popularity is on the rise.

Pandas

It is a very powerful library that is built using Python. It is used for data analysis and data manipulation.

Pandas comes with the provision of high-level data structures and an assortment of analysis tools. One of its best features is its ability to translate complex data operations through just one or two commands. Pandas even has several integrated methods for the grouping, combining, and filtering of data, including time-series functionality. Supporting processes like iteration, re-indexing, sorting, aggregation, visualization, and chaining is one of the highlights of the library.

Pandas data frames can handle large amounts of data and can perform manipulations like finding missing values, organizing data in specific formats like in date and time. It also enables the reading and writing of data from different file types and doing operations on them. It also makes file format conversion very easy. It is a very important library in Data Science and Data Analytics.

Matplotlib

- It is a very popular library that is used to create visualizations and graphs in Python. It is used to plot interactive graphs and figures in 2-D and 3-D. In machine learning and deep learning, data visualization plays an important role. Using matplotlib, we can easily create plots describing various properties of data, which helps us in formulating better models. Graphs are also helpful in comparing the performance of the model with time and to other models as well.

References/Further Reading

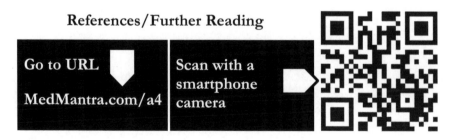

Go to URL

MedMantra.com/a4

Scan with a smartphone camera

CHAPTER FIVE

HEALTHCARE DATA

Before we start getting into the specifics, let us first understand what healthcare data is:

- **Healthcare:** This refers to the maintenance and restoration of the health of a person, usually by trained medical practitioners.

- **Data:** This is the word used for raw or organized sources of information. It can be in the form of spreadsheets, images, texts, etc.

Hence, **Healthcare Data** refers to the data that is obtained and used from patients and other related individuals to draw insights and maintain and improve the health of an individual or a group of people.

With that, let's dive deeper into the topic to find out how data-driven healthcare is transforming the industry at unprecedented rates.

Data

Data has been generated by human beings for ages undefined. Initially, the generated data was not digitized. However, with the introduction of modern computers, there is an exponential explosion of the amount of generated digital data from various sectors of the industry as well as individuals.

Classification of Data

Data can broadly be classified based on two sections: the format of data and the type of data.

Classification based on the format of data:

- **Text:** Text data refers to text-based articles or conversations. Basically, most of the data that is available on the web is text-based data.

- **Tabular Data:** This refers to columns and rows of data that may or may not have relational dependence among themselves, for example, patient medical records.

- **Image Data:** This refers to data that is present in the form of images or pictures, for example, X-ray scans.

- **Video Data:** This refers to data that is present in the form of videos, for example, camera-based laparoscopy.

- **Sound:** This refers to data generated from sound or sound-based imaging, for example, digital stethoscope

- **3D Imaging:** This refers to data that is generated from the three-dimensional imaging of objects or organs, for example, MRI/CT scans.

Classification based on the type of data:

- **Structured Data:** This refers to pre-structured data. Insights can easily be drawn from this kind of data with minimum pre-processing. Structured data is generally found in tabular format with relationships between the columns, for example, data stored in relational databases like MySQL, PostgreSQL, etc., or data stored in spreadsheets.

- **Unstructured Data:** This refers to data that is not structured in a particular way or that has no predefined model or schema. This type of data requires a significant investment of time and resources in terms of the application of pre-processing techniques, for example, unorganized text data, patient reports, and prescriptions.

Sources of Data in Healthcare

Now that we understand what data is and its types, it is important to understand where the data originates. In general, users across the world generate 2.5 quintillion bytes of data every day. However, healthcare-relevant data is generated primarily by patients themselves. This involves several medical wearables and IoT devices like fitness bands, digital medical records, patient demographic information, etc.

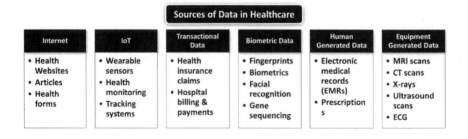

Internet	IoT	Transactional Data	Biometric Data	Human Generated Data	Equipment Generated Data
• Health Websites • Articles • Health forms	• Wearable sensors • Health monitoring • Tracking systems	• Health insurance claims • Hospital billing & payments	• Fingerprints • Biometrics • Facial recognition • Gene sequencing	• Electronic medical records (EMRs) • Prescriptions	• MRI scans • CT scans • X-rays • Ultrasound scans • ECG

Sources of Data in Healthcare

Big Data

Now that we have an idea about data, let's look into Big Data. In simple terms, the name is self-explanatory. Big Data is data in which the volume is quite large—larger than traditional data. Another definition of Big Data is that it refers to datasets that are too big to be stored or processed in a relational database system (e.g., MySQL). One of the common methods of storing Big Data is in a NoSQL database (e.g., MongoDB).

Big Data is known to have a few common characteristics to distinguish it from other normal sources of data. Interestingly, these keywords all start with the letter "V" and are popularly referred to as the "10 Vs of Big Data." Let us Look at them in detail.

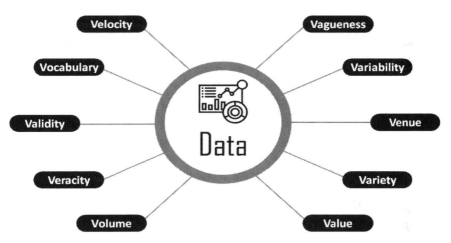

Volume

In the field of healthcare, data is generated by every patient and his/her concerned medical professionals (for example, doctors, hospital staff, etc.) at every second. All this data, whether digital or physical, is collected and stored. Out of this, the digitization of physical data has seen an increase in recent years, which contributes to a huge chunk of Big Data.

The sheer volume of data that is being created across the world at every step is astounding, to say the least. Storage, maintenance, authentication, and security are some of the major concerns that accompany such a large volume of data. Hence, many organizations are looking into storing and maintaining data in the form of decentralized network systems, also known as the blockchain.

The main concern is that most of this data is unorganized and is not effectively used by the healthcare industry. On the bright side, when institutions use this large available volume, some impressive results emerge. For example, an initiative in the United Kingdom was able to determine the prevalence of Type 1 diabetes through social hashtags and was able to map it to particular geographic regions.

Variety

"Variety of data" refers to the variation or variance in data. Due to digitization and the fact that digital devices are logging more data, there has been an exponential boom in the variety and type of data available to the healthcare industry.

More variety in data has both pros and cons.

Pros:

- More variety of data equates to more data, as more and more data is being generated by different sources. This brings us back to the "volume" of data.

- Greater variety ensures higher variance. This helps the analytical and machine learning models to be more generalized instead of being specific to a particular type of data. In the longer run, they can provide more accurate results.

Cons:

- More variety means more unorganized data. For example, data can be present in a structured form (e.g., tabular data—clinical records, forms, medical test results), semi-structured form (e.g., image and video data—X-rays, MRI scans, endoscopy), and unstructured form (e.g., communication/interaction with patients, patient history records, patient reports).

- Too much variety may reduce the quantity of data present for each format. This leads to analytics problems like class imbalance and insufficient data of a particular type.

Internet of Things - Wearables

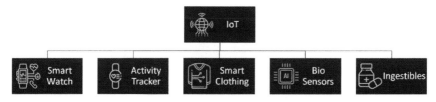

"Internet of things" refers to the everyday objects/electronics that are always connected to the Internet and that form a mesh network for such devices to communicate autonomously with each other. For example, in the healthcare section, fitness wearables like fitness trackers are one of the most common examples of the Internet of Things.

The Internet of things or IoT creates a lot of digital data, which are usually organized forms of data. This type of data has both Volume and Variety. This combination makes it ideal for analytics algorithms to draw meaningful healthcare insights/information from this data.

Let us look at some examples of IoT-based devices in healthcare:

- *Activity Trackers:* These are usually in the form of fitness bands that are connected to a smartphone via Bluetooth. These track and monitor a range of fitness activities like steps taken, movement, sleep patterns, heart rate, etc.

- *Smart Watches:* These have the same functionalities as a fitness band and more. In addition to being able to track the same activities like a fitness tracker, smartwatches often are self-contained and do not require a persisting Bluetooth connection to a smartphone to function and push data. They often have their own internet and GPS connectivity.

- *Smart Clothing:* There is an endless list of applications for smart clothing, from sleep tracking and heart rate monitoring to measuring blood pressure and other vital signs. Smart clothing can achieve everything an activity tracker can do and more.

- *Ingestibles/Implants:* These are more recent inventions and are more of bleeding-edge technology. Ingestibles are often tablet-sized devices that can be ingested through the mouth and remain within the body for a specific amount of time. They monitor certain specific functions and communicate with the outer world via Bluetooth or ZigBee connectivity protocol. Implants, on the other hand, are surgically inserted electronic devices that remain in the body for a longer duration, sometimes a lifetime. These also function primarily in health monitoring and tracking. Some implants, e.g., pacemakers, also serve as critical life-support systems inside the body of the patient.

Value

Simply put, "value" refers to the usefulness of data. In most domains, the value of data is calculated by both qualitative and quantitative analysis. The same is done in the healthcare industry.

Data without analysis is valueless. Data gains its value when it is converted to information after analytics are applied to it. Hence, it is safe to say that if any data cannot be converted to meaningful information by applying analytical techniques to it, then that data is valueless.

As an example, let's discuss how Google brought value to its search data to track flu symptoms in 2013. It is well known that Google's search trends are recorded and later analyzed. This is very useful data for the company for delivering targeted advertisements. However, during the 2013 flu crisis, Google decided to use the same data differently. In doing so, it managed to track searches for flu symptoms and identify potential flu hotspots. By doing this, Google was able to bring a lot more value to the board than its search data initially had. Hence, the value of data can be generated; it is not absolute.

Veracity

"Veracity" refers to the quality of data in terms of correctness or accuracy. Veracity is an important factor in Big Data because no real value can be created out of unorganized and inaccurate data. This is because inaccurate data will always lead to inaccurate insights, which will likely do more harm than good.

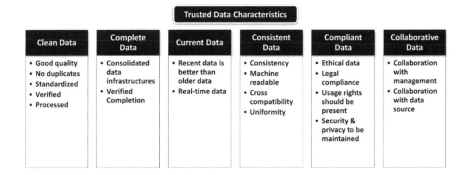

Trusted Data Characteristics					
Clean Data	**Complete Data**	**Current Data**	**Consistent Data**	**Compliant Data**	**Collaborative Data**
• Good quality • No duplicates • Standardized • Verified • Processed	• Consolidated data infrastructures • Verified Completion	• Recent data is better than older data • Real-time data	• Consistency • Machine readable • Cross compatibility • Uniformity	• Ethical data • Legal compliance • Usage rights should be present • Security & privacy to be maintained	• Collaboration with management • Collaboration with data source

Let us explore some potential sources of inaccurate data:

- *Generation of Wrong/Fake Data:* For certain indecent reasons, any person, group, or organization is capable of generating improper and inaccurate data. These usually do more harm than good. Hence, it is important to identify the same.

- *Error in Data Entry:* Most of the data that human beings generate is manually entered into the system. Error while entering data is quite common because human beings make mistakes. These errors can sometimes be corrected by processing the data before applying analytics to the same.

- *Staleness:* Staleness refers to the relevance of the data with respect to the current time and problem at hand. For example, some data that was updated on a viral strain 100 years ago might not be directly relevant to research if the virus has mutated significantly in the same time frame.

- *Usability:* The availability of data is not enough for extracting meaningful insights. The data should be relevant and meet the given problem statement requirements. It should also be ethical to use the data.

Validity

Conceptually, the validity of data is quite similar to the veracity of data. "Validity" refers to the correctness and accuracy of the data for the intended use. The primary difference between the veracity and validity of data is that veracity is absolute and pre-defined, while the validity of data is subjective and changes as per the context.

Variability

Variability is related to the change in data with respect to time. If the data is regularly changing, it is difficult to draw insights from it using analytics algorithms. For such kinds of data, "online learning" or live learning algorithms are required, which automatically update as new batches of data enter the picture.

Visualization

Visualization of Big Data may seem simple but is quite a complicated process. Visualizations are required to make Big Data more understandable and readable.

It also allows us to understand and make sense of high-dimensional data (higher than three dimensions). High-dimensional data can be reduced to lower dimensions for visualization and further processing using algorithms like principal component analysis, t-SNE, etc.

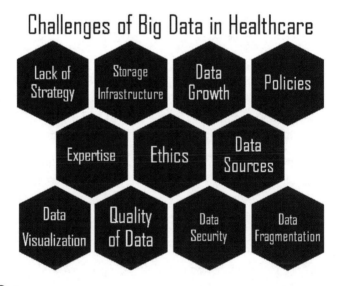

Small Data

Small Data is the exact opposite of Big Data. As is evident from the name itself, here, the volume of data is significantly less. Some examples of Small Data are medical records, biometric measurements, scans, prescription data, etc.

Healthcare Data - Applications and Case Studies

Now that we have the basics out of the way, let us look at some real-world applications of healthcare data.

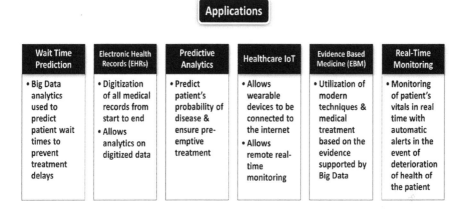

Wait Time Prediction	Electronic Health Records (EHRs)	Predictive Analytics	Healthcare IoT	Evidence Based Medicine (EBM)	Real-Time Monitoring
• Big Data analytics used to predict patient wait times to prevent treatment delays	• Digitization of all medical records from start to end • Allows analytics on digitized data	• Predict patient's probability of disease & ensure pre-emptive treatment	• Allows wearable devices to be connected to the internet • Allows remote real-time monitoring	• Utilization of modern techniques & medical treatment based on the evidence supported by Big Data	• Monitoring of patient's vitals in real time with automatic alerts in the event of deterioration of health of the patient

Predicting Patient Wait Times

Long patient wait times cause a delay in treatment and sometimes result in irreversible damage. This delay and improper management of resources cause many higher-priority patients to be neglected.

To avoid this, time series analysis can be used to look at past patterns and parameters in order to assess and prepare for a surge in incoming patients. This allows for shorter wait times.

One such example can be found in Paris, where four hospitals teamed up with Intel to analyze ten years of hospital admissions records and perform hourly and daily predictions of the number of patients who were expected to visit the hospitals in the near future.

Electronic Health Records (EHRs)

Much data is generated for each patient, starting from the medical history, continuing with medical trackers, the diagnosis, and test results, and ending with the hospital bills. All of this data is usually generated and stored in different formats, from hard paper to Excel sheets to X-ray images, etc. Due to this fragmentation, most of this data cannot be used for predictive analytics and/or requires digitization and cleaning before being used.

A solution to this problem is to use EHRs, which store all the patient information from start to end digitally. EHRs usually consist of patient details, medical histories, allergies, clinical results, demographics, etc. Because they are digital, the records can easily be shared with any concerned healthcare professional at any point in time over the Internet.

Though the maintenance of universal EHRs across healthcare organizations and institutions is still a concept at this stage, it is a promising approach toward bringing uniformity to the way patient data is handled and stored.

The United States of America is leading the race here, with up to 94% of its hospitals actively using EHRs.

Predictive Analytics

Similar to predicting patient wait times, predictive analytics makes use of static data to calculate readmission intervals and waiting times.

The EHR data for more than 30 million patients has been collected by Optum Labs, which created a database for predictive analytics. This allows for improved delivery of care for patients.

These 30 million health records proved to be quite robust and helped in training and validating models. Some of the parameters that were used to generate the predictive model were economic demographics, patient age, and other health biomarkers.

Hence, based on the given data, these models were easily able to find the patients who fit the predicted risk trends for diseases like Type 2 diabetes, metabolic syndrome, heart disease, and hypertension.

Healthcare IoT - Wearables and Real-Time Notifications

Simply put, wearables are connected (to the Internet) electronic devices that we wear on our bodies and that serve a function, primarily monitoring an event in our body. For example, activity trackers (like Fitbit, Microsoft Band, etc.) can measure sleep patterns, heart rate, and blood glucose level and count the number of steps taken. Furthermore, more advanced devices, such as the Samsung Watch Active Series, allow the user to measure blood pressure in real-time through sensors tied to a watch.

From the raw fundamental data that these wearables generate, more complex insights are drawn by applying real-time analytics right on our smartphones and the wearables themselves. For example, atrial fibrillation (irregular heart rhythm) can easily be detected in real-time by monitoring and detecting certain irregular patterns in the heart rate. Real-time and early detection of such diseases can potentially save the lives of high-risk patients.

Looking at a case study, the University of California Irvine allowed patients suffering from heart disease to return home with an IoT-based weighing scale, which would automatically alert their concerned physicians if the patient's weight crossed a certain threshold.

On the negative side, there is an estimated 30% abandonment rate of IoT-based wearables after a fixed period. This issue is being tackled through the development of more intuitive and engaging software for the user.

Evidence-Based Medicine (EBM)

Evidence-based medicine (EBM) is the use of modern, best evidence in making decisions about the care of individual patients. EBM is used to experiment with existing, proven drugs on new/unknown diseases, backed by existing research, which can potentially lead to a cure.

Initially, small-scale clinical trials are carried out to determine the effectiveness of the treatment and whether any side effects arise. This approach allows the healthcare industry to rapidly come up with new potential cures for any disease while delivering quality care and maintaining transparency regarding the outcomes.

Let us look at a very recent worldwide pandemic: COVID-19. We'll review how the World Health Organization (WHO) is using EBM to come up with a cure to the deadly disease.

Since the onset of the disease in late 2019, the virulence of the virus was evident. Thus, rapid coordinated drug testing across the world was necessary. To that end, the WHO announced the Solidarity program, in which any participating country and a medical professional could choose one of the few proven medical tracks of treatment and document the outcomes of the same on a central database.

These outcomes were later processed, and the success rate was determined for each medical track using Big Data analytics. This allowed for rapid prototyping on EBM for a large sample size across the planet, potentially leading to an optimal method of treatment, if not a cure.

Real-Time Patient Monitoring

Traditionally, a patient under treatment and/or observation in a hospital ward is attended by a nurse at a fixed interval to measure vitals. The main problem with this approach is that because the patient is not being monitored continuously if that patient's health status drastically deteriorates in between the nurse's visits, the result could be fatal for the patient.

A solution to this would be bedside wireless sensors that can actively monitor the patient's vitals and send a real-time alert to the concerned healthcare worker in the event of a drastic deterioration in the patient's health.

Deploying Big Data Project

Problem Statement	Skills and Technology	Implementation and Deployment
• Understand Problem Statement	• Identification and recruitment of the right skillset	• Identify the necessary requirements for collection of Data
• Determine if it is a right fit for your business	• Determining the technology stack requirement	• Practice Ethical Data Collection
• Quantitative Objective Identification	• Analyzing available resources	• Identifying Deployment Device – Cloud or Edge
• Determination of Return on Investment	Identify type of Data	
	• Identify type of Analysis	• Identifying deployment at scale

Conclusion

Big Data analytics is one of the most promising additions to the healthcare industry. It allows us to predict and anticipate the outcome of many events, which leads to lower mortality, early warning, advanced preparation, fewer readmissions, and much more.

Real-time patient monitoring using Big Data is also an important part of the entire stack, where we can get real-time or even early warnings about any deterioration in the patient's health condition.

This chapter shows that the AI applications based on healthcare data are plenty, the potential is unlimited, and the pros outweigh the cons by a large margin.

References/Further Reading

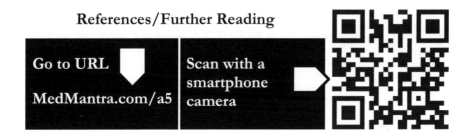

Go to URL

MedMantra.com/a5

Scan with a smartphone camera

CHAPTER SIX

THE AI BLACK BOX ISSUE AND EXPLAINABLE AI

AI is now an essential component of our lives. Practically, it is employed in almost every field. AI is involved in lots of decision-making. AI products are also marketed as safer alternatives because they lack chances of human error. In specific domains like healthcare, predicting diseases such as cancer and the development of new and better medicines is done using deep learning (DL). It is the human tendency to find the logic behind a decision that makes the decision more trustworthy. Most DL-generated results lack any logical explanation. Besides, most of us don't understand the technicalities related to AI. Sometimes, decisions are hard to trust; this is where the actual problem starts. Earlier, people were satisfied with the results they were getting from the implementation of AI; now, they want to know the reasoning behind the formation of results. Therefore, Explainable AI (XAI) is the next big thing.

The black box issue

Essentially, the black box issue stands tall because the workings of DL algorithms are difficult to understand. We feed DL models with vast amounts of training data so that they learn from it. After that, we input data at one end, and on the other side, we get the predicted output. But what happens in between remains a mystery. These models do not give details about how they arrived at any decision. These decisions are very opaque.[1] Conventional ML algorithms are transparent (white box); however, modern DL algorithms are opaque (black box).

Thus, it gets quite hard for professionals in the field to explain how these models do it, usually when presenting these ideas or results to different stakeholders or investors or the common public. No doubt, the DL models employ mathematical functions and values, which is not a mystery or magic. However, it is a bit harder to explain how they work to people who lack related technical know-how.

Why it is important

On the whole, people believe that they have the right to know how and why a particular decision was made. This is highly important in terms of the healthcare sector because patients want to know the answer to the question of how and why they're supposed to believe this information. More than that, the doctors wish to understand the reasoning behind the AI's decision.

The hidden problems

AI algorithms learn on their own based solely on the training data. This data may contain hidden biases and human prejudices. These hidden traits in data do affect decisions dramatically. Algorithms lack morale, which is a vital part of any human decision.

AI often predicts unfair or wrong decisions due to these hidden features of data. This has been observed several times. Its most prominent example is the *COMPAS* case.[2] **COMPAS**, an acronym for Correctional Offender Management Profiling for Alternative Sanctions, is assistive AI-based software that helped judges decide whether to detain a defendant before trials. Its creators ignored the biases contained in the training data. Its predictions in the case of black defendants failed utterly. The software labeled black defendants as being twice riskier than their white counterparts. Many US state jurisdiction authorities used it. The case showed that data must be carefully assessed and then fed into the model.

This is problematic not only for lack of transparency but also for the correctness of the decision. AI has a significant impact on various people's lives. Such biases can have disastrous effects in real life. They must be appropriately addressed, especially with the implementation of AI in the healthcare sector.

Why explainable AI?

If AI could explain the produced answer, this would add to its credibility. It will also help us tackle all the biases and prejudices hidden in the training data. Using XAI, one can know what went wrong. Then, software engineers can work that out, ultimately boosting the performance. We will also get insights into the workings of these systems.

From multiple perspectives, XAI seems promising.

There can be two approaches for XAI:

- Explanation by Design,

- And Black Box Explanation.

In the former, a model can be trained to produce an explanation along with the decision. The latter approach suggests developing models that can explain the results from a black box model perspective. Both methods are useful in their approaches.

Black box issues in healthcare

Trust is a massive factor in medical treatment. Unless we are sure of a particular decision or treatment, we cannot risk it. Believing the prediction or recommendation by AI algorithms without knowing why and how is hard. Lack of transparency in healthcare can have serious consequences. Healthcare professionals are very much answerable for their decisions legally as well; they cannot merely say that AI recommended it unless they know the reason behind it.

One such study was conducted by Riccardo Moitto and colleagues[3]; it was called Deep Patient on Electronic Health Records (EHRs). It aimed to predict the health status of its patients and help prevent further disease or disability. According to the study, it was quite successful in providing the right diagnosis to patients. While it was helpful to a great extent, it also proved to be a black box. It was able to predict the onset of mental disorders in patients. There was no clear explanation of how these predictions were made, but they proved to be true over time, leading to baffled doctors.

While AI is significantly helping in the healthcare sector, the creation of the black box leaves professionals utterly confused. Thus, there is a focus on XAI and creating more transparent algorithms for people to understand and work with.

Layer-wise Relevance Propagation (LRP)

This is a very appropriate method in explainable AI. It can be easily applied to pre-trained models. LRP uses layer-wise weights and activations to calculate their contribution to the overall prediction. Using it, we can inspect what made a model predict this output. LRP can be used on Convolutional Neural Networks (CNNs), Long Short-Term Memory cells (LSTMs), and other deep learning algorithms.

It can be easily implemented in most programming languages.

Other useful techniques

Several machine learning algorithms like decision trees and Bayesian networks are easy to interpret. They can be visualized easily, and we can explain their predictions. We can see what properties were used as a decisive factor and how much they affected the predictions.

Some XAI frameworks

What-if Tool:

This is made by the TensorFlow team. It is an interactive visual interface designed to visualize datasets[4] and better understand the TensorFlow model output.

DeepLift:

This assigns contribution scores to each neuron involved in the model, which is used for prediction. It considers positive and negative contributions differently and gives them scores accordingly. It can also reveal dependencies that other approaches might not detect.

Activation Atlases:

This is developed by the combined efforts of Google and OpenAI. It aims to visualize how neural networks interact with each other. It is developed to visualize the inner workings of CNNs so that humans can easily understand them.

Future of XAI

Explainable AI is a field of active research. New algorithms are being worked out to solve the black box AI problems. Model transparency and explanation are very much needed in this digital society.

References/Further Reading

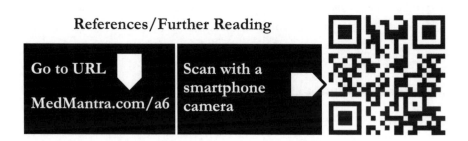

Go to URL	Scan with a smartphone camera
MedMantra.com/a6	

CHAPTER SEVEN

THE FUTURE OF AI IN HEALTHCARE WITH FEDERATED LEARNING

Machine learning (ML) is constantly evolving. One of the latest developments is federated learning (FL), which was introduced in 2017 by Google AI researchers.[1,2] Here is a complete guide to what federated learning is and the future of AI in healthcare with federated learning.

The Basics of Federated Learning

In conventional methods of ML, a data pipeline utilizes a central data server, which pools data from local data sources, and the local training nodes acquire data from this server to train ML models locally [see Figure 7-1 A]. The problem with this method is that the data must be transferred from the central server to the local training nodes. For that reason, the ML model is limited in its ability to learn in real-time.

There are two types of FL workflows: the aggregation server FL workflow and the peer-to-peer FL workflow.[3] In the aggregation server FL workflow, the most current ML model is downloaded and an updated model is computed in the local training nodes/computers using local data. These updated models are sent from the training nodes to the central (aggregation) server, where they are aggregated [see Figure 7-1 B]. Aggregation means that an improved global and consolidated model is computed and sent back to the local training nodes. In the peer-to-peer FL workflow, there is no central aggregation server and the aggregation is performed by each local training node (a peer). Initially, all local training nodes are synchronized so that they have the same, most current ML model [see Figure 7-1 C]. An updated model is computed by the local training nodes using local data. These updated models are exchanged by the participating nodes such that each node has all the updated models. Each node then aggregates these updated models so that each one has the same updated global model.

Because of FL, the ML algorithms gain experience from a wide range of data sets in different locations. In short, it allows many organizations to collaborate without sharing their sensitive data.

FL decentralizes the process of machine learning, as it removes the need for pooling data into a single location (the central server). Only the characteristics of the model are transferred, such as gradients, parameters, etc. The model is trained at different locations in different iterations. The process repeats for several iterations until a high-quality model is developed [see Figures 7-1 B and 7-1 C].

Here are the five most important benefits of FL[4,5]:

- Patient data privacy is maintained.

- The models are smarter – FL-trained models are superior and have incredible performance levels compared to models that see data from only one institute.

- It allows for better clinical decision-making. Clinicians can use their own expertise in conjunction with knowledge from other healthcare institutions to diagnose and treat diseases. Patients in remote areas can also benefit from such a model, as they have access to better care.

- Predictions are made locally, so latency is lowered.

- Once the FL model is successfully implemented in healthcare centers, it allows for unbiased decision-making without data privacy and governance concerns.

- When the FL model is used, it is much easier to become a data donor. This is because patients know that their data will remain safe and the accessibility can be revoked at any time

Now that you know the basics of FL, let's move onto understanding the future of this AI model in healthcare.

FL and Data Privacy Issues

The problem with conventional methods of ML is that they pose a risk to patient data privacy in the healthcare industry. Such a risk hinders the progress of AI in the life sciences and healthcare. However, FL can help in dealing with data privacy issues.

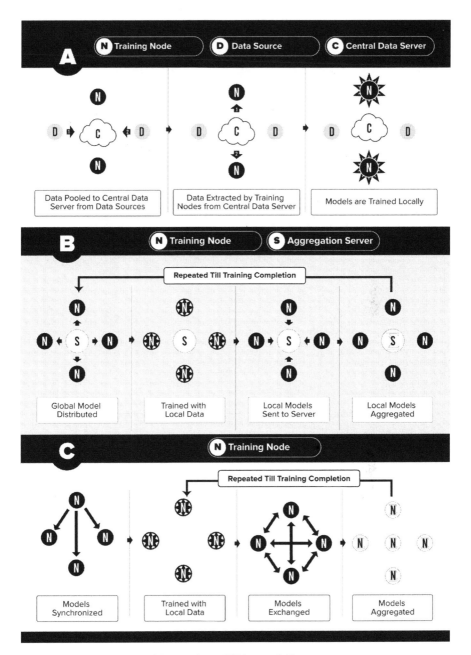

Figure 7-1. Federated Learning (FL) workflows

Previously, many researchers proved that even anonymized health datasets can be used to re-identify patients.[6] Other research has shown that MRI or CT data can help reconstruct the faces of the patients.[7,8] Of course, because of these possibilities, there are concerns with patient data privacy.

Many have wondered if one must compromise to benefit from AI models in healthcare. However, FL has changed the game entirely, as the ML algorithms in this model are trained locally. This means the patients' data is not shared outside the privacy of the hospital/institution. The model has privacy-preserving techniques, which include data being stored locally and neither leaked to a third party nor sent to the cloud/central server. Decision-making becomes better due to these privacy-preserving techniques. Also, real-time predictions are made possible because the process happens on the local device. Such a model has long been needed in the healthcare industry.

FL follows all compliance and consent requirements and regulations. These include the European Union's General Data Protection Regulation, HIPAA, and many others. Compliance is achieved by ensuring that all data remains within the network of the healthcare organization.

How FL Can Help Healthcare CIOs

CIOs (Chief Information Officers) are responsible for leading the IT (Information Technology) departments of healthcare organizations. Here are some of the key tasks they carry out:

- Assessing current and future technology needs

- Devising strategic initiatives to advance data-driven innovation

- Devising strategic initiatives to diversify revenue streams

- Managing and improving the technology spend of the healthcare organization

- Leveraging the organization's data for research and revenue purposes

The problem with achieving some of these aims is that a lack of resources prevents existing data from being made available for collaboration or used effectively. Leveraging data cost-effectively and efficiently is one of the most essential goals right now in the healthcare industry.

That is why CIOs should work toward unlocking the value of the existing data instead of focusing on gathering more data. They should seek out FL models that are capable of ensuring data security and privacy. Such security should be not only in the data but also in the code utilized to write the FL algorithms.

If CIOs implement such an FL system, they can foster collaborative data, diversify revenue streams, and achieve data-driven innovation for their healthcare organizations. Here are many other ways an FL system can help CIOs[9]:

1. *Accessibility and Security*

All data collected by the FL model is kept locally, which improves the physical data transfer speeds and reduces the risk of a data leak. People authorized to access the data can do so effectively and securely from any location. That is why the CIOs have more accessibility and everyone in the organization benefits from higher security.

2. *Compliance and Privacy*

Any FL model is created in compliance with various rules, regulations, and standards. These ensure that the data stay in the healthcare organization and are protected. Thus, using an FL model ensures compliance and privacy. The CIOs can then focus on other aspects of improving the healthcare organization.

3. *De-Risked Correlation*

One of the most important things in clinical research is the ability to correlate with various data sets. This is because local data sets are small and can be biased. Also, the correlating data can become de-anonymized and linked.

FL can encourage more secure data correlation. It can offer differential privacy, which allows for data sharing by describing patterns of groups within the data sets. All this can be done by withholding information about individuals and protecting patient privacy.

4. *Integration*

Healthcare data is vast and expansive. Patients have a long history of healthcare, and this data needs to be consolidated and integrated. Previous ML models did not achieve this aim well.

However, with FL, the existing healthcare databases can be integrated and organized. The structuring of data becomes easier, actionable, and searchable. All authorized persons can access integrated data to better understand the patients' medical history.

The FL model can help CIOs achieve these four aims so that their organizations can progress in terms of technology and revenue. After all, every healthcare organization needs to work towards achieving these goals to provide a better experience for their patients.

FL Applications That Are Being Used Today

Keep in mind that the FL model is relatively new as compared to the other ML models. It still has a long way to go before it can prove its validity in a regulated and productive environment. As of now, a few healthcare technology providers are rolling out and making use of this technology.

For example, the ML startup Owkin has come up with a new FL platform known as ***Owkin Connect***.[10] The platform gives data owners the capabilities to track their data usage and define their data authorizations. A ledger keeps track of the data being used by the model for training and how it contributes to the parameters of the model.

On the other hand, the ACR Data Science Institute is piloting a new FL framework for medical devices, known as ***NVIDIA Clara FL***.[11] It is a toolkit that democratizes AI by providing radiologists with the capabilities to develop algorithms using the patient data at their healthcare organizations. There is still a long way to go before FL becomes as common as the previous ML models.

Of course, many companies are working on the technology and we will soon see many applications being rolled out that will help healthcare organizations. The technology will put the patient or user in charge of coordinating their health data. More effective models will be built using the FL architecture. That is why it is likely the future of AI in healthcare.

Challenges With FL

All AI models come with a few sets of challenges that must be overcome. One of the main challenges of the FL models is communication. Because the FL models are trained using data generated by local devices, efficient communication must be developed.

That is because if there are too many communication rounds, it will require more time, effort, and resources. Besides that, small model updates will have to be sent as part of training instead of sending the entire dataset altogether. Developing efficient communication methods is key to building a successful FL framework.

Another challenge with FL models is the anticipation of low levels of device participation. That means only a handful of devices will be active at once. Few devices will be able to tolerate variability in the hardware that affects the communication, computational, and storage capabilities of each device in the network.

Lastly, communicating model updates during the training phase of the model has a chance of revealing sensitive information. Such information can be leaked to either the central server in the network or a third party. These challenges must be overcome for the model to be a success in the healthcare industry.

Of course, this AI model is relatively new, and research to test it is still being carried out. Once we know more about this model, researchers can devise ways to overcome these challenges for a better experience.

The Future of Digital Health With FL

Many studies and much research have been done on FL. Recent studies have shown that the models trained by FL can help achieve performance levels that are superior to older models that see data from only one institute.

There is high potential once the FL model is successfully implemented. It can lead to unbiased decisions, better patient privacy and data governance, and an accurate reflection of the physiology of each individual.[3] The FL model shows a lot of promise in overcoming the limitations of models that require centralized data from a single pool.

That is why it is said that the future of digital health lies with FL. It promises one essential thing that has been missing from previous ML models: patient privacy and data governance. Each data controller in the FL model:

- Defines its governance process

- Defines its associated privacy policies

- Controls data access

- Has the capability to revoke data access

All these aims can be met in the validation and training phases. That is why FL has the potential to create many new opportunities in the healthcare industry. It can enable much-needed research on rare diseases and allow large-scale institutional validation inside a healthcare organization.

The FL model can also scale naturally. It can grow global data sets without disproportionately increasing data storage requirements. That is why it can help healthcare organizations naturally scale in the long run as well.

FL now provides an opportunity to capture higher data variability and analyze patients across different demographics. For example, in the context of EHR (electronic health records), FL can find and represent clinically similar patients.[12] Besides that, it can make predictions of hospitalizations based on ICU stay time[13], cardiac events[14], and mortality.

The FL model has the power to create a direct clinical impact. For example, the *HealthChain* project aims to deploy an FL framework in France across four hospitals.[15] The framework will generate common models that make predictions of treatment response for melanoma and breast cancer patients.

The framework will help oncologists determine what course of treatment to take for their patients. It will demonstrate the response based on dermoscopy images and histology slides. That is just one of the examples of how FL is already affecting digital health.

Another promising example is that of *FeTS (Federated Tumour Segmentation)*.[16] This is an international federation consisting of thirty healthcare institutions using an open-source FL framework. This framework aims to improve tumor boundary detection from various myeloma patients.

However, the application of the FL framework in digital health is not just on treatment response or disease detection. Instead, the application extends to industrial translation and research as well. That is because FL allows for collaborative research.

One of the biggest initiatives of the FL framework for this purpose is the *Melloddy* project, which aims to deploy multi-task FL across data sets of ten pharmaceutical companies.[17] The pharmaceutical partners aim to optimize the drug discovery process by training a common predictive model. The model will infer how chemical compounds bind to proteins. The partners will be able to achieve the aims of this model without revealing their data.

Many clinicians have already improved diagnostic tools for imaging analysis through the use of FL models. Additionally, pharma companies are reducing their costs and saving their time to market with accelerated and collaborative drug discovery. In the future, the FL model has the potential to increase the robustness and accuracy of healthcare AI tools while improving the outcome for patients and decreasing costs.

In the coming decades, the FL model will improve medical care, diagnosis, treatment response, disease detection, and much more. We will just have to wait and see how it all happens.

Conclusion

That was your complete guide to the FL models being used across healthcare industries. It is the most promising AI model we have right now. However, it is still in its initial phase; more research is necessary to completely understand its potential.

It is showing much promise in the field of healthcare and we can't wait to see more companies coming up with the latest FL technology. It is the future of healthcare and might soon take over the industry.

References/Further Reading

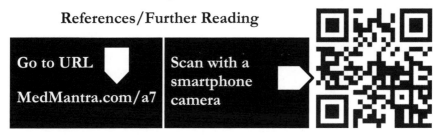

Go to URL

MedMantra.com/a7

Scan with a smartphone camera

CHAPTER EIGHT

NATURAL LANGUAGE PROCESSING (NLP) IN HEALTHCARE

Healthcare is on its way to universal transformation, and AI is the most significant contributor to this change. Natural Language Processing (NLP) will be one of the most significant catalysts, as it provides various opportunities to change the healthcare system for good.[1]

In the long run, NLP will aid in reducing costs, streamlining healthcare processes, providing the highest quality of healthcare, and much more.

Natural Language Processing Explained

NLP is one of the most specialized branches of artificial intelligence (AI) that emphasizes manipulating and interpreting written or human-generated spoken data.[2]

In simple terms, NLP dictates the manners in which AI policies assess and gather unstructured data from human language to extract patterns. The primary aim is to get the meaning and compose feedback about the data. Because of this, the healthcare industry can now make the best use of unstructured data.[2]

In the long run, NLP will help the healthcare industry provide high-quality healthcare and enrich patient lives. The latter aim will be achieved using real-time data to enrich the patient experience.

Applications of NLP in Healthcare

Following are the many ways that NLP will transform the healthcare industry:

1. Speech Recognition

Speech recognition is one of the top applications of NLP, and it has matured over time. Now, clinicians can quickly transcribe notes to offer useful Electronic Health Record (EHR) data entry.[3]

The most exciting part is that the NLP speech recognition technology detects and corrects mistakes in the transcription before passing it on. Because of this, clinicians receive accurate data for creating flawless EHRs. Keep in mind that many speech recognition technology players are in the market.

An advantage of having so many players is that many startups are transforming the speech recognition space through deep learning (DL) algorithms that uncover more possibilities for NLP.

2. Evidence-Based Medicine

NLP will significantly improve the quality of care for patients. It is set to do this through evidence-based medicine. This is informed by patient-reported outcomes. An example is negative effects retrieved with NLP from data created outside randomized controlled trials. In the long run, the data is set to transform many aspects of healthcare, including evidence-based medicine.[4]

3. Enhancing Clinical Documentation

The manual systems of EHRs consume a significant part of clinicians' time. Because of this, clinicians can't give more time to patients, which affects healthcare quality.[5] NLP's clinical documentation will help free clinicians from this laborious task. Speech-to-text dictation and organized data entry will allow clinicians to focus more on patients.

The technologies used in NLP help to bring out relevant data from speech recognition tools that modify the data for insights used to run population health management (PHM) and value-based care (VBC) efforts.[5] It will create optimistic outcomes for clinicians, as they can apply such NLP tools to determine the usefulness of health policies.

4. Supporting Clinical Decision-Making

Because of the lack of sufficient time and the fact that clinicians are busy with paperwork and patients, their decision-making is not strong. NLP technologies will work to support and improve clinical decision-making. More solutions will be formulated with NLP to boost clinical decisions.

For example, in the healthcare industry, many areas of improvement require better supervision techniques. Medical errors are one of the top areas of improvement, as mistakes cost time and money and affect the quality of care for patients. Much research is being done to understand the use of NLP to detect infections in a computerized manner.

Of course, such technology is still in its early stages. There is a long way to go before positive healthcare results are seen. However, one thing is a given: that NLP will transform clinical decision-making to ease clinicians' workload. For the hospital staff, this will save time and effort in the long run.

Currently, NLP is already helping clinicians check symptoms and diagnose patients. In the next decade, the technology will keep improving.[6]

5. Integration of Data Mining

Currently, in the healthcare industry, decision-making is subjective and can lead to mistakes. However, integrating data mining with NLP will decrease subjectivity and provide medical knowledge to staff.[7] If the healthcare industry integrated this appropriately, the result could be better medical knowledge discovery.

Such knowledge discovery can allow healthcare organizations to create better strategies and offer high-quality care to patients. There is no aspect that NLP will leave out, as it is set to change healthcare for the better. Once healthcare organizations implement and use such technologies in the right way, patients will trust the healthcare system more as they receive better and efficient care.

How Can Healthcare Organizations Make the Best Use of NLP?

It falls on the healthcare organizations to make the best of NLP and use the technology in the most advantageous way for patients. If this is done correctly, the healthcare industry can manage solutions in a better way by transforming the quality of patient care.[8]

For example, healthcare organizations can use machine learning (ML) to enhance patient workflows and outcomes. This is a win-win situation for patients and organizations in the long run. Here are the top ways that healthcare organizations can make the best use of NLP:

1. Enhancing Patient Health Awareness

EHR has many challenges in healthcare that NLP can overcome. One of the biggest challenges is that patients can access a part of their healthcare data, but many of them can't comprehend the information in EHR systems. Because of this issue, only a few patients can optimally use their healthcare data to make better health decisions for themselves.

If machine learning (ML) is applied in healthcare through NLP, patients will no longer face this issue. The technology will accurately transcribe and analyze medical data to help patients understand medical terms and enrich their knowledge.[8] Through this accurate and informative data, patients can make better health decisions for themselves.

2. Enhancing Patient Interactions with EHR and the Provider

NLP can help enhance patients' understanding of medical jargon and their health.[9] It can help curb the EHR distress that patients face when they can't understand their medical history and data. Many clinicians are using NLP technologies as an alternative to handwriting or typing medical notes.

As more healthcare organizations adopt NLP, it will streamline the workflow for clinicians and enrich patients' understanding of their health data. Such application and benefits will enhance patients' interactions with their healthcare providers and EHR data.

3. Improving Quality of Care

Of course, this is a no-brainer. NLP will improve the quality of care for patients because they will receive much more accurate data. In addition, the technology offers better ways to evaluate current care quality and develop strategies to improve on it.[10] To achieve this aim, healthcare organizations must measure and evaluate physicians' performance.

Evaluating the performance of physicians will help the healthcare organization understand gaps in the quality of care. They can work on various areas to bridge this gap and improve patient outcomes. The most exciting part is that NLP algorithms can also quickly identify potential mistakes in the quality of care.

If the healthcare organization combines the data from NLP algorithms and its own evaluation, it can quickly create better strategies. Organizations will have a full view of what can be done to improve patient outcomes. Once they apply these strategies, better quality healthcare will no longer be a distant future.

4. Identifying Patients' Critical Care Needs

People face many constraints and challenges in accessing healthcare. Sometimes, doctors diagnose illnesses when it's too late, or they don't identify the care needs of patients.[11] Fortunately, with its robust technologies, NLP can curb this problem.

For example, NLP algorithms can quickly and efficiently extract information from big datasets. Such extraction of information will give physicians the knowledge and tools necessary to treat patients with critical and complicated illnesses.[11] NLP will never replace physician care, but it will help physicians provide urgent and better care to patients.

Benefits of Using NLP in Healthcare

Here are the top four benefits of implementing NLP in healthcare:

1. Efficient Billing Process

The entire billing process at hospitals is haphazard. There are too many patients, and human error is always a possibility. NLP technologies can enhance the billing process and make it easier for physicians and patients.

For example, NLP technologies can extract relevant information from physician notes and assign medical codes to each aspect of this information.[12] This facilitates the billing process and reduces the burden on the healthcare administrative staff. In the long run, the administrative costs of the healthcare organization decline significantly.

2. Reduced Patient Risk

Analyzing the best surgical or treatment methods, predicting post-surgical complications, and other such evaluations are prone to human error, leading to high risk for patients. This is especially true when the illness is complicated and clinicians must make urgent decisions to provide care to patients. In this regard, NLP can transform the healthcare industry by improving patient outcomes and reducing treatment risk.

NLP can extract information from large datasets and analyze the best treatment methods while predicting post-surgical complications and how to overcome them.[12] If healthcare providers work with NLP technologies, their decision-making time will decrease and they will provide the best care to patients.

In the long run, patients will be less prone to the fallibility of doctors and medical errors. The risk of problems will greatly fall and more patients will trust the healthcare system.

3. Prior Authorization Approval

Administrative delays and errors can significantly increase the amount of time that patients wait before receiving care. People combating complicated illnesses don't have this time. This problem can be overcome by integrating NLP into the healthcare system. NLP technologies can leverage information from physician notes.

Extracting and analyzing such notes will reduce the number of administrative delays and errors. Patients will not have to wait long to receive care, as they receive accurate prior authorization approval through NLP technologies.

4. Streamlined Medical Policy Assessment

Public sources are always changing and releasing newer clinical guidelines and protocols. NLP technologies can compile and compare all the clinical guidance from each source.[13] Then, they can help healthcare providers define the best care guidelines for better quality care delivery to patients.

To that end, NLP will also streamline medical policy assessment. The process is not fully automated right now and is prone to time delays and human errors. NLP will overcome all these problems, thereby creating positive outcomes for medical staff and patients.

Conclusion

That was your complete guide to understanding NLP in healthcare. There are endless opportunities for NLP to transform the landscape of healthcare for the better. Currently, the healthcare system is overburdened and faces many problems such as errors, time delays, administrative challenges, poor patient care quality, and much more.

NLP is here to change how healthcare operates by overcoming all these problems and offering new opportunities for better care. We are just starting to discover the opportunities that NLP will create. Only time will tell how healthcare can positively transform.

References/Further Reading

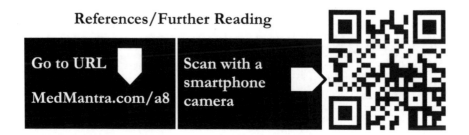

Go to URL
MedMantra.com/a8

Scan with a smartphone camera

CHAPTER NINE

MYTHS ABOUT AI APPLICATIONS IN HEALTHCARE

It takes at least a decade of hard work and experience to become a doctor, but still, they misdiagnose cases. Even the best of doctors make mistakes, and medical errors are now the third most leading cause of death in the US.[1] It's neither the doctor's fault nor is the deficiency in training; human nature is liable to make mistakes, and such mistakes in hospital settings might cost one his/her life.

This is where artificial intelligence or AI comes to the rescue. The ability of AI-enabled systems to work at super-human speed tirelessly has attracted billions of dollars of investment in the healthcare industry. Until recently, the healthcare industry has had little to no automation—and lacked predictive analytics—and complex protocols to reach a diagnosis. While AI models also need to be trained on a given set of data, just like doctors, they're far better at handling multiple variables at a time, providing logical reasoning and ceaseless analytics that is uninfluenced by sleep, tiredness, or long duty hours. This, in contrast, can provide a low-cost, highly efficient alternative to traditional health care.

As of now, the application of AI is best seen in diagnostic imaging and finding out specific patterns on microscopic slides in pathology. It can point out subtle changes that would otherwise be missed by a doctor, and that, too, in the blink of an eye. As a result of this, many healthcare organizations are attempting to take into account the most revolutionary uses of AI, such as automated diagnostics, MRI/CT/X-ray imaging analysis, histopathological identification of tumors, differentials of dermatology, and automated robotic surgery.

The learning of human-to-human interaction with robots can eventually train the AI model to perform optimally in hospital settings. The implementation of this process can help automate various processes, including referrals to specialists based on a diagnosis, issuing a warning for medicine allergies, automated treatment plans, and claims processing.

AI can help hospital management achieve 'Optimal Operational Performance' and ensure that facilities and equipment are always in use and never scarce, the right number and type of staff are present, and appropriate medical supplies are in hand. AI can also aid in analyzing data from many sources and compile them to increase the quality of health care while keeping the costs low

Myths about AI

Although the implications of AI in health care are vast, certain myths need to be busted before we continue the journey to the era of automated diagnostics.

Myth number 1: AI will replace doctors

Visiting a doctor is expensive! And the added burden of hospital charges and diagnostic costs makes sure that you're just one illness away from bankruptcy. AI, on the other hand, follows the 'zero marginal cost' trend, meaning that the first copy of the software is expensive, and the rest of them are just free. This can eventually make health care affordable and accessible throughout the globe, at least in theory.

Bots have been replacing human jobs since the rise of technological marvels. One report says that almost half of the jobs people are doing right now can be automated by augmenting currently available technologies. Between now and 2030, 400 million persons are estimated to lose their jobs to automation.[2] The AI has already replaced jobs that require repetitive tasks such as those of cashiers, secretaries, travel agencies, video stores, and many others. Here's a breakdown of the job routines in a healthcare setting:

Repetitive	Routine	Optimizing	Complex	Creative
Pharmacology	Hematology	Radiology	Medicine	Interventional Radiology
Medical Reporting	Histopathology	Research Analytics	Surgery	Plastic Surgery

AI is to completely replace the repetitive and routine jobs in coming years, such as those of histopathologists and hematologists. These jobs require a specific pattern recognition or image analysis to reach a diagnosis, and an AI model cannot only outperform but can also notice subtle changes that would otherwise be ignored by a human eye. But an AI-powered system will take more than a decade to autonomously perform more complex procedures and highly skilled jobs. Even with that level of tech development, AI can only perform in a specific niche, and General Artificial Intelligence is still a way off.

Expert doctors working with intelligent software to augment decision-making will perform significantly better than either of them alone. AI algorithms are currently being employed to diagnose minor medical conditions that general practitioners look into and, if proven accurate, can potentially assist the clinical accuracy of doctors.

But what's keeping AI from knocking down doctors on their own turf is the dependency of algorithms on data presets. Machine learning (ML), a branch of AI, requires a lot of data to be fed into the system for an algorithm to analyze and create a logical outcome. This data includes patients' electronic health records (EHR), radiological imaging, blood test values, and so much more. The unavailability of this huge number of processed medical data is the biggest hurdle to AI development.

No two patients are alike. There is even a difference in the anatomical landmarks and disease progression in different people. Although AI can take a 'guess' of possible differentials, it cannot precisely diagnose a case that has never been fed into it, requiring a human expert to tackle such cases.

Training the algorithms is an arduous process. It requires close interaction between the clinicians and the developers to make sure medically authentic data is fed into the training models. While the medical research data doubles every two years, it's hard to imagine an AI system is able to cope up with new trends without a doctor chewing up data variables for it. These tools can get better over time as they learn, which enables them to evolve with new medical research.

AI can, however, augment safe medical practice by helping doctors reach an accurate diagnosis promptly so a timely intervention can be done to save precious lives. AI will be a tech that assists doctors, not substitutes them. It will aid physicians to get more knowledge about the patient's ailment to make an accurate diagnosis and better-informed decisions, enabling the physician to spend more time winning the patient's trust and making emotional bonds. Just as a stethoscope augments a doctor in making a clinical diagnosis, AI is the latest tool that will further enhance the quality of health care.

In a nutshell, doctors will continue to do jobs that require creativity, decision-making skills, and human interaction. Characteristics like sympathy, judgment, creativity, compassion, and analytical reasoning are lacking in bots, so in the areas where human empathy is fundamental, AI-powered robots won't be a replacement. The aforementioned AI tools will continue to automate small repetitive tasks performed by doctors and allow them to focus on the doctor-patient relationship and patient-centered care.

Myth number 2: AI models are biased

What is bias? Bias in medical practice can influence a doctor's diagnostic accuracy and can lead to errors in clinical management. A number of biases can limit rationality and logical reasoning, which a doctor gathers and uses as evidence in making diagnoses. These biases are not limited to the medical field but, rather, are illustrations of suboptimal reasoning people are liable to.

The AI model can be biased if the data it's learning from is biased. This biased AI model can be potentially more harmful because of its vast scale of operation versus a couple of patients a doctor is checking. The art of medical diagnosis is so intricate that a biased AI system can go unnoticed for a long time. There are many subtle ways in which a model can go wrong and pick-up bias that is harmful. Therefore, more fundamental research needs to be done on data used in machine learning to avoid a catastrophe.

Fortunately, a biased AI-model is easy to fix, with correct logical data and retraining the machine algorithms. This continues to be an ongoing topic of research to identify ways of detecting and correcting biases and unreliable data sources.

Myth number 3: AI is too risky to use in healthcare

The scope of AI implementations in health care is tremendous—from diagnostics to research data collection to augmented surgeries—for revolutionizing the delivery of healthcare in the modern era. The AI implementation in clinical settings poses a greater risk to the healthcare facility. The stakes of getting the right diagnosis are much higher in this field.

The diagnostic accuracy of AI far exceeds that of top board-certified doctors. So, the risk of AI misdiagnosing a case is at least less than what we have in specialist care institutions. AI is only as good as the data upon which the model is trained, so the success of the AI model is not based much on algorithms but on the data provided to it.

In a head-to-head competition with senior radiologists in China, The BioMind AI system developed at the Beijing Tiantan Hospital made correct diagnoses in 87% of cases in about 15 minutes, while a team of 15 senior professors achieved an accuracy of only 66% in 225 total cases.[3]

Babylon developed an AI-powered app to help diagnose minor ailments or refer to a nearby healthcare facility if symptoms point to a serious condition.

"Babylon's latest artificial intelligence capabilities show that it is possible for anyone, irrespective of their geography, wealth, or circumstances, to have free access to health advice that is on par with top-rated practicing clinicians."

Dr. Parsa – Founder, Babylon

The Royal College of General Practitioners (RCGP) conducts an examination to grant practicing licenses to passing students. The company made its AI take the exam for MRCGP, in which it scored 81%, whereas the passing score is 72%.[4]

So, the advancements in AI can significantly improve the healthcare industry, promising improved patient care and more accurate diagnosis while slightly increasing the associated risks.

Myth number 4: Robotic Process Automation (RPA) will fix data problems

The biggest challenge in the healthcare industry is the sorting of data received from various sources. The new patient forms, medical prescriptions, handwritten notes, medical claims forms, and radiographs all exemplify the challenges of managing disorganized data and implementing its use in research and analytics. There's a misconception that AI will correct the data flow with its 'magic wand.'

AI developers and data scientists need organized, complete, and accurate data—not to mention metadata—to train AI algorithms on how to identify a red flag and return useful results only. Such data is not yet available, and even AI can't solve it.

There is a dire need for smart input software that can collect and organize data from different sources into one place, which enables record stratification and data extraction. This structured data combined with RPA can enable healthcare organizations to deliver data for machine learning. This organization of data can be achieved in the following ways:

- The implementation of one data entry point into the healthcare system. For example, instead of manually inputting data by asking patients every time, the data is automatically populated into the system with identity codes.

- The extraction of metadata from patient forms, ensuring that the concerned information filled out in the form is thoroughly validated and processed by Electronic Health Records (EHR) system.

- The incorporation of unstructured content such as X-ray and prescription information included within relevant forms for processing.

Myth number 5: AI means the end of privacy

There's an argument that AI can be worse than humans when it comes to privacy and security. Unauthorized access to databases containing critical health information can be more damaging than any other data breach in this modern era.

Artificial intelligence exposes us to a wide range of challenges concerning data security and privacy, along with the fact that AI models need massive amounts of structured data for training.

Although machine learning models are trained on anonymous data, some people are still concerned about their personal illnesses being revealed to others who have access to the system. In a study[5], around 90% of data experts said that patients should be concerned about their data being potentially misused when given to healthcare organizations for analytics.

For the coming years, AI development will depend on its access to even bigger and populated medical and healthcare datasets. The tools we have used up until now to protect people's privacy and identification while making the data available for research and analytics cannot be used to secure datasets used for AI development. To make the data available while maintaining privacy, there is a need for the development of modern privacy-enhancing technologies (PET). This will ensure privacy protection in the working environment of AI.

Conclusion

The potential benefits of AI implementation outweigh the risks associated with bringing automation to the medical field. While artificially intelligent robots are not yet there to replace doctors, they can augment doctors' jobs in the healthcare delivery system by taking up repetitive tasks such as analyzing tests, x-rays, MRI and CT scans, data entry, and loads of other tedious tasks. The preliminary progress is promising, but the data privacy and non-availability of massive structured data are stumbling blocks in AI development. In the upcoming years, AI models will get more mature to bring a revolution in the way we diagnose and treat ailments.

"AI is serendipity; it is here to liberate us from monotonous jobs and make us more human."

References/Further Reading

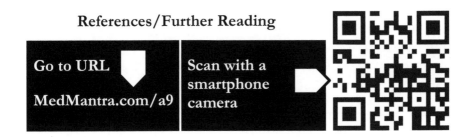

CHAPTER TEN

AI RESEARCH IN HEALTHCARE: A PRACTICAL GUIDE

ABCD...AI (anybody can 'do' artificial intelligence)

Artificial intelligence (AI) can be harnessed to detect patterns and associations in large datasets. In no other domain are these advancements more acutely needed than healthcare. With our health systems under unprecedented strain and with health inequalities increasingly becoming a global problem, the healthcare domain has pinned great hopes on the AI revolution. The utilitarian healthcare challenge is to provide the highest quality care, to the greatest number of people, for the lowest possible cost. In recent years, we have started to see the hope that AI may be up to the challenge.

Machine learning (ML) has revolutionized healthcare research as clinicians and academics realize the huge value of healthcare data in improving patient care and clinical working. Specifically, deep learning (DL) is now the gold-standard AI technology and is already showing an astounding ability to perform tasks more quickly, accurately, and cost-effectively than humans.[1,2]

The wide application of ML in healthcare, along with a rich community of support and the rapidly reducing cost of computational power, has enabled more casual researchers to ride the waves of this revolution. No longer is AI research reserved for computer 'geeks' or non-clinical data miners. For the first time, clinicians and academics around the world who find themselves with access to interesting datasets can ask themselves, *"What machine learning can we do with these data?"* and realistically achieve meaningful goals that, until recently, would have been prohibitively resource-intensive.

In this chapter, we present a practical guide to conducting ML research in the healthcare domain. We will focus on the specific challenges of healthcare projects and the limitations of healthcare data, including ethical and governance considerations. We will not cover ML theory or delve into deep detail about specific architectures, for which an abundance of alternative sources is available. After reading this chapter, the reader should have a good idea about the healthcare questions to which they could apply their data, as well as how they could process and augment their data, and a broad appreciation of the bigger-picture issues that are specific to the healthcare domain [see Figure 10-1].

What do you want to achieve?

One of the most common pitfalls of ML research in healthcare is that it is too data-focused at the outset. While this may be appropriate for some domains, it could not be less so in healthcare. Attempting to invent a research question solely to shoehorn the data you possess will risk wasting resources developing technologies that have limited clinical applicability and that are destined for failure.

The ultimate aim of healthcare is to provide high-quality care to users. This may be achieved in many different ways, such as improving disease detection, developing new treatments, increasing efficiency, reducing costs, or freeing up time for clinicians to focus on more valuable tasks.

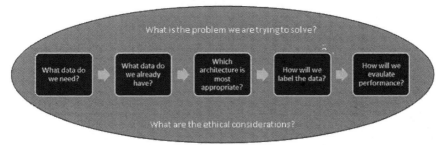

Figure 10-1. A schematic for practical steps and considerations when conducting AI research in the healthcare domain

From the very start of the project, the overall goal should be set—*what do you envision as the ultimate purpose of your algorithm?* This should, in the first instance, be discussed and agreed upon by the research team *without* looking at the currently available data. Later, the already-available data can be reviewed to fine-tune more realistic sub-projects and tasks. By doing this, you will stay true to the overarching clinical goal rather than trying to write the questions that your data might answer. This will enable an objective and critical appraisal of your data, identify gaps, and inform your strategy for data processing and augmentation.

Questions to ask yourself at the outset of the project include:
How will this project improve patient care?
How will this project improve the working lives of healthcare practitioners?
How will this project reduce healthcare costs?
How will this project increase healthcare efficiency?
How will this project advance the state-of-play in the field?
What is the current 'pain' that we are trying to overcome?
How quickly does the solution need to be delivered?
How much time, money, and human resources are available?

In more practical terms, it is important to hone into the specific objectives of the algorithm(s). This will determine the ML architecture, ethical considerations, and timeline. Consider the range of applications below, with landmark examples from the literature:

- *Diagnosis/disease identification* – Clinical services are overwhelmed by the number of patients to manage and the volume of data to interpret. Computing this manually and quickly is impossible for humans to do. Given the right data, machines can now learn within hours to detect the same diagnostic patterns that humans have learned throughout years of experience. This enables diseases to be detected more accurately, earlier, and at a faster rate than humans can manage. Ultimately, this reduces waiting times for patients and enables more timely treatment (and, in some cases, prevention of disease). In a landmark study, convolutional neural networks were able to detect skin cancer from photos with comparable accuracy to that of board-certified dermatologists.[1]

- *Risk prediction* – Whilst humans are trained to recognize early symptoms and signs of diseases, machines are increasingly capable of recognizing a pre-disease state that, if identified early enough, can change the course of progression. Doing so requires an ability to learn deeply subtle patterns from huge data that would be impossible for humans to detect. In DeepMind's seminal work, deep learning algorithms identified subtle changes in the macula before conversion to age-related macular degeneration and outperformed the majority of expert predictions.[2]

- **Decision support systems** – With the sheer volume of data available for constant interpretation, clinicians can suffer from information overload. Decision support systems enable users to input data from disparate sources and receive an output of risk, treatment advice (if the user is a clinician), or behavior prompts (if the user is a patient). ML models have recently been used to triage COVID-19 patients for hospital admission[3] and risk of death[4].

- **Drug development** – Deep neural networks can rapidly review entire repositories of molecular structures to identify chemical similarities pointing to potential new drugs. This would take entire teams of researchers years to process. These techniques have recently led to the discovery of a novel antibiotic, halicin—the first in over a decade.[5]

- **Personalized medicine** – Patients and clinicians are increasingly demanding individualized (rather than population-based) care recommendations. ML enables the grouping of patients based on similar characteristics, which enables highly bespoke healthcare. This is more likely to effect a desirable behavioral change. Applications include boosting the appropriateness of shingles vaccination alerts[6] and combining ML with patient-derived stem cells to determine a personalized epilepsy management strategy.[7]

- **Perform a procedure** – ML can be used throughout surgery and interventional treatments to determine the appropriate procedure[8], automate suturing[9], improve the dexterity of surgical robots[10] and evaluate surgical skills[11].

- **Reduce costs/increase efficiency** – ML techniques have shown considerable success in the sub-field of healthcare management. Examples range from time-series algorithms in order to manage inventory and predict shortages in Taiwanese blood banks[12] to predicting patient punctuality in outpatient clinics[13].

- *Clinical research and clinical trials* – Some of the greatest costs when conducting clinical research are human resources screening patient records for eligibility, manual data collection, data labeling, and statistical analyses. This pulls experienced clinicians away from high-level clinical research tasks such as follow-up consultations and research strategy management. ML has shown great value in automating many of these tasks, such as image segmentation and feature extraction from text radiology reports.[14]

This list is by no means exhaustive but can act as a reference for categorizing the early stages of your project.

What sort of data do you have?

One of the most unique and exciting features of ML research in healthcare is the sheer variety of data types on offer, creating an almost limitless possibility for high-quality, meaningful research that can change the way we experience healthcare and interact with healthcare professionals [see Table 10-1]. However, this also presents a challenge because clinicians and researchers often find themselves working with a mix of data types toward a highly specific goal, for which there is limited precedent and support. This challenge is unique to the healthcare domain, and, as a result, there is a slower progression in AI research and technology due to this heterogeneity. Table 10-1 summarizes the main data types within healthcare ML research, examples, and possible applications.

Each data type will require specific steps to process and analyze and will lend itself to specific architectures. When considering which data type(s) you require for your project, be mindful of how the question or problem is currently answered. If this is by a human (as most healthcare paradigms are), they are likely assimilating and computing a large amount of disparate data, which are of different types. Therefore, to emulate these highly nuanced behaviors, the algorithm must reflect the range of data types required to make the decision in question. It is entirely possible that in practice, you will require multiple algorithms, which input a particular data type using a specific architecture, later joining up into a hybrid ML structure to achieve your goal. Bearing this in mind, broadening your team with data scientists and ML engineers alongside clinicians is highly recommended.

Table 10-1. Common data types in healthcare ML research, examples from healthcare, and possible clinical applications

Data type	Examples	What can I do with it?
Image	X-ray, CT, MRI, patient photographs (e.g., skin)	Lesion classification Segmentation of regions of interest Next image prediction (real-time scan planning) Surgical planning (e.g., orthopedics)
Video	Ultrasound/Echocardiography	Inducible ischemia detection from cardiac wall motion
	Footage of patients	Detection of movement disorders Posture correction during physiotherapy
Text	Radiology reports	Diagnosis extraction Uncertainty modeling
	Discharge summaries	Automated clinical codes reimbursement
	Clinic letters	Medical to lay language translation
Numerical	Clinical outcomes (e.g., death)	Risk of death stratification Automated analysis of endpoints in clinical trials
	Blood test results	Decision support systems (e.g., AKI/sepsis)
Categorical	Urine analysis	Medication compliance monitoring
	Molecular structures	New drug development (e.g., antibiotics)
	Gene sequences	Pre-implantation genetic diagnosis
Time-series	Continuous ECG monitoring	Arrhythmia prediction
	Invasive blood pressure	Real-time vasopressor titration in ITU
	Blood glucose	Wearable insulin reminder device

PRACTICAL TIPS: Limitations of healthcare datasets

In most domains, the ML application is at the forefront of data collection and may even be the reason why the data are being collected at all. By contrast, healthcare data are a by-product of other medical, clinical, or research activity. For these data to arise in the first place, patients had to be treated, proteins pipetted, insurance companies invoiced, or some other activity conducted for a purpose entirely separated from (or even unaware of) the machine learning algorithm that you will be developing.

As a result, the data you find yourself in possession of are likely to be noisy, unstandardized, and incomplete. Take care to understand your data deeply, warts and all. You may find that the project cannot proceed further until the data gaps are filled, perhaps by revisiting the data source and manual extraction. Resources will need to be committed to this. In other cases, gaps could be filled by averages (e.g., of the other scalar values) or excluded. There may be a variable that is central to your algorithm but that was not collected from the source of your data. You must consider whether the reward of including these variables is worth the cost of extracting them.

Obtaining datasets within healthcare takes time. Usually, you must *take what you get*. Allow at least double your initial estimates for data gathering. Think two or three projects ahead so that you are requesting the correct data with all variables of interest in time for the project to start. Invest time and resources into developing clear data pipelines to streamline future research. In practical terms, this involves studying who the stakeholders are, fulfilling all information governance requirements, setting up and testing hardware such as servers and user interfaces, and developing a close working relationship with your institution's IT department.

Picking the right architecture

A detailed discussion about ML architectures is beyond the scope of this chapter. However, it is important to be mindful of the algorithm's architecture early in the project because this will impact your data requirements, explainability, resource allocation, and timeline. Below is a summary, with examples, of the key architectures used in healthcare ML research.

Supervised vs. unsupervised learning – Supervised learning requires a dataset of ground-truth labels, which are used to train, validate, and test the algorithm. Unsupervised learning does not require labeled data and relies on the algorithm finding its own patterns and features *de novo*. Whilst unsupervised learning has a wide range of applications, its need for huge amounts of data (which are hard to come by in the healthcare domain)[15] and tendency to make spurious (and potentially clinically meaningless) relationships result in it being rarely used in healthcare ML research currently. This chapter focuses primarily on practical tips for ML healthcare projects involving supervised learning architectures.

Artificial neural networks (ANNs) – These are the most ubiquitous and versatile architectures for ML in healthcare. They can be used with images, text, video, and time-series data. They are relatively intuitive and can be created by novice programmers but require large amounts of labeled data.[16,17]

Convolutional neural networks (CNNs) – A type of ANN that averages features in high-dimensional space using kernels. These are extensively used in medical image analysis tasks.[18] They are highly powerful and boast superior performance compared to many other architectures but can be difficult to interpret and are computationally expensive.

Recurrent neural networks (RNNs) – these networks feature hidden layers that are informed by previous information.[19] They are, therefore, used in particular for time-series healthcare data but are computationally slow and suffer from long-range dependencies (the loss association between information that is temporally separated).[20,21] They are increasingly being superseded by transformer architectures (see next paragraphs).

Generative adversarial networks (GANs) – These networks can generate new data with similar statistics to the training dataset.[19] Currently, they have limited use in healthcare research[22,23] but are likely to become increasingly relevant, given their obvious application to augment spare healthcare datasets.

Encoders and transformers – These are increasingly being used in medical natural language processing (NLP), with the advent of sophisticated transformer encoders such as BERT.[24] A key benefit of this is that pre-training on a large corpus of unlabeled data can be conducted. Then, only fine-tuning with a much smaller labeled dataset is required for good performance.[14]

PRACTICAL TIPS: Playing to your strengths

For the most part, the research question and data available will determine the most appropriate ML architecture. To a certain extent, this will also be influenced by the expertise within the research team. While ANNs and CNNs are now well-established and offer plug-and-play functionality for relative novices (such as TensorFlow by Google and PyTorch by Facebook), some of the latest transformer architectures are evolving so rapidly that they require specific expertise to be able to program. In practice, the difference between architectures may be only a few performance points. If this is the case, it is usually preferable to select an architecture that your team is comfortable and experienced with programming and troubleshooting rather than one that will require constant external technical support.

Labeling data: What are the options?

High-quality, accurately labeled data are the cornerstone of effective supervised ML algorithms. Consider a child learning the alphabet by seeing a deck of cards picturing different objects. They will learn by (i) repeatedly being shown the cards, (ii) being told which letter each picture represents, (iii) having the opportunity to guess what the objects are, and (iv) being told whether their guesses were correct or incorrect. Similarly, for an ML algorithm to be able to 'learn,' it must first be "told" the correct answers for a set of examples. Next, it must guess or predict the answer for a set of examples it has never seen before and receive feedback regarding its performance.

These examples are labeled data points or "annotations." By repeating this process iteratively, the algorithm will learn associations and stands a good chance of converging on acceptable performance levels. When an ML algorithm fails to perform well, usually at least one of three things has occurred:

There are insufficient labeled data

The data are labeled inaccurately

The labeled data are unrepresentative of the population

Ultimately, the algorithm will be only as good as the labeled data that were used to train, validate, and test it, so it is entirely intuitive that investing time and resources into high-quality data labeling is of the utmost importance.[25] But where do the labels come from?

Domain expert labeling – The majority of labeled data within the healthcare domain will have arisen from routine clinical activity (e.g., a radiologist entering the diagnosis of "pneumonia" into the electronic health record after reviewing a chest radiograph; this is called "classification") or a clinician specifically reviewing the data point and manually assigning a label to it (e.g., a tissue viability nurse tracing around ulcers in a set of photos of patients' shins; this is called "segmentation"). In both cases, considerable time and effort have been spent on deriving the labels. Furthermore, the labeling has been done by highly trained individuals, drawing from years of experience and practice.

There is a trade-off for expert data labeling. On the one hand, this usually leads to highly accurate and representative labels, much to the benefit of the downstream algorithm. On the other hand, these labels are extremely time-consuming and expensive (consider a surgeon's time labeling techniques from operation notes versus spending the same time performing procedures, or an intensive care nurse determining whether a set of blood pressure trends is septic, hypovolaemic, or anaphylactic shock versus treating critically unwell patients). In practice, it is likely that only a limited number of labels could be derived from experts and maybe an order of magnitude smaller than that needed for training ML algorithms. Employing a team of expert labelers may be highly desirable but prohibitively expensive, and the opportunity cost of lost time engaging in more clinically urgent tasks may be too great. This is what makes high-quality, expert-labeled medical datasets so valuable in the research (and commercial) marketplace.[26]

Automated labeling – Computer power can be harnessed to carry out data labeling, which then feeds into the ML algorithm. This could be using programmed rules (e.g., whenever the ejection fraction in an echocardiogram report is <55%, assign the label "left ventricular failure") or using ML itself (e.g., a natural language processing transformer, which assigns diagnosis labels from free-text echocardiogram reports and appends them to the image files that will then be used for the main ML classification algorithm).[14]

The former is quick and computationally light and does not require any pre-existing labels. The downside is that rule-based labeling techniques are rigid and require the data to be clean, homogenous, and highly stereotyped (which is uncommon for medical data). The latter (using ML to generate labels) is powerful and flexible but still requires a set of manual labels in the first place and is more time-consuming, expensive, and computationally intensive.

Non-expert and crowdsourced labeling – An increasingly popular alternative to domain expert and automated data labeling is "non-expert" or "crowdsourced" labeling.[27] This aims to balance the accuracy of human labeling against the cost of highly trained experts. Many medical labeling tasks that appear insoluble at first glance can be adapted into more manageable prospects for people without medical training. The recent rise of the "gig" economy and the demand for flexible and home working has led to an upswing in crowdsourced data labeling platforms. This enables a much higher volume of labels to be generated quickly for a fraction of the cost of a domain expert, thereby freeing up their time for higher-level tasks.

The gamification of medical data labeling has also increased recently[28], inspired by trends in other domains[29]. In this technique, the medical labeling task is slightly adapted to appear as a game to the non-expert labeler and has been shown to have higher degrees of uptake, attention, and accuracy.[30] There are important limitations to the appropriateness of outsourcing data labeling to the crowd, namely, the anonymization of medical data and whether patients and the public would be willing to entrust their care to an algorithm that has been trained on data labeled by non-clinical experts.

Data augmentation – Sometimes, you are stuck with the data you have. Labeling more data (by any method) may be impossible or impractical. This is usually the case when the project timeline is highly urgent or no more data exist for further labeling. In these cases, techniques can be used to augment the existing data. In computer vision (image analysis tasks), the dataset can be multiplied many-fold by incorporating flips, scaling, transformations, and random rotations to the images.[31-33] The algorithm will regard these as new unseen data, but no extra work is required for labeling, as they will retain the label of the original source image. This can also be used to even out class imbalances in datasets (e.g., if your skin cancer dataset is lacking in malignant melanoma, add several augmented versions of your existing melanoma images).

This is also possible for other data types; for example, (i) time-series data of test results can be padded out by adding interim data points based on trendlines, extrapolations, and averaging, (ii) text data can be augmented by changing the order at the word, sentence, and paragraph levels, and (iii) video data can be trimmed, sheared, and transformed much like still image data. There is a wealth of literature and programming support on this topic, and, additionally, plug-and-play programming libraries that enable these features with a few additional lines of code.

Overall, the importance of high-quality, accurate, representative, and abundant data labels cannot be overstated in the ML healthcare research domain. It is unlikely that a one-size-fits-all approach will be appropriate for your task. Careful time and attention should be taken to identify the data requirements for your project, the needs of the algorithm, and your own time and resource constraints.

Evaluating performance

After selecting the appropriate architecture, training, and validating the algorithm, its performance must be evaluated against a set of data that is previously unseen (the test set). This will ultimately determine the extent to which the algorithm has achieved its goals. There are myriad ways to evaluate the performance of an ML algorithm, which are heavily influenced by the type of algorithm, the research question, and the clinical application. Exhaustive lists of performance metrics and how to calculate them are readily available in the literature and are beyond the scope of this chapter. Some of the most common performance metrics in the healthcare domain and their key implications are mentioned below. Many are intuitive and will be familiar to most clinicians with a basic knowledge of epidemiology or medical statistics. Take the example of an image classification algorithm aiming to differentiate between COVID pneumonitis (CP) and idiopathic pulmonary fibrosis (IPF) from chest CT scans:

	Algorithm classification (prediction)	
Ground-truth	COVID pneumonitis	Idiopathic fibrosis
COVID pneumonitis	True positive (TP)	False negative (FN)
Idiopathic fibrosis	False positive (FP)	True negative (TN)

The classification (prediction) made by the algorithm can be classified in relation to the ground-truth ("real") diagnosis in a binary fashion, resulting in a 2 x 2 grid known as a confusion matrix. This can be done any number of times separately for each class, in cases in which multiple diagnoses' predictions are outputted by the algorithm. From the confusion matrix, we can define four groups:

True positive (TP) – the algorithm correctly predicted a true case of CP

False positive (FP) – the algorithm predicted CP, but it was actually IPF

False negative (FN) – the algorithm predicted IPF, but it was actually CP

True negative (TN) – the algorithm correctly predicted a true case of IPF

From these groups, we can derive the following common performance metrics [see Table 10-2]:

- **Accuracy** – the overall number of correct predictions compared to the entire number of predictions made.

- **Sensitivity** (recall) – the algorithm's ability to correctly predict all cases *with* the label of interest.

- **Specificity** – the algorithm's ability to correctly predict all cases *without* the label of interest.

- **Positive predictive value (precision)** – how many people predicted to have the label of interest by the algorithm truly have the label. *This metric focuses on how useful the algorithm is in clinical practice.*

- **F score** – the harmonized average of precision and recall. *This metric captures the trade-off between other metrics, which is very relevant to the healthcare domain and widely used in the healthcare ML literature.*

- **Precision recall curve** – As the name suggests, this is a plot of the positive predictive value (PPV) and sensitivity (recall) over the range of possible values that the dependent variable(s) can take. The curves can be studied to determine the optimal value of the variable at which the precision and recall are maximized. *In healthcare ML research, this is particularly useful for determining the threshold for a classification algorithm.*

- **Receiver operating characteristic (ROC) curve** – Similar to the precision-recall curve, the ROC plots sensitivity (true positive rate) and specificity (true negative rate) at all values of the dependent variable. The area under the curve (AUC) can be easily calculated to determine the aggregate performance of the model across all possible classification thresholds.[34] A high AUC is desirable for most algorithms. *This metric is widely used in the ML healthcare literature, in particular when comparing algorithms' performance to that of human experts (human vs. computer experiments).*

Table 10-2. Common performance metrics for evaluating ML algorithms in healthcare

Performance measure	Alternative name	Formula
Sensitivity	Recall, TP rate	$TP/(TP + FN)$
Specificity	TN rate	$TN/(TN + FP)$
Positive predictive value (PPV)	Precision	$TP/(TP + FP)$
F score	F1 score	$2 \times (\text{Precision} \times \text{Recall})/(\text{Precision} + \text{Recall})$
Accuracy		$(TP + TN)/(TP + FP + TN + FN)$

Carefully choosing the most appropriate performance metric(s) is of great importance to ensuring that algorithm evaluation is well-matched for the desired clinical application. For example, a population-wide fecal occult blood detection algorithm for bowel cancer screening may aim to maximize specificity over sensitivity to avoid inappropriate investigations and avoidable anxiety for false positive cases, while an algorithm to determine which lesions should be biopsied during colonoscopy may rest the balance in favor of sensitivity, to avoid missing cases at this key diagnostic stage.

Ethical, legal, and governance implications

ML research in healthcare operates within a minefield of ethical and governance implications. As clinicians and healthcare researchers, we have an ethical duty to do no harm, act in the best interests of patients, ensure that patients' autonomy and confidentiality are respected, and uphold the key tenets of justice. With the advent of AI in healthcare, the previously well-marked ethical boundaries are increasingly being blurred within a world of black boxes, trade secrets, and commercial competition. This chapter does not aim to exhaustively discuss the numerous ethical conundrums. Rather, a selection of relevant questions is presented below, which should stimulate reflective thought when planning your algorithm and presenting your research [see Table 10-3].

Table 10-3. Key ethical, governance, and legal questions arising from practical research in healthcare machine learning

Ethical questions	Is our algorithm safe to use in clinical practice? Is our algorithm explainable to users and non-experts? Can users trust our algorithm's output? Do we understand why/how our algorithm made its output? Is our algorithm biased against particular groups? Does the algorithm reduce or increase health inequalities?
Governance questions	Who owns the data used to develop the algorithm? Do we have permission from stakeholders to use the data in this way? How will the data be stored? Who has access to it? Do the data need to be anonymized? If so, how? How will the algorithm be audited?
Legal questions	Who owns the algorithm? Is the algorithm intellectual property? Do we require patent protection? Should the algorithm be open source? Who is ultimately responsible for the algorithm's decisions? Where does liability lie if the algorithm makes a mistake?

Conclusion

Owing to technological advances and a wealthy community of support, anybody can now "do" AI research in healthcare. The overall goal of the project (how will it improve healthcare?) should be the central focus from the outset. Healthcare data are sparse, noisy, and expensive to label, but also highly versatile and powerful. Choosing the most appropriate ML architecture for the data and your research team is one of the key steps in the research journey. Finally, being mindful of the ethical and governance implications of your research at every stage will deliver a successful project that improves healthcare and progresses the literature in the field.

References/Further Reading

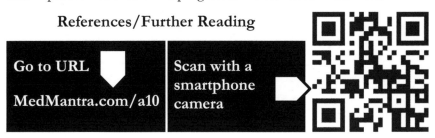

Go to URL

MedMantra.com/a10

Scan with a smartphone camera

"Whenever I hear people saying AI is going to hurt people in the future I think, yeah, technology can generally always be used for good and bad and you need to be careful about how you build it … if you're arguing against AI then you're arguing against safer cars that aren't going to have accidents, and you're arguing against being able to better diagnose people when they're sick."

- Mark Zuckerberg

Section 3

ETHICS OF ARTIFICIAL INTELLIGENCE IN HEALTHCARE

CHAPTER ELEVEN

ETHICS OF ARTIFICIAL INTELLIGENCE IN HEALTHCARE

We are living in a data-driven world. From the advertisements we see to our social media feed, everything is powered by data-driven algorithms. Of course, the role of artificial intelligence (AI) goes even further as these algorithms are now being used in every industry.

Entertainment, finance, business, and all other sectors are experiencing growth because of data and AI. This is because the information derived from these algorithms is priceless to decision-making.

All of this may seem necessary for growth, but what does it mean for us? What are the moral and ethical consequences of creating these highly intelligent systems? Let's find out.

Technological Advancements in Healthcare

Before we move on to understand the ethical consequences, let's first understand how the healthcare industry has changed in the past decade as a result of AI. Here are some of the most notable advancements that have been made:

- Foot Concerns: Any problem related to your foot such as bruising, ulcers, diabetes[1], and much more can now be detected early thanks to machine learning

- Bioprinting: This technology allows 3-D printing to facilitate the reproduction of skin cells and blood vessels for healing.[2] This is especially remarkable for patients who have burns

- Blood Glucose Level Management: Many tech companies are developing AI to determine the blood glucose level in the body[3]

- Digital Communities: Patients can now find support from other patients experiencing the same illness from anywhere in the world[4]

- Open-source data sharing: Data is shared openly within a healthcare organization[5]

Of course, as years are passing by, even more advancements are being made when it comes to AI in the healthcare industry. This is because there is a big gap in healthcare. This gap can be seen with the ongoing pandemic. There is a shortage of professionals, resources, and much more.

So, AI and machine learning are trying to bridge this gap to fulfill the healthcare requirements of people. According to some reports by the World Health Organization (WHO), there will be a global shortage of healthcare workers in the next fifteen years.[6] This problem can easily be solved by AI and technological advancements.

AI is predicted to replace all the professional abilities of healthcare workers as they will be driven by data. They will provide much more accurate, precise, and accessible healthcare.[6] This will reduce the cost of healthcare for people and prevent diseases before they even occur.

However, the big question is, will you take the advice of an AI over a human? What are the challenges we will face as a global community?

The Basics of Ethics

In simple terms, ethics are principles that are guided by our moral compass. These principles shape our behavior and help us make decisions. Our moral compass is the way we see the world morally.

This means what is good/bad or right/wrong for us since this is subjective. Our moral compass is the code of conduct we have made for ourselves. You can see this in institutions too. For example, a school or university has its own code of conduct that the students have to follow.

Apart from that, you can see these ethical codes being implemented in organizations as well. Our focus will be ethics in the field of data science.

Ethics and Data Science

There are ethics when it comes to data as well. This is because data is sensitive information, and it needs to be protected in the right way as it is destructive in the wrong hands. So, the branch of ethics in data science is concerned with the sharing of data, the privacy of data, and decision-making.

There are three main branches of ethics in data science[7]:

- **Data**: This is concerned with security, ownership, transfer, and use of data
- **Intelligence**: This is concerned with the predictive analysis that is developed by data
- **Practices**: This is the morality of intelligent systems

These principles guide the ethics in data science. However, do people follow these guidelines? Is there room for error? There might be because these principles are followed by data scientists, and they can make errors too. The problem is that these errors can have grave consequences.

Implications of Data Ethics in the Real World

Did you know that humans produce 2.5 quintillion bytes of data every day?[8] Yes, that is right. With the growth of technologies available to us, we are constantly creating data even if we are not aware of it.

Our phones track our digital activity, our smartwatches track our health, and every gadget that we own has some sort of data about us in place. This is why companies are now paying more and more money to derive this data.

Even the apps that we use have so much of our personal data that is developed to produce insights and predictions about us. This is why the question of ethics in data is a fundamental one. After all, no one likes being this transparent, but we are giving it all away to companies who exploit us without realizing it.

There have been many real-life cases of data ethics as well. The biggest example to date has been the Cambridge Analytica case. This data leak was concerned with Facebook providing demographic and behavioral data of their users to Cambridge Analytica.[9] This data was then used to influence the U.S elections of 2016.

This was a major breach of security, and the most shocking part is that this leak was reported two years after it happened. Such an incident just goes to show how our privacy is being breached, and data is being sold. The Cambridge Analytica case is just one example that came into the limelight.

Imagine the amount of data sharing that happens daily among tech companies. Our data is revenue for tech companies. This is the time to address the ethical consequences of data. How it is used, where it is used, and if it is reliable.

Application of Machine Learning and AI in Healthcare

The future of healthcare can be transformed through the application of AI and machine learning. However, are we ready to give this much information to intelligent systems? You first need to understand the different ways through which AI and machine learning can be applied in healthcare.

The most important use of such technology will be to effectively diagnose and treat patients. This also means diagnosing early so the onset of a disease can be prevented. Such technology will help doctors diagnose patients more accurately, especially in cases where rare illnesses are involved.

Biosensors are the key innovation in the healthcare industry. This is because these sensors are responsible for converting our biological processes into electronic data that computers can analyze and store. These biosensors can be used to understand our underlying health.

For example, through these biosensors, your heart rate, your blood sugar levels, your food consumption, and everything else can be connected to your medical records.[10] This will allow technology to diagnose you before you even know there is a problem with you.

Of course, this technology has a long way to go but where it is heading right now is powerful. The data from these biosensors can also be linked to your health insurance. So, the implication of this technology is multi-faceted[10] as it will develop a chain reaction that will be hard to stop.

So, of course, this kind of technology also comes with its own set of moral and ethical problems. These are related to the machine learning models that utilize data. The problem is that these systems are so complex that it is extremely difficult for humans to understand them as well.

However, it has the ability to do some actual good in the world. For example, these systems can provide diagnosis and treatment at a fraction of the cost that we are paying right now to healthcare professionals. Another good these systems can do is that they can provide healthcare to highly inaccessible areas. This can change the dimensions of healthcare available in third-world countries. Of course, this is a farfetched scenario right now, but it is entirely possible.

Machine learning and AI can also determine the right dosage of medicine that a person needs.[11] Apart from that, it can also determine the medicine that is best for a certain individual. Biosensor data will help them to effectively respond to individual medical needs.

As data becomes more available, medications for rare conditions can also take into account individual needs and factors. This way, treatment will be customized to suit the patient (personalized medicine). Of course, while all of this is great for us and the healthcare industry, there are ethical and legal hurdles too that need to be addressed.

Machine Bias

Humans are not the only ones who are biased in their predictions and decisions; machine learning models are biased as well. This is due to the way a model is created, and the data used to train the machine learning model. Do remember that the bias that occurs in these models comes from the creators and not the machine or the algorithm itself.

One example of this is that there has been software that predicts future criminals. This software is not accurate because it shows bias towards black people and marks them as criminals.[12] Of course, this just means that the developers of the learning model of the software entered biased data.

So, if we are judgmental and biased, then the systems we create will reflect that too. If these models are created correctly, then they can bring a wave of positive change globally.

Human Bias

We are programmed to be biased. This is because we are constantly judging other people. The first thought that comes to us when we look at anyone is judgmental. So, of course, the machines and systems we create will include this bias too.

A prime example of this is when Tay (a chatbot) was created by Microsoft three years ago. Tay had many interactions with a variety of different Twitter users. However, the problem began when users started interacting with Tay in a racist and sexist manner.[13] A few hours later, Tay also started tweeting such posts. In a nutshell, if AI can learn from human behavior in this way, then it is not safe.

Data Bias

Even the data has a bias. If the data itself is biased, then this will lead to biased predictions, analysis, and outcomes as well. This is why data scientists need to understand how different types of bias show up in their data.

Once this has been identified, then some form of data governance and check can be established that can be utilized to remove this bias from the data. The impact of biased data needs to be reduced; otherwise, it can lead to catastrophic consequences.

Intelligence Bias

When biased humans develop these machines, these models have the tendency to amplify this bias even further. This is because AI and machine learning have much higher capabilities than us. This has led to data scientists discussing ethics when it comes to AI and machine learning.

When machine learning models were in their early stages, they used to be built on population data. However, this ultimately showed bias on many different things regarding the population, such as social issues, social class, race, ethnicity, sex, and other factors.

The implications of this bias can be seen in the criminal justice system. The COMPAS (correctional offender management profiling for alternative sanctions) algorithm was brought forward in the court regarding its use. This is because the model of this algorithm showed a bias towards black people.[14] Such a bias can wrongly accuse people and profile people based on factors that are not in their control.

Even algorithms used by home insurers to assess home insurance risk show bias towards people living in a certain area. So, in the long run, these algorithms have the ability to amplify our bias, and this can lead to minorities being underrepresented.

This is why bias needs to be removed, and data needs to be normalized. However, even after that, there is a risk that the AI model can learn biases the same way we do.

Overcoming and Correcting Bias

There has to be a way to remove this bias and correct it in machine learning models for better analysis and outcomes. There are two types of ethical agents that come within the sphere of machine learning. These are known as implicit and explicit agents.[15]

Implicit agents have an inherent purpose and programming because of which they are ethical. On the other hand, explicit agents are examples to learn from in uncertain circumstances to make ethical decisions.

So, to overcome and correct bias, one should start by collecting an unbiased data sample. This is not easy, but it can be done to improve the quality of data that goes into these machine learning models.

Machine learning models should be diverse and inclusive. This means that the people making these models should also reflect these values; otherwise, bias will show up one way or another.

The Philosophical Conundrum of Bias

We assume that biases are bad. This raises a philosophical question of bias being a good or bad thing. However, bias can be helpful too. For example, machine learning models that are built on classification have a tendency to show bias towards higher accuracy[16] in classes that are overrepresented in data.

So, if you are building on such a model and you need to ensure that there is high accuracy in some classes, then you can collect more data on those classes. So, the process of collecting data can be optimized, and the cost of collecting data can also be reduced.

Of course, this is just one example. Bias can also lead to inaccurate data, poor decisions, and poor results. The question of bias being good or bad can only be answered by the individual dealing with the machine learning model.

What is Informed Consent?

When talking about informed consent, it mainly refers to the consent from the patient to use their data. It is mainly the communication that is present between the healthcare practitioners and the patients.[17] It represents whether the patient gives the go-ahead to perform a particular medical procedure on them.

Mainly, the concept behind informed consent is being able to decide between undergoing a medical procedure with a clear understanding of what it is. Practitioners need to provide you with all the relevant details that entail a particular procedure before giving them consent to move forward with it.

Let's take a look at some of the cases where you would require informed consent:

- Surgeries

- Blood transfusions

- Vaccinations

- Anesthesia

- Radiation

- Blood samples

These are only the major parts of healthcare where you will need informed consent. There is a range of other possibilities that would also require informed consent from the patient.

What is Freedom of Choice?

When talking about freedom of choice, the concept revolves around the patient's ability to make decisions for their medical procedure. With the rise of the data being used in third-party applications, the once-clear line of freedom of choice remains a bit hazy.

For instance, a person who might be suffering from a disease might have to ensure that they are keeping their bodies in control before going on to carry out any particular activity. All these details are easily available from simply the smartwatch you might wear to track your fitness and health records.

With the rise of artificial intelligence and its use in the healthcare industry, the possibility of freedom of choice seems a tad bit difficult.[18] While this is something ideal and should be practiced in the system, but doing so isn't possible in the situation. Why is that?

Well, if a person seems to be in an emergency where they're required to undergo a series of screenings, the emergency team seeking any possible methods to get data about the patient seems inevitable. Given that there is a range of devices that are easily available for storing data, there's no coming back from it. You either make effective use of these devices to plan your livelihood and take control of your choices, or you live obliviously, without knowing what your body might need in the future.

The Ideology Behind Overturning a Person's Data Consent

Now, when it comes to what the patient chooses when it comes to sharing their data, some situations might require the opposite. So, let us take an example of a woman who might have refused consent to medical teams to access her data. When the time comes, and she is in an emergency, medical practitioners might opt for overruling her decision and going on to make use of her data to heal her. Now, had the woman been able to make this decision, what do you think she would have done?

- *Emergency Situation*

  If it isn't obvious, the woman would want medical practitioners to make use of all her data to make her feel better. Who wouldn't want that? But does this mean that the professionals in the industry can access any data even if the patient hasn't consented to it? Not entirely. This mainly depends on the circumstance put forward. In the case of an emergency, the consent may be overturned to save the patient's life. They will surely be grateful for it later on.

- *Criminal Activity*

  When it comes to overturning someone's data consent, a person involved in criminal activity is highly likely to get their consent overturned. There

have been cases where a person was convicted of committir
as rape, based on the data found on their phones.[19] The he
a person's daily activity is monitored helped track the pers
culprit. While the person in question didn't openly offer the code to uicii
phones or any kind of consent, their consent was involuntarily overlooked
because of the gravity of the situation.

Public Awareness About Data Consent

It is high time that people start learning about the essence of informed
consent and freedom of choice. Doing so will limit the wide range of
problems that arise because of consent-related issues. How can there be
public awareness about this, though? Well, there are a series of platforms
that can be used to help the general public understand the importance and
relevance of data consent. Let's take a look at some of the major ways
through which this is possible.

- Social media campaigns

- Advertisements

- Public outreach programs

Finding people where they're spending most of their time is the best way
to get them to understand the importance of consent. Stimulating a better *or anything else*
understanding of data consent will help them know the right details when
it comes to applying their consent.

Who Does the Data Belong to?

We are talking about data and consent, but where does all this data go? Who
owns all of this data? There is no short answer to this. There is a range of
mechanisms at play here, and you should be aware of where your data is
going once you add it to any of your smart devices or other applications.

One thing that you need to understand is that there are data controllers
present in the system that monitor and manage your data. So, no matter
what type of data you might have, these controllers are the ones handling it
on their parts. Moreover, they are the ones that are making use of your data
as well. While on the exterior, it may seem like the data is yours, data
controllers are the ones making use of it at the backend.

Things That Data can be Used for

All of this data is being collected for one reason or the other. So, when there is sufficient data available, then what can be done using it? There is a lot that users can make out from the data. Almost every business or industry is trying to maximize the data available to them to maximize their profits while also making sure to satisfy their customers to the maximum. Getting hands-on relevant data also ensures that you understand the risks involved in a particular field and work your way to minimize them.

Let's take a look at some more ways that data can be utilized:

- Track customers

- Create applications

- Get information on competitors

These are only some methods through which your data can be used by other organizations. There is a long list of other ways through which your data is utilized further. So, how does this relate to the healthcare industry? Well, the healthcare industry has an immense need for data to understand their patients better. For instance, medical practitioners should diagnose a disease when they have all the relevant data displayed right in front of them.

However, this doesn't mean that your data is always used in the right manner. You want to make sure that you understand the risks of sharing data with third-parties that shouldn't be trusted.

Who Gets Access to My Data?

Now, let's understand who gets access to the data that you are giving away. One of the main things that you will have to focus on is that you are approving the right authorities and granting them access to your details. You don't want everyone to know everything about you. So, as you go about giving out your data, you should know who you are giving it to and how trustworthy they are.

For instance, once you access Facebook through a third-party app, you are always asked approval from the social media platform. Here you get asked whether you allow the third-party app to make use of your specific data.

Once you hit allow, your data is in with the stream of many others.[20] This goes to the specific platform that you have allowed to view your data.

When it comes to the healthcare sector, however, you will find that the majority of people have a positive attitude when it comes to sharing data. But why is this? This is mostly because people may use your data to their advantage. So, you want to make sure that you are sharing your data through secured channels.

Data's Impact in The Long Run

As people go about sharing their data, a pool of adequate data accumulates, allowing the healthcare system to optimize their future services. So, how do they do this? Let's have a look at how data collection adds to future healthcare.

- *Focusing on Treatments*

  One of the main things that data collection helps with is getting the right input about the patients. For instance, through data collection, there will be enough information to create predictions and analysis of various patients.[21] Moreover, this will also allow practitioners to understand which of the treatments will be more successful than others. That is not all; with this, there's also ease of understanding which patient might develop a disease and start with their treatments beforehand. This will make life much easier for those suffering and curing both.

- *Giving Way to New Treatments and Management*

  With the number of researches that are carried out, there is a range of data available for professionals to focus on developing new treatments that actually work. No longer do they have to stick to old routines and management as the data offered helps them to improve their management skills while also focusing on new treatments for various diseases.

  Data through various forms of collection not only helps ensure there are new treatments under process, but you also get to make sure that you're creating a more efficient recovery system for the potential patients.[21]

- ### *Access to More RWE*

  Real-world evidence is crucial to develop mechanisms that are well-suited for the patient's needs. This is where the importance of data comes in. Since patients are already providing the system with data, there's a better understanding of what goes on in the real world.[22] People making use of applications that determine their fitness and health levels prove to be some of the most highly beneficial platforms that one could have.

- ### *Drug Development*

  One of the best things that enhanced data and research has to offer the healthcare industry is the development of new drugs.[23] With the right details, creating much more effective drugs to help people get better becomes easier. Since the creation of drugs takes a lot of time and research, already having ample amounts of data enables researchers to quicken the process and present treatments that would help patients get better much quicker than using old drugs for the same diseases.

Is There a Limit on Optimizing Pathways Through Connectivity?

Now, let's talk about what the main uses of machine learning are. Essentially, the idea behind this is to get hands-on better data analysis while also being able to predict what goes on in the future. Doing so helps gather enough data that proves to be highly beneficial for the industry. But to what limitation does this operate with? Or is there no limit placed on the application of this?

Security

A grave concern that is posed by this entire system is what happens if the security of the system is breached? All the data and everything else with it will be at the hands of parties that will be able to use it for malpractice.[24] How is the possibility of this happening controlled? What are the ways that this is taken care of?

Well, the possibility of security breaches can be easily avoided if adequate measures are taken. What are these measures? These include the following:

- Establishing strong passwords for data storage

- Encrypting all the data

- Making use of a viable firewall system

- Securing smart devices in the best way possible

- Regular monitoring of the system

While there is a range of methods available for keeping check of security, there is always a chance that these may get breached. However, by making sure that you're keeping a regular check on the security and making sure to update the systems, then the risk subsides exponentially.

Prediction Ethics

While there is a range of advancements taking place in the machine learning aspect, it gives way to something much bigger. Now, you get much more accurate results and predictions of diseases or any other issues while also developing the relevant hypothesis for it.

In the healthcare industry, you will find the use of machine learning exceptional. A range of images and other things are assessed through these devices that help understand what might be wrong.[25]

- *Understanding Predictions*

    Understanding the depth of machine learning is not easy. You will find a range of complexities here. If one chooses to overlook the necessity of machine learning at this stage, then they would be putting themselves at risk of making use of wrong or insufficient data when the time comes.[25] It is essential to understand that data and the concept of machine learning prove to be highly essential when it comes to getting to the right answers.

- *Keeping Mistakes Minimum*

    When it comes to making mistakes, humans and machines are equally prone to making them. But what helps them do better is the possibility of learning. This is why there are a series of steps associated when it comes to developing an algorithm for machine learning. Nothing is put forward in one go, there is a range of validity tests done, and models run to get a more accurate result from it. No one wants to have to deal with informing patients of the wrong diagnoses because of the machine learning model.

- *Validating Machine Learning Models*

   Making sure that the machine learning models are run without mistakes requires a lot of verification and validation from the right sources. To minimize the possibility of mistakes and increase the possibility of accurate results, a series of tests are conducted on these models to assess their viability. If there aren't enough validation tests done, then there is a high possibility that the model might end up giving inaccurate results.

- *The Possibility of Algorithms Becoming Immoral*

   There is a high chance that algorithms don't follow the same ethics because of how they are designed. This brings them to make decisions that aren't always considered normal or moral enough when it comes to treating patients or dealing with any other clients.[26] Therefore, heavy audits need to be implemented to make sure that these algorithms are in check rather than letting them run however they are.

- *Consequences Developing from AI*

   When it comes to making use of AI for the healthcare sector or perhaps any other industry, there is little understanding as to what these machines have to offer. Also, given that most people have biased views about incorporating machine learning or artificial intelligence into practice, it is best to make sure that you're managing it the right way. There are large possibilities of things going south if you're not keen on managing your AI using the right measures.

Regulation and Policy Making for Machine Learning

With every emerging industry, regulatory powers have to step in to monitor and control the activities. The sole purpose of such regulation is to prevent misuse of the product. Similar is the case for AI. With AI being increasingly important for every sector, governance and regulation are in great need.

When talking about ethics in AI, it is always assumed that AI should be put to good use. However, no one can ignore how it can also be used for malicious purposes. AI has been used as technological warfare ever since its existence.[27] Therefore, it is critical that policies are in place that make such uses limited. But it is also used by state agencies alike for the same purpose, which proves that limitations should remain open. By open, it means that the use should be up to an ethical judgment call with several uses restricted.

Maneuvering back to the healthcare sector, AI's usage in every department will only increase because of its necessity. Regulating AI in such an environment isn't a simple task but rather requires many stakeholders to be actively involved in the process. The key goal is to make sure that AI is not over or under-regulated.

In order to do this, policymakers should apply an inter-disciplinary approach. This means including AI engineers, lawmakers, people in the healthcare sector, humanitarians, and every key player that relies heavily on AI. Additionally, to make sure that the law does cater to everyone, lawmakers should ensure that global communication is done. This can influence the presence of leveled global platforms that encourage competition and innovation within the realms of AI. What's more, is that this type of regulation can easily restrict certain AI activities and encourage the ones that are ethical.

For the healthcare sector, the personnel should adopt a holistic approach so that they can instill proper policies. When they understand the mechanics behind AI algorithms and their uses, it will be easier to implement such a law. The need for regulation in AI will always remain until a set of appropriate laws is established.

Governance Policies for Data and Information

Data and information governance policies are sets of rules that govern data and information, respectively. However, why is there a need for such guidelines? It is because the healthcare sector can face a lot of problems due to the ethics of data use. Many times, when AI is deployed with training comprised of incomplete data, the healthcare professionals suffer. This affects their systems, their fiduciary relationship with patients, and their care.[28]

These sets of governance policies can help manage data in a way that AI transformation is facilitated. This is because the policies are designed to manage four aspects of data. This includes availability, usefulness, reliability, and security of the information and data. Most data governance policies

se business process management (BPM)[29] and enterprise risk
RP), but it depends on the policymakers. In the end, it clearly
demonstrates the institution's intentions with the use of AI.

Can AI be Overregulated Through a Lot of Policies?

Strict policies limit growth for any area that they are applied to. For
encouraging innovation and to ease barriers of entry in any field, policies
should be made less stringent. That has always been the common rule. For
the implementation of ethical AI, engineers and data scientists should be
given sufficient room to innovate.

Plus, start-ups are currently the frontier for AI. To continuously adapt to
the changes and the field that governs AI's direction, policies should have
enough room for compromise. The motivations for stakeholders should
always be the first consideration when designing the policy. Over-regulation
would not be the way to go.

International Standards for the AI Industry

Currently, there is an obvious absence of international standards for the AI
industry. This negatively impacts every area that actively uses AI, especially
the healthcare sector. The accuracy of AI predictions cannot be measured
unless standards are developed and established. If not, AI results will often
be based solely on the data provided and might vary everywhere. With the
absence of standards, measurements are difficult. Not to mention that the
predictions may begin to become unreliable with the lack of evidence.

A minimum criterion should be set for all AI systems. The first requirement
should be consolidation between the ethical code for AI systems and
schematics. They should not differ so much that it makes unethical behavior
okay in different areas.

This lack of standardization also slows down major processes and updates.
With AI being a quick development structure, the absence of standards can
cause material delays in the healthcare industry. Clinical acceptance is urgently
required within hospitals to treat many patients. This delay in implementing AI
systems can often have high and irreversible costs. Mislabeling of patients is
also a common phenomenon that might occur due to this issue.

Humane Treatment of AI – Ethical or Objective?

When it comes to the deployment of AI and its use, the treatment is a very important factor to be considered. The ethics of AI requires this area to be explored, and it is an additional question people must decide the answer to. It can be debatable. Since AI mirrors humans, should AI also be treated in a similar fashion?

Artificial intelligence systems are known to react to stimulus, but inherently it is considered to be objective. Humans can feel and perceive different stimuli, which is why everyone has a moral and ethical responsibility towards each other. Does this responsibility of treating AI in a human way exist too? It might. A common example of this could be the reward and punishment system. When humans make mistakes, they are punished and rewarded if they perform well.

If AI is treated in the same way, it might help AI to become more human-like. Except the rewards and punishments would be digital. Therefore, it truly depends on the intention of where everyone wants to go with AI. Treating AI with humanity seems to be the ethical response here. After all, it will contribute to improving human lives too.

Ethical Code and Conduct for Data Within Organizations

A code of conduct is established to maintain ethical behavior within organizations. It is the most effective way to govern and convey how one should act within (and sometimes outside) the bounds of business. Framing an ethical code of conduct isn't the only step, but the implementation of it is a huge responsibility too. Employee training is the most basic way to achieve this. Let's talk about the ethical code.

Code of Ethics

It may seem like everyone knows the difference between right and wrong, but that's not true. There are always grey areas within organizations. This is why a code of ethics is a basic requirement. An ethical code is a document that lays down how employees should act such that it is morally correct. This code can ensure that the work environment is ethical and provides assurance to stakeholders.

Businesses are required to perform their functions in a way that they are free from wrongdoings. This is easily preventable with the implementation of an ethical code. However, there are some elements that must be taken care of when formulating the code. This requires that the code does not have any jargon that employees would have difficulty understanding. The more difficult the language – the easier it is to misinterpret it. Everyone should understand what acceptable behavior is. This acceptable behavior doesn't simply have to be legal, but it should also be ethical in societal norms.

All employees must understand the consequences of violating the code of conduct. The code could especially be crossed when developing new technologies or new products. This is why it should always be consulted beforehand to avoid any moral issues down the road. With respect to AI, it is also important to set boundaries. Ask yourself the following questions to determine what the ethical code for AI should look like.

- What are AI ethics? What should be its goals?

- What benefits of AI should the organization strive to achieve?

- What consequences must be avoided with regards to AI?

While asking these questions, you should also measure how effectively the code helps in making decisions. This would help assess if the code is useful or needs improvement.

How to Form Ethical Codes and Frameworks

In the healthcare industry, there is accountability for everything. Because the sector relies on patient data for relevant diagnosis and billing etc., there is a great risk of breaching privacy. Patient data could easily be manipulated or misused. Therefore, when forming ethical codes and frameworks, a couple of steps should be used to make the code airtight.

- *Collect only the relevant data*

   While AI functions perform in the best way when they have more information, that should not be the case for the healthcare industry.[30] In case you need to admit a patient, their medical history and contact information are the only necessary items. Billing information could be collected as well when the time comes. However, in such cases, other information like the past purchases or credit history of the patient should not be required. Similarly, for a bank, the medical history is not relevant at all.

- *Treat sensitive data with security*

  Oftentimes, hospitals and clinics will have access to sensitive information about the patient. This must be secured properly. Following the ethical rules for data protection, the authorities must ensure that the sensitive data isn't treated the same way as the name of the patient is (non-sensitive). AI could be deployed in a way that sensitive data is identified and scrubbed.[31] This would lead to the data being stored on external drives for security and accessibility.

- *Comply with data ethics laws*

  In many areas, it is essential that data ethics laws are complied with. However, these laws often require healthcare sectors to self-accredit. This means that while there is no requirement, the submission of proper documents will give some places an edge. If anything, it improves the reliability of many hospitals. The General Data Protection Regulation (GDPR) and International Organization for Standardization (ISO) standards require compliance with data management. Make sure that these conditions are met.

Oaths for Physicians and Data Scientists to protect information

A Hippocratic oath is often signed by physicians when they begin their practice of medicine. It is an ethical oath that mandates them to act in a morally responsible way. The term could be used for data scientists as they also have a similar requirement to fulfill when they begin their practice.

Because all data scientists have access to sensitive data, they are required to sign relevant documents. These documents mandate the professionals to protect the data and have the necessary precautions in place for security. This ensures top ethical conduct within the world of AI in the healthcare sector.

Reviewing Ethical Codes

The simple formation of an ethical code is not enough. Ethical conduct must be held at the same standard as the changes require. AI is a fast-paced industry where changes take place every second of every minute. This is why ethical codes must be reviewed and audited regularly. Implementation of ethical codes usually sheds light on the practical implications of the code. Data scientists can observe how the codes impact the AI and the effects of the AI. Many other employees also observe the effect of the code. This can highlight many shortfalls that the code might have.

However, these shortfalls can always be improved upon. To do this, feedback is the best way to go about it. All employees must have opinions on ethical conduct and the effectiveness of the code.[32] Furthermore, observations could also help in the proper identification of any places of overregulation. Tightening and loosening of the ethical code and policies will always be required.

Additionally, with the ever-changing AI, these reviews could help the ethical framework become more transparent. This will not only build trust but also veracity.

Humanity Versus AI: Who's in Control?

As we establish the importance of ethics while using the technologies of artificial intelligence, one question remains: who shall be in control? Humans are the ones who developed AI in the first place – yet they remain conflicted upon whether or not machines could be more effective decision-makers than humans themselves.

By nature, humans are driven towards control. This can be attributed to the human cognition abilities that allow the brain to function in mysterious ways. In the 1950s, psychologist J. P. Guilford was able to divide the thinking process of humans into two different categories: convergent thinking and divergent thinking.[33]

Convergent thinking refers to answering questions based on facts, logic, and memory.[33] This makes convergent thinking extremely objective in nature, making it less susceptible to margins of error. Divergent thinking, on the other hand, is the humanistic ability to be creative.[33] This includes being able to come up with multiple answers to the same question – showing traces of subjectivity and much relevance to one's own experiences.

While artificial intelligence is particularly well-equipped with convergent thinking, it lacks any form of divergence. This means that an AI healthcare system might be extremely efficient with its facts and figures but maybe helpless when it comes to using uncommon antidotes to combat a disease.

However, AI is now evolving and becoming increasingly intelligent. With recent ground-breaking developments in technology, AI-agents are becoming equipped with the ability to process divergent thoughts as well.

For humans, this may not sound like great news. While humans have the innate need to be in control, they may have to pass their ruling on to AI machines that could potentially be smarter than humans. The problem with this, however, is that an AI machine that is smarter than humans cannot be given any specific boundaries to operate in.

The Interaction between AI and Human Beings

As AI becomes more intelligent, it also becomes more integrated into our lives. As mentioned earlier, ethics are significant when it comes to integrating AI in the lives of people – especially when it concerns matters related to healthcare or medicine.

But what ethics shall AI machines follow? What are their priorities?

What we must not forget is that AI machines are developed by human beings – and that they too have flawed priority hierarchies. The debate on whether an AI should be protecting one victim in an accident or the other is complicated. It requires far more evidence than is currently available to researchers, thus making it difficult to determine the pathway that an AI machine should take in case of a medical emergency.

Another way that AI machines are slowly making their way into our everyday lives is the introduction of virtual assistants, such as Siri, Cortana, or Alexa. By constantly interacting and engaging with humans, AI machines are now becoming smart enough to replicate conjunctions of human speech[34]. While the voice of the AI is still computer-generated, the machine picks up humanistic characteristics of speech such as pauses, flow, intonation, and tone variation. This makes it increasingly difficult for humans to actually recognize the difference between another human being and a virtual assistant.

However, this interaction is widely condemned as deception. People are led to believe that they are interacting with a human, but in reality, they are only engaging with a man-made machine. This is one of the biggest examples of why ethics remain important in the development of AI – with people constantly vouching for practices such as informed consent or debriefing after interacting with an AI machine.

Regardless of the backlash, there are certain positive elements to this covert interaction with AI for humans. Unlike other human beings, virtual assistants are smart enough to instantly recognize changes in the style or content of speech. This means that during a normal conversation, an AI will be able to detect any changes in mood or behavior that may otherwise be ignored. By adopting this approach towards healthcare, it could become easier to identify the emotional wellbeing of people[35] without forcing them to reveal more about themselves.

However, the consequences of determining the emotional state of people through the use of AI also have their fair share of pros and cons.

A Glimpse into the World of Smart Healthcare

Similar to how AI machines could detect instances of deteriorating mental wellbeing, there are many other uses of smart technology for the purpose of healthcare. The health industry continues to expand, and with expansion comes the dependency on computers. Healthcare organizations are responsible for handling exceptionally large chunks of information and need efficient computer systems that are able to process, store and organize information effectively. For this purpose, AI serves as the perfect tool.[36]

AI also makes significant contributions to the industry of healthcare services by making it easier to diagnose health conditions. It also helps conduct quick and smart research for the purpose of pharmacology, or the development of new medicines through research and testing.

However, as smart healthcare becomes a reality in our world, there are increasing concerns of the public regarding adherence to ethical considerations. Healthcare data is highly confidential, and AI machines must be smart enough to understand the privacy of patients. Additionally, before smart healthcare is introduced to the masses, it is important to develop systems that are in line with this new technology as well as identify the potential risks involved with integrating AI into healthcare.

Legal Concerns: Matters of False Reports

With artificial intelligence, healthcare professionals will be able to bring vast improvements to the entire medical system while improving integral systems such as diagnoses, treatment, and costs. Human beings can only process a limited amount of information in one moment – be it test results, samples, or clinical imaging. Despite all of the efforts of healthcare professionals, there are still huge margins of error while diagnosing patients with serious health conditions.

AI, on the other hand, can be far more efficient and accurate. AI machines in healthcare are smart enough to process an infinite sum of data within seconds, allowing them to make informed decisions much quicker in comparison to human beings.

But what if there is a false report?

To combat such problems, an optimal approach of combining human diagnoses with AI is developed. This means that both a healthcare professional and an AI machine will be consulted simultaneously before concluding a patient's condition – in hopes of making their diagnosis more accurate.[11]

But this isn't all that simple. Even if the healthcare professional deemed his decision final, it would still be a compulsion to consult the AI machine since it can compare the current patient's case with similar ones from the past.

However, this becomes more complicated when legal matters become involved. In case there is a misdiagnosis – who is to be blamed?

The answer is nobody. Neither the healthcare professional nor the company that developed the AI will be willing to take full responsibility for such a careless mistake. The main reason behind this is the legal complications that may follow, but it can also be attributed to the fact that none of the parties involved are solely responsible for the mistake.

As a result of these newfound complications in the world of medicine and technology, there will be fewer professionals willing to join either field in the future. However, upon the concern of ethical adherence, it is necessary to hold the AI company responsible for such an incident in order to avoid such instances in the future.

The Problem of Human Psychology

As we consider ethical guidelines for the integration of AI in healthcare systems, it is important to consider human psychology as well. The further development of artificial intelligence basically means that coded machines are now able to predict the future – or underline the risks of developing a certain disease.

AI that can detect illnesses such as type 2 diabetes[37], hypertension[38], and even cancer[39] have already been developed. These machines consider lifestyle habits, genetics, and the physiology of a person with their extensive range of data and determine whether or not a person is likely to encounter a disease in their lifetime.

However, this has dire consequences for the mental health of individuals. As humans become more reliant upon technology, they have also begun to trust the words of machines far more than fellow humans. If an AI agent were to tell them that they are not at risk for developing lung cancer, it is likely that the person could become involved in unhealthy and risky behaviors such as cigarette smoking. On the contrary, if the AI tells somebody about their high likelihood of developing cancer, they may become prone to depression and intrusive thoughts.

This increased information regarding the risks and probabilities of developing certain illnesses can be harmful to the mental health of people. While the long-term effects of such predictions have not yet been studied in-depth, preliminary research does suggest that AI predictions affect the behaviors of people significantly.

Using AI with Caution: Behaviors, Addictions, and Ethics

Human behavior is complicated and is now influenced by advances in technology. All humans have become mere rats in a lab to the world of technology – especially as user experiences become optimized and customized through the collection of information. Regardless of how unethical this practice may be, it has been fairly successful in grasping the attention of millions of humans.

In order to protect the privacy and rights of individuals, AI development organizations must follow ethical guidelines. This means to censor certain pieces of data for vulnerable groups of society such as children, the disabled, or the unwell. While behavioral experimentation continues to exist across all bases of technology, it is important to adhere to a fixed code of ethics in order to avoid further complications.

Internet addiction is also a negative behavior that is driven by the integration of AI in our everyday lives. With virtual assistants in our homes and on our phones, people are becoming increasingly dependent upon technology to carry out basic everyday chores that help them sustain their livelihood. Since children are highly gullible, they are most at risk for developing internet addiction early in their lives.

The physiological consequence of internet addiction is the damage caused to the prefrontal cortex of the brain.[40] The psychological consequence is a rapid decline in normal human behaviors such as socialization or productivity.

In order to avoid such dire consequences of integrating AI within the healthcare systems in the world, it is necessary to adhere to ethical guidelines and considerations.

Can Healthcare Specialists Become Obsolete?

Long before artificial intelligence came, the processes of automation – or when organizations replaced huge masses of labor with efficient machinery, occurred. With AI now becoming part of the healthcare system, the same could be true of healthcare specialists.

With AI, hospitals will require less staff to handle paperwork or even consult patients. Most diagnoses could be made with the use of AI-agents, and further treatment processes could also be detailed through virtual assistants or automated machinery. This means that a large number of healthcare specialists may become redundant due to the lack of demand for their skill – thus being replaced with AI.[11]

However, healthcare organizations are trying to remain as ethical as possible. Instead of making their employees redundant instantly, organizations are trying to retrain their staff in ways that align with the usage of AI in their systems.

While AI is highly efficient in carrying out practices such as identifying symptoms, analyzing test reports, and even providing informed diagnoses – they can never be humans. In order for AI in healthcare to be ethical and considerate, it is important for them to remember that while an AI agent can be consulted, it is not the equivalent of human knowledge and experience.

The Public Confusion Regarding AI

The biggest reason why the public is so afraid of having AI take over their lives is the constant reinforcement of this idea through various media channels. There is a great deal of confusion amongst the public regarding whether or not having AI in healthcare would be beneficial since many people are increasingly concerned about the consequences that may follow.

Conclusion

AI and machine learning models will completely change the healthcare industry in the near future. However, we don't know yet if this change will be good or bad. Only time will answer this once the industry is transformed.

The challenges that come with it will also not be easy to overcome, especially the ethical challenges of this change. This is why there needs to be more governance in this aspect. Data is sensitive information that should not be exploited or used for sale.

However, this conversation is one that no one wants to have as the exploitation of this data is revenue for many big companies. Once AI and machine learning models advance even further and mature, it will be too late to have this conversation.

Ethical concerns need to be eliminated so that we can have a better healthcare system in the future. If these challenges are not overcome now, then they can have disastrous implications for our future.

References/Further Reading

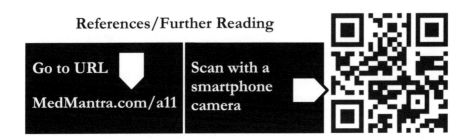

"Most of human and animal learning is unsupervised learning. If intelligence was a cake, unsupervised learning would be the cake, supervised learning would be the icing on the cake, and reinforcement learning would be the cherry on the cake. We know how to make the icing and the cherry, but we don't know how to make the cake. We need to solve the unsupervised learning problem before we can even think of getting to true AI."

- Yann LeCun

SECTION 4

IMPLEMENTATION OF AI INTO CLINICAL PRACTICE

CHAPTER TWELVE

IMPLEMENTATION OF AI INTO CLINICAL PRACTICE

Introduction

Even non-clinical laymen can hardly fail to be impressed by the rate at which artificially intelligent software algorithms and systems are having an impact on their day-to-day lives. The contextual image processing available—for free and without asking—in the Google Photos classifier is a salient example of the potential power of AI. Little surprise, then, that the AI techniques are being explored, understood, developed, and made accessible to a whole range of business sectors—including the medical sector.

Medicine can hugely benefit from AI techniques. Hardly a day goes by without the announcement of another advance or insight enabled by the large-scale multivariable data crunching capability of the AI revolution (enabled by big data, affordable cloud computing, open-source algorithms, and high-speed computer networking). Only today (November 13, 2020), amid the COVID-19 pandemic, a Swedish study[1] has highlighted Baricitinib (Olumaint) as reducing mortality by 71% in admitted, moderate/severe COVID-19 patients. Of course, the clinical trial was undertaken using tried and tested techniques, but the initial identification of Baricitinib as a candidate substance for the efficacy trial was undertaken by BenevolentAI, a London-based company[2] leveraging and developing advanced AI techniques for a variety of clinical research purposes.

Taking research to one side, the subject of AI use within the treatment workflow of clinical environments is also very active. The supplier ecosystem is stuffed with established traditional giants, boorish consultancies, pushy start-ups, and open-source initiatives. Some areas, such as clinical imaging interpretation, in which deep learning convolutional neural network platforms are applied for diagnostic image interpretation, are toward the front of the pack. However, this is just one sector where AI techniques are rapidly gaining traction. Pathology, oncology, cardiology, dermatology, psychiatry, ophthalmology, and other fields are also being addressed using AI approaches.

The scope is huge. The number of applications with an AI potential probably exceeds the number of professionals able to work effectively in these sectors; the laws of supply and demand have kicked in, and remuneration packages for AI professionals have skyrocketed in recent years. Dual-skilled (clinical with data science (DS)/machine learning (ML)/AI competencies) professionals are actual unicorns and command even more of a premium.

So, mirroring many other industries, expectations of AI are high for delivering a radical transformation in medicine and patient outcomes. Consideration within many healthcare organizations now turns to the specific areas in which these techniques can be best applied and the mechanisms for doing so safely. Within the profession, the application of ML/AI techniques is often considered more appropriate in some clinical settings than others. For example, in fast-moving acute care environments (such as emergency/trauma rooms and operating theaters), clinicians often prefer rapid, experienced, intuitive assessment-based practice, so the space for AI directly in the workflow may be limited. Contrast this with more rigidly structured, transactive diagnostic regimes, in which an ML/AI platform informed by complex DS techniques can be a useful tool for improving diagnostic capacity, accuracy, and patient outcomes.

Parallel technologies such as Assisted and Virtual Reality (AR/VR) are often discussed in the same context as AI/ML/DL. It can be argued, however, that these are merely beneficiary technologies rather than AI technologies in their own right. AR and VR leverage advances in computing, edge processing, IoT, and display technologies to render visualizations whose source data may be (but is not necessarily) derived having been processed from the AI repository of techniques. Notwithstanding that position, using AR and VR technology to visualize biological structures, both in context (AR) or with enhanced contrast and detail, is becoming very valuable in the clinician's armory.

However, healthcare in general, more than many other industries, is an area that is highly regulated, risk-averse, bound by territorial patient data privacy regimes, and (again, territory-dependent) highly litigious, with many lawyers, administrators, and patients being nervous of AI.

The burden of evidence required to introduce AI into the clinical environment is high, and well-established, traditional trial frameworks can struggle to incorporate AI technologies into the process. Amongst the many evolving frameworks for AI adoption, the FDA "Good Machine Learning Practices"[3] provides a useful framework, with a baseline set of strategies to manage the adoption of these new technologies. GMLP guidelines are intended to align with the existing guidelines for Good Clinical Practices (GCP) and Good Laboratory Practices (GLP). The FDA's position[4] is that GMLP *"would be analogous to good manufacturing practices (GMP)"*, but *"specifically focused on the unique challenges for machine learning."* Although there is a lot of experience and proprietary approaches in this space, there is a standards deficit in the acquisition and curation of ML data sets, but *"it would make everyone's life easier if they did"*!

The FDA approach to defining "good practice" is a precursor to incoming regulatory frameworks in what has been defined as Software as Medical Devices (SaMD), where SaMD are software tools leveraging AI and ML.[5] This regulatory framework will be explicitly focused on addressing the capability of AI/ML software platforms to continuously learn from experience and improve their results.

So, many clinicians are keen to embrace the potential of AI techniques in their fields, but the above referenced risk-averse nature of healthcare regimes, coupled with the need to fit new practices within long-established clinical workflows, is a significant barrier to adoption. This article discusses these barriers and provides some pointers to approaches that may ease the journey.

Data, AI, and the Challenges of Medical Data

If there is one thing that underpins the success and accuracy of AI in all (not just clinical) environments, it is the availability of accurate representative data sets. Whole fields of the DS discipline deal with the challenges of acquiring, validating, formatting, segmenting, cleaning, ingesting, storing, and interpreting relevant data into the AI.

The FDA Good Machine Learning Practices framework contains guidance in this respect. Of course, the FDA is only one authority, and local regulations may be more or less stringent. Nevertheless, the FDA guidance below can be taken as generic good practice:

- Ensure the relevance of the available and collected data to the clinical problem at hand.

- Ensure that the data is acquired in a consistent manner and aligns with the intended use and the modification plans submitted to the FDA.

- Ensure appropriate separation between training, tuning, and test datasets.

- Ensure clarity in the output and the algorithm used.

From this succinct set of guidelines flow numerous project delivery requirements, which makes the acquisition and preparation of data not just important, but a major and absolutely critical component of the delivery program.

In any established industry, there are huge challenges in acquiring and preparing data sets for use in AI training—some common to all industries and some unique to the sector.

Regulation, Privacy, and Trust

Healthcare data is universally acknowledged as being sensitive and highly private. Systems processing or transferring patient data, and particularly those with access to EHR, require protection against data breach, exposure, and loss. Given the sensitivity of the data, EHR are bound by stringent governmental regulation on the collection, processing, handling, and storage of this data.[6] The regulation, of course, varies by territory, but commonly GDPR (European)[7] or HIPAA (North American)[8] standards apply. It is an essential part of any AI/ML project that the territorial privacy regulations are understood and complied with.

This regulatory constraint can be both onerous and frustrating for data scientists; however, it must be remembered that trust is a core principle of healthcare. Patients must be comfortable that not only is their privacy being respected, but that their data is processed only in a manner aligned with their consent, and that only the patient data relevant to their conditions and treatment is collected. When data is accessed or sold in a manner in which consent is not present, the patient's view will be that a privacy violation has occurred. This view will be considered valid by the patient even if no harm occurs as a result of the breach.[9]

This field and the considerations around the validity of consent or unconsented anonymized use are complex, a study in themselves. The above reference poses several ethical test cases to tease out the complexities around this subject, but the core message is that the maintenance of trust is essential to both the healthcare and platform providers. The regulation exists to protect the patient and maintain this trust. Acquisition and use of patient data must be undertaken ethically and within the terms of the local regulatory environment, and these requirements form a mandatory part of any project. Therefore, any project instigated to deliver an ML/AI platform into the clinical environment MUST have resources assigned to ensure strict compliance when acquiring and processing this patient data.

Structure and Format

The ability of a platform to consume data is underpinned by context and association. Medical health record collection standards[10] have varied through the years in formats, including free text and often handwritten notes, test results, and typed reports stored in vast localized file systems—often unique to the healthcare provider and over several institutions. With increases in population mobility over the last several decades, paper-based systems struggled to cope with the requirement to provide a single, transportable patient history. The accuracy, integrity, and, occasionally, the security of this format does not well support assimilation into AI/ML models. The interpretation of these different formats can be assisted by advances in Natural Language Processing (NLP) techniques[11] for the interpretation and normalization of unstructured data into structured information. Assessment of medical notes is fraught with subject-specific jargon and abbreviations. Of course, for the hand-written form, we have the perennial issue of physicians' handwriting! Nonetheless, research continues into NLP techniques to enable this rich archive of medical data to be exploited.

The advent of highly structured electronic health records should have been the bellwether sounding for releasing knowledge from accumulated medical notes (along with enabling simple sharing of data between clinicians and institutions). They should be a transferable, single, consolidated view of the patients' entire medical history, including baseline data, history of diagnosis, treatments, prescriptions, vaccinations, allergic reactions, medical imaging, and lab results.[12] However, again, this area has been subject to differential technical standards, the same privacy concerns as well as constraining regulation.

One principal issue[13] is that the primary purpose of EHR is to support existing clinical workflows rather than to support the normalization of data for assimilation with AI/ML contexts. This does not mean that all EHRs must be revised to a new primary purpose, but rather that, looking forward, developments in EHRs should have a common goal in enabling (appropriate) AI/ML data extraction. In the meantime, many EHRs suffer from the same issues as some of the more manual approaches used in the pre-EHR era, such as jargon-filled free-text fields requiring the application of the same NLP techniques referenced above—though the challenge of recognizing clinician handwriting should now be obviated!

Accuracy and Completeness

Medical error is the third leading cause of death after heart failure and cancer in the USA.[13]

Of course, the accuracy of data is an issue across all industries and beyond AI applications. Data-driven IT architectures have been common for many years. Examples include SCADA control systems in a factory or network environments or stock and order management applications in warehouse or retail; woe be to the system that orders more stock due to the belief that stock is low, only to find that no one has correctly updated the stock levels. Data is most useful when it is complete, accurate, and accurately described.

Even in the presence of a unifying EHR, the completion and correct data filling of the record still depend on fallible humans, which provides an opportunity for omission as well as error. It is well understood that a trained AI is a sophisticated encoding of the data with which it has been fed. It does not think or make abstract value judgments in the way a human does. Conversely, it is capable of tracking massive multivariate data sets in ways a human cannot. Using inconsistent training data will not cause an AI to pause for thought; it will cause the AI to make the wrong diagnosis. This is one area in which the feedback loop capability of DL algorithms comes into play.

So, given the criticality of correct training for meaningful outcomes, in any AI environment, the cleansing of data prior to AI training cycles is imperative to develop the most accurate possible network response. The classical data science approach providing representative data sets separated into training, tuning, and test batches is a critical element of the program workflow.

Volume - The Big Data Challenge

"Big data" (BD) is one of the buzzword technology domains that has been feeding consultancies across various sectors for many years. The term refers to technologies designed for storing, processing, and accessing very large data volumes of (either structured or unstructured) data while avoiding the performance limitations that were imposed by many of the more traditional database technologies.

Originally developed and adopted by large internet companies (like Google and Yahoo) for their search indexes, the field extended beyond internet search as many other sectors saw the potential of these indexing techniques to leverage value from the very large quantities of data their sector produced. Off the back of these movements, several open-source technologies were developed (such as Hadoop[14] and MapReduce[15]), as well as modified, adapted, and pressed into service.

Many sectors (astro and particle physics, for example) were quick to adopt BD techniques for data storage and processing. Medicine was also considered to be an appropriate sector.[16] Imaging and genetics naturally generate huge amounts of data. Patient records in aggregate present a sizeable processing challenge, but other, less obvious data sources can provide valuable data at a scale that becomes problematic to manage unless specialist techniques are adopted.

The massive adoption of IoT devices in recent years has seen healthcare and assisted living devices providing significant extra valuable data. In some cases, the smartphone itself becomes a sensor, and a smartphone-coupled smartwatch can provide highly dense patient biometric data. With some very low-cost devices providing a multitude of indices (temperature, heart rate, SpO2, blood pressure, movement) measured tens if not hundreds of times a day. A few hundred kB a day, over an extended period, over a large population, provides both a data management challenge and excellent fodder for medical professionals and data scientists.

Leveraging big data sets is, of course, a technical challenge that the architects of AI/ML platforms must face. However, whereas researchers in less regulatory constrained areas (such as astrophysics) would traditionally (in this relatively new field!) address them by implementing a set of cloud services from one or another of the traditional cloud providers (Google, Amazon, IBM, etc.), in medicine, there are additional constraints to be considered[16], which may mean that more secure, more highly segmented, and higher reliability cloud solutions are mandated—and these, of course, come at extra costs compared to those incurred by sectors operating with less critical, less private data, in less regulated areas.

Barriers

Data, of course, is a big issue in its own right. However, aside from the regulatory, integrity, access, and acquisition issues discussed above, numerous other barriers to the adoption of AI in a clinical context are present.

Acceptance and Maintenance of the Output

To be valuable, AI-generated diagnostics must be accepted by several entities throughout the process. The clinician, the patient, and the regulatory bodies all must accept that the AI is acting in the patients' interest.

At the most simplistic level, clinicians must trust that the AI is providing results that at least assist them in improving individual patient outcomes and, ideally, assist them in treating patients optimally—meaning more patients with less clinical effort. Continuously monitoring the accuracy of AI output in the diagnostic environment, though, becomes a task in itself, and particularly so with DL-enabled products whose AI schemes are predicated on evolving and refining outputs based on cumulative data sets and feedback. This is analogous to the behavior of many clinician practitioners who are often heard to say, "I am always learning." The same is true of AI, only in this instance, programmed learning is a built-in, bought feature, and the machine learns very quickly from one example to the next.

It is this learning and map revision that requires careful monitoring to ensure its evolution still returns valid results.

Whether undertaken administratively, by the supplier, or by clinical staff themselves, the preparation and presentation of test data, followed by verification of the results, is an activity that will provide both reassurance and proof of performance to all entities in the process. It could be argued that the challenge of overseeing the machine learning state (elements of which must be undertaken by a clinician) denudes and could demolish the business case for using an automated diagnostic in the first place ("I spend more time checking the AI than it saves"). And the overhead of AI maintenance is indeed a factor that must be realistically considered in the implementation business case.

Strategies for mitigation against the overheads of constantly "checking the machine" in the diagnostic workflow could be adopted by, for example, having the AI assign a certainty score to each case and inspect based on a sliding scale. The workflow could, for instance, mandate that 1 or 2% of high-certainty assessments be human-checked, whereas all low-certainty assessments will be reviewed by a competent human. In addition to adding complexity to the clinical workflow, this approach, of course, brings with it its own disadvantages as unintended consequences. Like the surgeon who takes on only the most challenging cases and procedures, the human diagnostic expert would be faced with diagnosis only of the very challenging cases—which would, of course, place a downward weighting on their own accuracy/success rate. This must be recognized when measuring performance.

Trust - For Everybody

Alongside being able to prove the efficacy of the AI practitioner, gaining and maintaining patient trust is an activity that may be considerably more complex, as the majority of patients are simply not familiar with AI and, worse, might be biased against trusting it due to a perceived lack of experience in their daily lives. These perceptions could be false.

An in-car satellite navigation system is AI, particularly when supplemented by radio data traffic reports. A system's ability to locally calculate and determine a route, track your progress, and then suggest time-saving route alterations in near real-time depending on real-time traffic conditions would have been nothing short of miraculous only a few years ago, yet it is now more than commonplace. It is commonplace to the extent that motorists have been judged to be losing map-reading skills due to the near-total reliance on Sat-Nav.[17]

Similarly, Siri, Alexa, Google, and Cortana voice recognition are well accepted and are all AI. They perform well and accurately interpret not just voice but intent and context in many cases. Not five years ago, this would have been akin to dark magic.

That Alexa plays the right song or turns on the lights when asked is trivial but provable and familiar; however, it is also low-impact. Alexa may play the right song 19 times out of 20—and the twentieth is often amusing and easily fixable but low-impact. Conversely, an AI saying, *"That is not a glioblastoma,"* when it is, in fact, a glioblastoma is high-impact, never amusing, and almost certainly not fixable.

And finally, the regulation comes into play yet again. The European GDPR legislation brought into being the right of explanation.[18] The actual intent of the legislation in this context is subject to very technical legal arguments (see reference). However, the impact is to enable the patient to request a detailed explanation of the algorithmic reasoning that contributed to the subject's diagnosis.

While physicians can supply a justification/explanation of any given human-derived diagnosis and/or treatment, and this justification will often be present in the patient's medical file, in practice, these decisions are based on a human-capable set of inputs (symptoms, scans, tests) leading to an output. In contrast, a comprehensively trained neural network is capable of basing decisions deterministically on many thousands of independent input variables, each with an individually described "weight" derived from the training data. Not all of these determinants will be obvious (or palatable). While they can "log" their reasoning, the logged data may not be easily consumed by a human physician, much less a patient or advocate.

Finally, hysterical "special interest groups" cannot be totally ignored when looking at reasons for trust being undermined. While no major conspiracy theories directly address AI in healthcare, recently (November 2020), we have seen "5G rollout causes COVID-19" dramatically undermining the rollout of new cellular networks and leading to actual physical attacks on infrastructure and staff. Also, with the announcement of (long-awaited) new vaccines for COVID-19, the anti-vax theorists are having their day on YouTube. Both of these spread problematic amounts of ill-informed and incorrect information, but in an unignorable and influential manner.

Resource Issues

The actual competencies required to deliver a full AI project are in short supply. Project team resourcing is discussed in some detail later, but DS/AI/ML is a subject area currently in very high demand across multiple industries.

AI and ML courses and subject matter are easily accessible and routinely available for consumption. However, the field is complex and time-consuming. Clinical personnel with the inclination, capability, or time to pursue these studies may well be those more aligned with research and development than patient practice.

In graduate recruitment events, it is a sellers' market. Graduates trained in data science who interview well are competed for and are paid very well. The aligned fields tend to be mathematics, engineering, and software engineering.

Similarly, medicine is a serious study. To develop competence and accreditation is a multi-year dedicated undertaking.

Noting the aligned fields above, the intersection between life sciences graduates and those with advanced machine learning competencies are vanishingly small

AI and data sciences are not subjects taught to the required levels at medical school. This is not to say that clinicians are not capable of being data scientists—far from it. Rather, medical school syllabuses have not evolved to take account of this relatively new field. The inclusion of DS/ML is probably something that should be considered as a strategic initiative; however, it is not a short-term fix. The bald fact is that qualified, competent resources for these projects are in short supply and, therefore, a price premium is typically paid.

Workflow

Traditional clinical workflows in diagnostic environments were not created with the introduction of AI in mind. That said, it is impossible to deliver any new system or capability into an operational environment without changing to accommodate it.

All IT systems deliveries (AI or not) are expensive and require a business case of some form to justify the expenditure. The business case for the introduction of AI into the workflow is valid only if it delivers on its business case goals. Typically, these are one or both of:

- Sustainable improvements in patient outcomes—more consistent, accurate diagnoses with fewer mistakes.

- More efficient treatment of patients—more patients with fewer clinical resources.

Both of these must be measured to be considered successful.

That said, few "off-the-shelf" AI diagnostic platforms have been explicitly designed from the outset to accommodate all the variations in the clinical workflow that may be found in the field. Typically, with very advanced platforms, much of the design "thinking" will have gone into the "novel" components. However, in retrofitting any platform into an existing operation, systems and process integration work will need to be undertaken. These components must be considered as part of the requirements gathering for the platform.

Execution

Choosing and deploying an AI for the first time in a clinical environment is a daunting task.[19] At one level, this is simply a process and system integration challenge. At another, a completely new sort of capability is being retrofitted into an in-flight operational process. It's a bit like landing on the moon and building the rocket on the way down.

Lots of systems and process delivery frameworks are defined, some more appropriate than others. However, delivering an AI into clinical operations probably requires a more nuanced approach. This means doing more rather than less—and spending a lot of time looking inside the organization first—before getting the vendors in

The examples given below draw from a generic approach to operational program management, with some additional emphasis on those areas required for AI/ML/DS.

Consider

Consider the challenge the organization wants to address. It should be very specific and relevant to improving the clinical workflow.

All relevant, senior stakeholders must have read, debated, and agreed on the challenge. It is often helpful to:

- Rewrite the agreed-upon challenge as a specific mission statement, mandate, or scope.

- Agree on a budgetary envelope that denotes the funds available for investment (should the business case stack up and an agreeable solution be found).

Build a Team

Define a senior team to work on approaches in the agreed-upon challenge/mission statement

As well as the typical program management roles (sponsor, program board, program manager, program administrator), it is important to ensure that the program team is built to include lead representatives of:

- All areas impacted by the changes
  - Clinical
  - Clinical process design
  - Legal and regulatory
  - IT architecture/network/security

- All areas required to deliver the changes
  - Financial
  - Procurement/supplier management
  - HR
- Specialist resource to contract in, if required
  - AI/ML/DS specialist advisor

Build a Plan

Not the whole plan, but a high-level plan that defines the next few stages (to the end of the approved tasks) and sets out expectations of:

- What must be done?
- Who must lead on each task, and who will contribute?
- How long are these tasks intended to take?

Include specific tasks/decisions around:

- Is the intent to run a trial/proof of concept (PoC) of a commercial-off-the-shelf (COTS) software deployment sufficient?
- What is the end-state high-level operating model?

Evaluate and Prepare

Having assembled the team, look hard again at the mandate. If the mandate is wrong, now is the time to challenge it with the board.

- Is it right for the organization?
- Is the expectation realistic?
- Is the scope credible (too big or too small)? Do not try to "eat the elephant."

Undertake an AI readiness study. Frameworks for this exist[20] and will provide an objective assessment of the organization's capability to introduce and utilize AI-enabled applications within the clinical workflow.

Determine the approach to AI model validation that the organization will need to take.

Determine the regulatory compliances that the delivered project will need to attain.

The learnings from the exercise will additionally inform the requirements, the deliverables, the project success criteria, and the evaluation process.

Define success in a specific and measurable way:

- Define how success will be measured—what are the measurement points?

- Measurements should be based on business outcomes and linked directly to the mandate.

Set a detailed project scope:

- This should be driven by the success criteria.

- Understand the dependencies.

- Detail the inputs, outputs, and deliverables

    - Not all of these are technical—legal, ethical, regulatory, financial ... all have a bearing.

- Define the workflow within which the project sits.

    - It may simply be a component within an existing workflow.

    - It may require a wholesale change to the workflow—best to know this now.

- Set solution requirements.

    - Do this in such a way that the requirements can be traced back to the success criteria.

    - The requirements should be expressed as simply as possible.

    - The organizational data structure constraints should be a part of this model.

Before looking at any solutions, decide how the project will select a solution.

Create a high-level requirement set to evaluate companies to engage.

Break Cover

Only now entertain detailed contact with vendors. Literature search, trade shows, and colleague recommendations all form a part of this activity.

Undertake internal reviews to determine the shortlist of vendors. Use the project AI resource to give detailed, informed feedback on the promises and potential of various solutions.

Draw up a shortlist and issue the requirements through the supplier management team.

Choose

This is where the pre-work in evaluating responses pays back. There is a response evaluation framework set out, and the normal supplier management practices apply.

- Evaluate the responses according to the model already created.
- Down-select the suppliers and deselect others.
- Undertake deep-dive engagements with the pack leaders.
    - Cheapest is not always best (in fact, it seldom is).
    - The most expensive is not always the best (in fact, it seldom is).
    - Deep-dive into the customer references.
        o Understand how the claims were delivered.
    - Understand the training model, the datasets, and the target accuracy.
        o Training data.
            ▪ Used to build the AI model.
        o Validation data.
            ▪ Used to validate the model.
        o Test data.
            ▪ Used to determine the accuracy of the model built.

- o The data MUST accurately reflect the data that the organization can provide as inputs.
    - Data formats.
    - Accuracy.
    - Completeness.
- Shortlist and engage a preferred vendor.
    - o Make sure the preferred vendor knows that they are not the winner until signing.
- Tie the partner's success to the organization's.
    - o Make sure the partner understands YOUR ORGANIZATION'S SUCCESS CRITERIA.
    - o Make sure that the partner understands the organization's intent to publish and discuss the results of your project.
- Negotiate.
    - o Agree on a structure that delivers good value to both parties, and that gouges no one.

Approve

Comprehensively document the decision of the program team and present it to the board for approval.

Deploy

All the normal good program and project management practices apply here.

Of key importance (for both parties) is the initially agreed-upon proof of value (PoV)/proof of concept (PoC) phases of implementation to show that they will address the issues that the project set out to achieve in the mandate.

Review

A post-implementation review of the entire project, including technical, operational, maintenance, quality, and workflow processes, should be undertaken here.

A review of the deliverables against the mandate, the requirements, the project plan, and, most importantly, the business case is undertaken.

Improve

The board considers the post-implementation review and makes recommendations for future work (if any).

Conclusion

Looking like they might actually live up to some of the hype, AI techniques are gaining traction and undoubtedly have the capability to address many clinical situations, significantly improving, if not transforming, many patient clinical outcomes.

AI platforms for healthcare are not technically distinct, and the implementation technologies and approaches are already used successfully across many other sectors. Nonetheless, organizations seeking to utilize AI continue to struggle with issues around the adaptation of clinical workflow, resource, diagnostic traceability, regulation, privacy, trust, data availability, and preparation. These barriers to adoption are predominantly non-technical; therefore, the approach to implementation must address and consider these at the outset.

Traditional program delivery techniques still have relevance. However, the program structure, sponsorship, and resourcing capable of delivering AI into this sector must be built into the program right from the start.

References/Further Reading

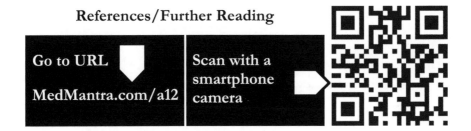

Go to URL

MedMantra.com/a12

Scan with a smartphone camera

CHAPTER THIRTEEN

IMPLEMENTATION OF AI INTO RADIOLOGY WORKFLOW

A. Introduction

Radiology today is facing a storm of conflicting developments. As the imaging technology itself improves and scanners generate higher resolution images and richer data sets, demands upon clinical imaging departments are likewise burgeoning. The volume of requests for imaging studies is exploding; at the same time, radiology departments are seeing a shortage of available trained personnel, to the extent that in many territories (especially the UK), bursaries are offered for training, and international migration is offered with preferential visa schemes. Radiologists, therefore, find themselves with an ever-increasing volume of tasks. The key to managing this situation is supporting the radiologist workforce to be more productive and to maintain or improve the standard of diagnosis and decision-making. AI is frequently proffered as a possible solution to this issue, and numerous AI-capable products are marketed to address this need. But how are these products best adopted in an existing clinical environment, already stretched and operating at a critical patient workflow?

It is regularly asserted that, eventually, computers will largely displace humans in medical imaging interpretation, in much the same way that satellite navigation systems have displaced map reading (and look set to do so with automated driving cars). Every year, more and more AI products come to market, offering to apply advanced AI techniques to clinical imaging diagnosis.

Several research papers have compared the performance of AI-augmented clinical imaging against humans undertaking the same tasks. A well-trained AI can return results that compete with experienced radiologists. This paper[1] showed, in an AI-assisted mammography study, *"The performance of the AI system was statistically non-inferior to that of the average of the 101 radiologists." The AI system had a 0.840 (95% confidence interval [CI] = 0.820 to 0.860) area under the ROC curve and the average of the radiologists was 0.814 (95% CI = 0.787 to 0.841)."* The machines' performance was at least in line with, if not very marginally better than, that of the radiologists when compared against this narrow task.

However, just because a company has a cool AI application, which appears to perform really well and provides a great diagnostic benefit (based on the sales material/case study), this does not mean that every new tool is a great fit for all departments or that the mechanism for integration is as obvious as the salesperson may infer.

The key to success in delivering benefit through AI in radiology is understanding in advance:

- How does the department's existing workflow operate, and what are the challenges (technically and from work and process management perspective)?

- What benefits are expected from AI?

- What could the various modified target workflows look like, and how can these support the expected benefits?

B. Barriers and Limitations

Systems and Process Integration

It's not a problem just in healthcare; it's a problem across all sectors. In almost every case, systems that look great in the brochure must be inserted into an existing technical and human process workflow. As attractive as the brochure might paint the system to be, if it cannot be efficiently used within the operation, it cannot be (successfully) acquired. "Efficiently" covers a number of angles.

Delivery of any change into existing workflows is complex—more complex than most imagine. As the radiology work process is ongoing, and in many cases, cannot be interrupted, that delivery must be as seamless as possible. Integration into surrounding systems, process design, data transport, security and storage, staff training, systems failover, maintenance, and support all must be considered, designed, tested, and delivered. Often, periods of parallel running are required to both minimize disruption and validate outputs.

All of this is expensive, and those costs escalate if the platform designers have not considered interoperability—the technical process of interfacing systems together with common networking and data formatting standards—such as DICOM. Any element of the process that requires the manual rekeying of data from one system to another is ALMOST CERTAIN to reduce productivity and introduce both delay and error, which must be avoided.

Thankfully, standards exist, and most platform developers are both aware of and make efforts to comply with these standards. However, extensive validation and testing are required. More on this later.

Trust and Regulation

The experimental capability of AI in many settings exceeds its practical utilization—that which is demonstrated in the lab or published in Nature (journal) is exciting but mostly not yet commercialized. Trust is a key component of healthcare delivery. With the impact of errors being so serious, physicians, patients, and regulators would not accept AI being allowed to operate unchecked without extensive verification and monitoring. Therefore, the introduction of AI will always lag significantly behind experimental headlines.

In the execution of this task, the FDA and other regulators have moved to provide frameworks for the introduction, maintenance, and operation of AI[2] in clinical practice. While this could be interpreted as a barrier to entry, such frameworks are essential in building and maintaining trust in AI operations.

An area in which AI applications can make an immediate contribution is in the support of human radiologists. Notably, AI does not (yet) take coffee breaks, hang around the water cooler, argue with its partner or colleagues, or get bored and burned out by repetitive work. Screening, flagging, and checking tasks undertaken by AI in support of existing workflows have the potential to improve the consistency of results (by, for example, screening a very large number of scans for critical findings that require a priority read by a radiologist) and avoid radiologist burnout while retaining the oversight of humans. These approaches can significantly increase the productivity of the human team, thereby reducing costs and improving efficiency.

Data Relevance, Data Privacy, and Availability

Like its human predecessors, AI makes decisions based on the sum of its experience—with the notable difference being that an AI is a learning machine and does not require several years at medical school. That said, AI is only as good as the data it is trained with[3]—that data must be complete, annotated, verified, relevant, representative, appropriately formatted, and clean. Data preparation must separate the data into three distinct data sets:

- *Training*: Data used to populate the AI model.

- *Validation*: Data withheld from training and used to tune the parameterization of the trained model.[4]

- *Test*: Data withheld from training and validation and used to finally validate the output of the trained and tuned model.

The requirement to ensure both the consistency and the relevance of training data is onerous—the variability of subject structures is huge[5], but, additionally, variability in scanned images (obtained from different machines), different scan settings, etc., all contribute to the variability of data. This is often addressed by seeking ever-larger training data sets, but all this contributes to the complexity of acquiring training data.

The regulation also plays a role. A further key and non-optional step in acquiring data is the "de-identification" of the model data. Simply removing obvious patient identifying metadata (name, address, any patient reference number, social security number, insurance details, etc.) may not be sufficient. Regulatory support is required to ensure that the local regulatory regime data privacy regulation surrounding the acquisition and use of the data is provably met.

C. Systems in Play

More than many other areas, radiology generates, interprets, and distributes a huge volume of diagnostic data. The volumes of data generated by imaging systems are so large that they present storage issues for non-specialized platforms and require specialist platforms for review, analysis, annotation, and distribution.

When considering the impacts of AI implementation, there is sector-specific terminology to be aware of. Also, typically, several major systems must be considered, and a couple of standards are regularly found in these environments.

PACS - Picture Archiving and Communication System

PACS acts as a specialized store, inventory, and analysis system for medical images. They are technical workflow systems, directly managing the image reception and analysis tasks.

PACS platforms receive images from various scanners as a series of files. Radiologists use the PACS platform to search for and retrieve images, view them for analysis, identify lesions or other structures, highlight these, and annotate them for use in diagnostic reports or treatment plans.

The image files themselves are in a sector-specific data format (DICOM—see below) and contain both pixel and metadata relating to the scan. PACS may be cloud-based or on-premises solutions. The use of digital media obviates the need for printing, distributing, and storing physical films and reports. PACS also mitigates the handling errors related to the misfiling or loss of patient data.

PACSs are often large-scale multi-user enterprise platforms. Rather than being monolithic, systems are often split into multiple functional components:

- PACS archives store all DICOM format files.

- PACS viewer terminals provide a native user interface for viewing, analyzing, and annotating images.

- PACS interfaces provide a set of Application Programming Interfaces (APIs) for enabling interactions to and from external enterprise systems.

VNA - Vendor Neutral Archive

An imaging server that also receives DICOM data but is not a vendor-specific PACS platform. It may be implemented to enable intradepartmental sharing of imaging data without impacting the PACS

RIS - Radiology Information Systems

RIS can be viewed as the departmental detailed workflow platform within the radiology team. Meeting interoperability requirements with the RIS is a core consideration when introducing new systems into a working imaging department.

Typically, while managing appointments and scheduling, staff availability, and access to and recording of the utilization of scanning resources, they also support advanced functionality such as repetitive appointments, scheduling moves and changes, etc. The RIS may also allow secure data sharing with other systems within the hospital environment.

RISs consolidate radiology reports across a patient treatment cycle, allowing current and historical images and radiology reports to be viewed in one place and making it easier to track the progression of a condition and treatment plan.

The benefits of RIS are typically centered around information management and removing the administrative burden of scheduling, rescheduling, and chasing appointments.

Electronic Medical/Health Record EMR/EHR System

The Electronic Medical Record or Electronic Health Record is a single logical data structure that encodes a single consolidated view of a patient's entire medical history.

The EMR/EHR platform typically contains:

- All elements of patient identification (name, address, date of birth, gender, etc.)

- Other medically relevant metadata (weight, height, smoking/drinking habits, sexuality, religion, etc.)

- Allergies

- Immunizations

- Tests

- Scans

- Diagnoses

- Treatment plans

- Prescribed medicines

Typically, inputs from PACS and RIS are combined into an EMR/EHR—although, often, medical imaging studies are so large that source imaging data is not included directly in the record. Rather, a reference is provided that links to the information stored on PACS/RIS. This avoids duplicating data (storage costs = money).

CIS - Clinical Information System

CIS is a generic composite term that may refer to one system or a federation of several.

CIS platforms consolidate all patient information (radiological and otherwise) into a single patient view. Similarly, they may also include patient workflow/scheduling functionality. Thus, CIS systems may incorporate a RIS and may also include EMR/EHR management systems.

DICOM

DICOM (Digital Imaging and Communications in Medicine) is not a system, but it is a hugely relevant interoperability standard for the encoding and transfer, storage, retrieval, and display of medical imaging data.[6]

Adherence to DICOM standards ensures that medical images are not only of the correct format but are encoded with the correct quality necessary for clinical use. DICOM is an international standard registered with the International Standards Organisation—ISO 12052.

The standard exists primarily to facilitate information sharing between different manufacturers' systems and practices. It specifically addresses medical imaging and metadata related to medical imaging. For example, patient ID, name, and other attributes are encoded within the DICOM file alongside the pixel data.

Implementation of DICOM is almost ubiquitous across radiology imaging devices (X-ray, CT, MRI, ultrasound, PET, etc.)

Workflow, Architecture, Organization, and Integration

The architectural approach to AI integration is ultimately a discrete choice of each individual project and organization, but one that is not stand-alone, in that it sits within a spectrum of options and constraints.

Large-scale healthcare organizations, possibly those that operate either large facilities or across multiple sites, will/should have an enterprise architecture that will incorporate:

- *Enterprise platform strategy*—a strategic set of specific enterprise platforms (like PACS and RIS) that change programs must work with and accommodate within their plans.

- *Systems interoperability strategy*—a set of data formats, security standards, and data interchange standards that projects must work with and accommodate within their plans. There may even be a specific enterprise platform whose function is interoperability—this is typically termed an Enterprise Service Bus.

- *Enterprise data models*—an organization-wide descriptive data model, probably pivoted in this instance around the EMR/EHR platform.

- *A long-term target architecture*—an aspirational architecture, toward which (rather than away from which) it is anticipated that successive projects would iterate.

Organizations put these strategies in place for several reasons:

- Constraining (or hopefully reducing) the number of systems that need implementing and supporting.

- Consolidating costs into fewer larger supply contracts (taking economies of scale from the suppliers as a result).

- Simplifying the systems integration challenges.

- Enabling multiple, disparate platforms to communicate and exchange information via a hopefully single, but more often smaller, set of common standards (an enterprise service bus architecture may even be defined).

- Reducing the costs of ensuring regulatory compliance across the estate.

- Simplifying the task (reducing the cost) of securing the platforms against both accidental and deliberate data breaches and malicious interference and ultimately (although it may not feel like it) making the task of evolving the IT systems estate easier, quicker, and cheaper ("conform to these standards and it should just click-in").

A comprehensive and well-formed Enterprise Architecture strategy will encompass data storage and archival (PACS/EMR/EHR/RIS), as well as compliance.

There will almost certainly be preferred vendors and, quite likely, a preferred platforms integration and delivery partner (likely to be from one of the larger IT companies or a consultancy) and a mandated project and business case approach.

This overarching strategy may feel burdensome and constraining, but having all these guidelines and frameworks in place will also increase the chances of delivery success. The project may be expensive to execute successfully, but this will still probably be less expensive than implementing it unsuccessfully several times.

So, the enterprise platform strategy will likely be the primary determinant of the approach to integration—and may even limit the ultimate choice of AI augmentation that is available for integration to those supported by the platform partner. However, the chances of a successful delivery are higher with its presence.

Conversely, smaller single-site organizations, or dedicated radiology specialist clinics, may have fewer overarching corporate constraints and a more flexible approach to clinic workflow and be better able to support a more manual process. This will also open the door to implementing AI systems that are not immediately supported by the large platform integrators.

Discussion

PACS and RIS are implemented to support the radiology department by automating many of the administrative tasks associated with the workflow, such as by providing advanced tools for visualization, easing storage, and making collaboration simpler by enabling the sharing of data through common standards, platforms, and data formats. This support has reduced cycle times, enabled significant improvements in individual and departmental productivity, and improved patient care.

Integration of AI into this pre-existing workflow must deliver only positive impacts into these established environments—not replacing the human workforce, but utilizing the qualities of an AI (infinite attention spans, no coffee breaks, no burn-out, algorithmic consistency of approach) by taking over repetitive and simple tasks from humans. An example includes processing a very large number of scans to identify and make preliminary observations (including measurements) of all lesions and other notable structures. This approach enables the human radiologists to focus only on the areas of concern, consult with colleagues, and draw conclusions without spending hours in preliminary identification.

The choice of platform and mechanism of integration may not be wide open and may be constrained by the existing technical architectures and interoperability standards enforced by the organization.

D. Modalities of Operation

Extensive consideration has been given to the technical approach to the integration of AI in imaging workflow. While the diagnostic application of AI is wide and varied, the modalities of operation break down into relatively few operational types. A discussion of some of the principal operating modes of AI in a clinical setting is also worthwhile when considering how any specific platform is applied.[7]

Flagging Lesions and Other Notable Structures

The AI surveys entire scans and highlights lesions or other structures with concerning features (e.g., critical findings). The AI may or may not provide analytical measures (a score or series of scores for each flag) to provide reasoning to the alert.

A radiologist examines all flagged items and makes the final diagnosis. A subset of non-flagged imaging studies may be quality checked to ensure that the AI is not missing notable features.

This is a cautious approach that presents the clinician with several potentially false positives for consideration. However, it does provide a consistent baseline for the evaluation of each lesion and increases the productivity of the radiologist team, whose time is spent evaluating identified and scored lesions rather than searching for them.

AI Evaluates and Prioritizes the Workstack

The AI examines entire scans and highlights lesions or other structures with concerning features. It scores each flagged lesion/structure and triages/prioritizes the workflow for attention with AI-scored high-risk cases to be evaluated by the radiologist first.

This can be a useful approach for triaging workflow into low and high risk—with low- and high-risk cases being presented in order of AI assigned priority—but the final assessment remains with the human radiologist.

Optionally, this scheme could be extended such that scans with no abnormally scored structures may not be reviewed in their entirety and passed back to the referring clinicians (although most clinics would likely review a sub-set of these).

AI Requesting Second Opinions

In this modality, the AI and the radiologist operate in parallel. Both assess and score the same scans, with the AI cross-checking the radiologist. If the opinion of the AI differs significantly from that of the radiologist, the AI generates workflow items to request a second opinion from another radiologist within the team.

While not delivering an improvement in productivity, this is an inobtrusive mechanism of using an AI to "catch" cases that may otherwise be inadvertently passed over.

Targeting Within Large Scans

Some scan types can return a very large number of images within which there are no notable abnormalities—for example, whole-body MRI scans for metastases or CT scans for trauma.

Examining very large scans can be tiring and error-prone for a human radiologist, as the limits of the human attention span are tested. This is especially a problem when reporting CT scans of trauma cases at night.

Letting an AI take the lead in these instances can dramatically improve productivity and mitigate the likelihood of missing critical findings.

Typically, the AI would flag and optionally score for attention only those sites with structures worthy of attention.

Discussion

There are several different mechanisms in which an imaging AI can be inserted into the radiology workflow to assist the human workforce. These modalities vary as to the extent to which the AI is used to either prioritize and cross-check/augment the consistency of departmental output or increase the productivity of each individual radiologist. The workflow solution and, therefore, system integration and process change approach for each of these are very different.

This highlights the importance of understanding the desired outcomes of an AI implementation before selecting and attempting to deliver a particular platform/algorithm.

It is also important to be aware that while AI programs find good application in addressing the narrow task for which they are trained, radiologists are often more adept at consolidating a more complete view of the patient from several different data sources other than the raw images and the metadata.

E. Workflow and Integration

In the same way that there are different approaches to supporting radiologists with AI-enabled image analysis, there are several approaches to AI platform and workflow integration.[8]

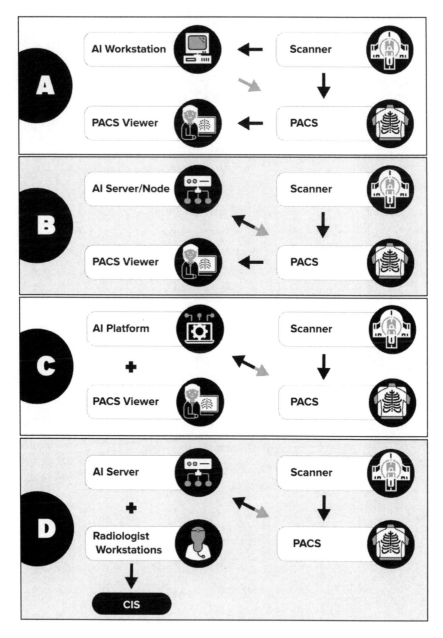

Figure 13-1. AI implementation in radiology workflows (A to D)

The basis of making a choice in this regard is established by determining the status of current workflows. This involves mapping existing workflows and considering which will be affected by the introduction of AI algorithms, as well as those actively targeted for change. There are two broad types of workflows to consider: those between people and groups of people, and technology workflows, which map the flows of information and dependency between different technical systems.

No Integration [see Figure 13-A]

At its simplest level, an AI platform could simply be bought and installed. Clearly, from a project perspective, this is likely to be the least expensive approach. Simplistically, the AI would be installed on a bespoke workstation or co-installed in an existing workstation. Radiologists would likely need to be physically in the same location as the workstation, and, similarly, only a single radiologist could access the workstation at any time.

This approach would provide a greater level of individual control and autonomy for users. Use could be expanded through multiple installations, allowing for concurrent access, although this would almost certainly incur extra licensing and support costs and, depending on the AI, may increase the burden of administration and management, particularly if the AI components use a continuous deep learning approach. Each AI will "develop" according to the specific cases it processes, which may impact the consistency of results generated from workstation to workstation unless all AI is using a central model.

There are significant workflow considerations with this model. Radiologists could adopt a "file-based 'cut-and-paste' integration" in which analyzed results are simply added to their final report. However, this would seem to be both manually intensive and open to considerable error.

The potential lack of any PACS storage and workflow integration would not support any consistency of approach between colleagues operating within the same department. However, in small practices, this may not be enough of an issue to justify a more involved integration.

Deep and Seamless Integration [see Figure 13-B]

In this model, the AI engine acts as an interim post-processing engine. An automated workflow is established between the scanners and PACS (this may already be in place). All images deposited into the PACS are sent without human interaction to the AI that processes the images. AI-enriched and annotated images along with the AI-generated report are appended to the scan archive and returned to the PACS.

At this stage, either with or without radiologist interaction (depending on the defined workflow), the AI-augmented results are returned into PACS/RIS for onward workflow.

Within this mode of operation, the report format is likely to be standardized and rigid. Clinicians can find this approach useful to inform the diagnosis. However, the automated workflow means that scans are interpreted by the AI without routine input and review from a radiologist. Therefore, the AI performance must be diagnostically excellent, consistent, and subject to continuous monitoring.

This architecture is least flexible for change in future workflow operations, as it builds systems dependencies into the flow and may restrict future workflow enhancements.

Multi-AI Platform Host [see Figure 13-C]

Several larger medical platform vendors operate a "host platform approach" whereby a single computing framework can host multiple AI technologies within a single interface. This is essentially a "wardrobe" into which can be hung multiple potentially host vendor and third-party AI technologies, accessed via a single user interface. It may be that the organizational enterprise architecture mandates this approach to minimize the number of systems that require support. Nuance AI Marketplace (nuance.com) is an example of an AI platform (like Google Play Store or Apple App Store for smartphone apps). Other similar AI platform providers are Blackford, Philips, GE, Siemens, etc. For details about various AI application vendors, please visit: https://medmantra.com/aih

This approach effectively supports macro-level workflows in which different, task-specific AI may be in play. As identified above, AI tends to be narrow in its focus of application. Therefore, having several AI within a single framework simplifies the task application.

The platform vendor is also very likely to offer additional support, maintenance, compliance, and quality control services across all vendors inside the kimono—simplifying internal support processes.

However, the downside of this approach is that the host platform vendor becomes a mandatory component of all AI integration projects, which may constrain the choice of future AI applications to only the algorithms and vendors that the host supports. Some future desirable product vendors may not "play nicely" with the specific platform integrator and, thus, be effectively unavailable to the department without a major architectural anomaly or strategy change. Additionally, the host platform vendors will be in a powerful commercial position and will typically try to extract value (cash) from all eco-system participants.

There are multiple workflow, data integrity, and operational efficiency benefits to be taken from this approach. However, the choice of platform vendor requires careful consideration and close involvement from the supplier management team to ensure that they do not become either an onerous commercial overhead or a barrier to development and innovation.

Multi-Department RIS Integration [see Figure 13-D]

This approach extends yet again the level of workflow and technical integration. Having been processed according to the platform hosted model, AI-augmented and reviewed results within the integrated PACS are distributed via the CIS for access. Actual images are not contained within the EHR; rather, the EHR contains a link to the AI-augmented image files and the final report within the PACS or the VNA.

Full RIS integration carries with it many of the benefits, shortcomings, and commercial risks of the multi-vendor platform approach while extending the integration beyond the radiology team and making the data more widely available within the organization.

Advanced Functional Options

Alongside the more "traditional" image-based analysis and annotation offered by AI components, some platforms can offer additional advanced functions, further leveraging the environment's support of the drive for increased productivity and diagnostic capability.

Voice integration for data capture: The typing of radiologist reports can be time-consuming and laborious. Platforms are now beginning to offer additional voice transcription for reporting services, allowing radiologists to dictate their reports to the PACS analysis platform for rapid capture of results—Super-Alexa, if you like.

Radiologist feedback used to improve the training model of the AI: Some products allow radiologists' feedback to be captured and used to enhance the training model used by the AI. This, of course, requires careful monitoring to ensure that the AI model is not degraded by the feedback or that additional biases are not created.

Re-submission and revision: Occasionally, radiologists may determine that the AI must revisit the evaluation of a particular structure with a different set of configurations. The ability to tune and re-submit images for revaluation is a feature that can improve both productivity and the consistency of output.

Research-based and feedback-augmented workflow[8]: This workflow is most suitable for academic and research institutes with large radiology department(s) and allows continuous improvement of the AI algorithm. Initially, research is done to develop an AI algorithm in-house [see Figure 13-E]. After adequate training, when the algorithm reaches an acceptable level of accuracy and quality, it is deployed in the production environment [See figure 13-F - grey arrows and shapes]. At this stage, a feedback loop is also created so that the AI model is continuously improved by periodic retraining using feedback data from the radiologists [see Figure 13-F - black arrows and shapes]. The radiologists check AI-generated annotations (stored in the annotation database) along with images, and if found incorrect, edit those. The edited annotations and the corresponding images are then used for retraining the AI algorithm (in the AI training server). The AI server is then updated with the latest retrained and improved algorithm.

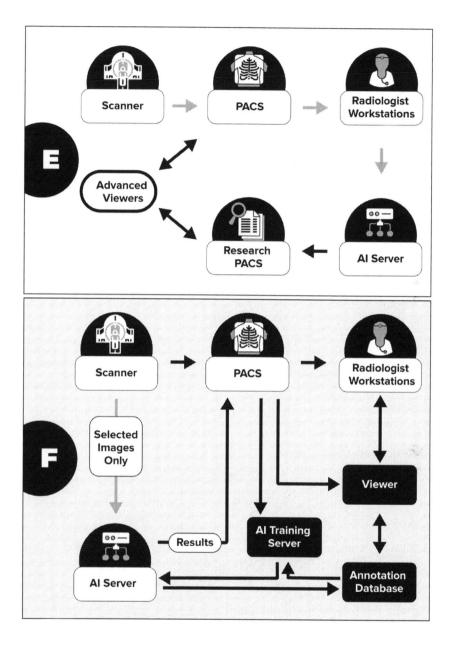

Figure 13-2. AI implementation in radiology workflows (E and F)

F. Non-Interpretive Uses of AI in Radiology

Here are the top non-interpretive uses of AI in radiology:

Enhancing Radiology Workflow

One of the most important things regarding enhancing the quality of radiology reports is optimizing the radiology workflow. This allows routine tasks to be carried out more effectively and reduces time and effort.[9,10]

Here are the most significant non-interpretive uses of AI in radiology that enhance the workflow:

1. Worklist Prioritization

Each radiologist has a worklist that is divided based on priority. The worklist has a set of rules that relate to the urgency of diagnosis, presence of an abnormality, location, subspecialty focus, examination type, and many other variables. Each rule has a different priority.

AI can help modify these rules and alter priorities to optimize the radiologists' efficiency in their practice. For example, deep learning approaches can be used to help radiologists by assigning a higher priority to cases containing abnormalities.[11] AI can alert the radiologist of critical findings so that turnaround time can be improved.

2. Study Protocols

During scanning, most CT and MRI examinations follow specific study protocols that ensure patients go through the optimal study that is best suited to their clinical diagnosis.[12]

The only issue is that this process is time-consuming, tedious, and prone to human error. Automating this entire process with the help of AI can reduce examination time and errors made by radiologists/technologists.

A properly trained CNN (convolutional neural network) can change the entire game for radiologists to create optimum study protocols. It will greatly enhance the number of sequences that can be obtained while reducing the time needed to execute these.

3. Hanging Protocols

A hanging protocol is a series of actions performed to arrange images for optimal softcopy viewing. When a hanging protocol is efficient, it can help with the radiologist's workflow in many ways. For example, it can significantly reduce the lag time between study selection and image viewing. Many automated hanging protocols are out there, but more efficient tools are required to optimize the radiologist's workflow.

Many challenges are involved in creating an optimized hanging protocol. That is because there are inconsistencies in metadata, differences in individual preferences, and differences in vendors. The use of AI can help overcome these problems to create efficient hanging protocols and enhance workflow.

Image Quality Control and Production

The most important task of a radiologist is to produce accurate imaging and results for each examination.[12]

That is why image quality and production are among the main tenets of radiology. AI is widely used in this aspect to reduce image production time and much more.

Here are the top non-interpretive uses of AI in radiology in this regard:

1. Reducing Contrast Dose, Radiation, and Scanning Time

In recent years, many concerns have arisen regarding the radiation doses associated with PET and CT imaging.[13,14] Radiologists worldwide are working to reduce exposure by utilizing updated protocols and technological solutions. This is an area in which AI can also help.

For example, AI algorithms can create high-quality imaging using low-dose raw sensor data. These can turn low-quality imaging into high-quality in no time. Besides that, AI can help reduce the need to use contrast agents in MRI.[13,15,16]

Deep learning techniques are quite effective in this respect because they can create high-quality MRI images using only ten percent of the standard dose of gadolinium (contrast medium/dye).[17]

2. Noise Reduction

Previously, deep learning techniques were used to reduce artifacts and noise in the images. They were also used to enhance visualization and contrast.[14] However, this led to the images being too smooth, and many details were lost.

Recently, this problem is being overcome with the use of newer techniques utilizing CNN and GAN (generative adversarial networks). These networks have led to noise reduction in images without the loss of essential information critical to the imaging.[12,18-22] In the long run, imaging quality can be significantly improved by transforming raw data into crisp images.

A post-processing stage can also be included to reduce the noise and artifacts in the images. The less noise there is, the better the image quality will be, and the more accurately radiologists can diagnose problems. AI can help with this in no time.

3. Automation of Image Quality Assessment

Medical images are routinely screened by the technologists to ensure optimal quality while they are being obtained. The images are checked for exposure, penetration, coverage, presence of artifacts, and much more.[23]

Besides that, sequence repetition and image retake are assessed.

Such image quality control is one of the core components of clinical imaging. If the quality is inadequate, the patient will have to be recalled for repeat imaging, which can be tedious and time-consuming. That is where AI comes in to help.

Deep learning models can be trained to recognize problems with the image quality so that they can be overcome during the imaging process.[24-28]

This will prompt technologists to rectify any issues before the examination is complete. Automation of image quality assessment can significantly improve diagnosis.

4. Reducing Scan Time and Increasing CT and MR Image Quality

Deep learning models have been used to enhance many aspects of MR and CT image quality. These include removing MR banding artifacts and CT metal artifacts, selecting specific MRI sequences, and much more.

Automation of all these processes will lead to a more individualized sequence selection that can enhance general radiology protocol selection. Currently, this is done manually and is a tedious process.[29-31]

The use of AI can reduce scan time for these sequences while simultaneously improving MR image quality. CNNs can be used to work on these aspects, as they have had previous success in such tasks.

Research Applications

When it comes to healthcare, research is the most important thing. AI can be used to enhance research applications in the field of radiology. Here are the top non-interpretive uses of AI in radiology in terms of research applications:

1. Image Quantification and Radiomics

Radiomics is the extraction of various features from medical images to support decision-making. It is widely used in oncological scenarios to identify image features that predict various grades and subtypes of tumors.[29-31]

AI models that use radiomics can be utilized to predict the severity of the disease. The imaging data can be quantified using AI, and the progression and severity of the disease can be quantified. This will help healthcare professionals produce an accurate diagnosis and offer optimal treatment to patients.

2. Image Labeling, Segmentation, and Annotation

For a long time, radiologists have been using annotations such as circles, arrows, flags, and various markings placed on images. Segmentation involves partitioning an image into different segments. Each of these segments represents an organ, abnormality, or area of choice. During labeling, text labels are assigned to each of the segments in the image. These three components are useful to radiologists in referring to findings for treatment planning, research, and education.[17,32]

These are currently performed manually under the supervision of a radiologist or by the radiologists themselves. AI can be utilized to automatically detect, localize, annotate, segment, and label many organs in the body.[33] One of the challenges is that the annotations can be permanently embedded in images, impacting their use for other cases or projects. These challenges can be overcome using deep learning models, as they can perform quantitative analysis, track changes, and help predict prognostic endpoints. AI still has a long way to go before it can completely and successfully replace these manual tasks.

3. Search Engines

Many search engines utilize images as input in academic and commercial use. These types of search engines perform a search utilizing the visual content present inside an image. Such searches can provide accurate results, as they are not limited by the text present in the images.

Radiology can benefit significantly from image-based search engines. They can provide the best opportunities to researchers and individuals who want to educate themselves. This will allow for ease of comparison and discovery while learning radiology, doing radiology research, and interpreting radiology images.

Text-based searches are not always accurate and don't always allow for ease of comparison. In this regard, there are endless research opportunities for learning more about radiology.

4. Explainable AI

A common challenge that many people face when it comes to AI is the lack of transparency in understanding how AI systems do their decision-making. Because of this challenge, healthcare personnel resist adopting AI, and there are significant delays in regulatory approval of AI. Healthcare professionals and patients don't feel that they can completely trust AI.

Also, evidence in non-medical fields shows that AI can make problematic decisions based on biased training data that includes gender, age, ethnicity, and many other factors. If a medical deep learning model makes an error, it is essential to find out why and how it happened to eliminate the same mistake in future models.

The European Union (EU) has introduced many guidelines and laws to ensure principles of transparency when it comes to AI decision-making.

Because of this, much research is being done on understanding explainable AI.

Business Applications

Finally, we have business applications in radiology. Here are the top non-interpretive uses of AI in radiology in terms of business applications:

1. NLP (Natural Language Processing)

NLP involves conversion of an unstructured text to a structured format. The conversion allows for easy facilitation of the automated extraction of information. The primary application of NLP is to enhance the quality of radiology reports while enhancing communication with patients and clinicians.

Currently, many radiology practices have adopted the use of speech recognition software. This allows the radiologists to use templates with subheadings. It is also reported that many clinicians give preference to itemized reporting, as it is easy to find many things in such reports.

There is no consistent pattern for the adoption of itemized reporting, as it depends on the radiology practice. That is why NLP can be a promising way to generate automated radiology reports. It can also be utilized to convert jargon into standardized terminology.

Incorporating NLP into radiology will make it easier to find and understand reports without hindrances. Imaging data can also be easily analyzed and applied using NLP.

2. Collections and Billings

In the end, any healthcare facility is also a business that must generate revenue in order to continue providing services to people. Insurance claim denials can lead to a three to five percent loss of revenue. Employing AI tools, the likes of NLP can optimize billing and collections.

In many healthcare facilities, the process of billing and collection is time-consuming and tedious. The use of AI and NLP tools can reduce these hindrances and ensure that the process becomes smoother. If that happens, healthcare managers can focus on other tasks.

Final Words - Non-Interpretive Uses of AI in Radiology

While AI has many non-interpretive uses in radiology, these are the most important ones that can quickly transform the field of radiology. Many of these uses are being applied in various healthcare facilities to improve the field of radiology. However, there is still a long way to go before these AI techniques are fully implemented.

The primary aim is to improve outcomes for healthcare professionals and patients. The non-interpretive use of AI can help both patients and healthcare professionals in this regard. Much more research remains to be done and implemented before AI can fully transform radiology for everyone involved.

G. Conclusion

AI applications have a very significant and developing role in radiology. However, the technology is developing fast and is further impacted by developments in parallel in associated technologies such as Cloud Computing, Networks, and Virtual/Augmented Reality. It must be noted that AI, in particular, is a group of aligned technologies, all the subject of intense technical focus is currently moving through a hype cycle, at various rates.[34] Several technologies currently near the peak are very relevant to this sector (Machine Learning, Deep Neural Networks, Natural Language Processing, AI Cloud Services, etc.). Therefore, claims made within any sales cycle that are related to these technologies must be significantly tested before commitment.

At this stage of their development, AI applications are marketed as being capable of enabling substantial improvements in productivity and a more consistent delivery of quality care—and there are some impressive case studies to indicate that this is feasible.[35] Yet, many AI applications are currently trained to undertake only a specialized subset of tasks and lack the wider patient view and the ability to consolidate information from multiple possibly unintegrated data sources into a diagnostic conclusion—all skills at which a human expert is adept. That said, the practically infinite attention span and tireless work capacity of AI are well placed to undertake time-consuming and boring radiology department activities in which humans become error-prone after a period.[36]

The principle challenge in selecting, adopting, and leveraging AI in a clinical context lies in understanding how it is to be applied in such a way as to extract maximum benefit. Inserting it into the workflow without harmful disruption takes consideration and careful planning, involving multi-disciplinary stakeholders from across the organization. Not only the clinical teams, but IT, HR, supplier management, and legal resources have critical roles to play.

Future developments in AI, supported by advances in computing power and communications, will enable much more capable AI, able to make inferences at levels not yet currently understood. Human radiologists will be able to confidently surrender more of their workload to the AI assistant and focus instead on delivering highly personalized, precision care to the patient.

References/Further Reading

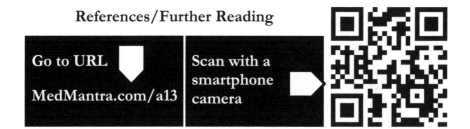

Go to URL

MedMantra.com/a13

Scan with a smartphone camera

CHAPTER FOURTEEN

IMPLEMENTATION OF AI INTO PATHOLOGY WORKFLOW

Artificial intelligence systems are no longer abstract ideas for the future, as the field continues to grow at a rapid pace, with cascading effects in all industries. Its impact on healthcare and diagnostics has the potential to truly revolutionize the speed and accuracy with which reports can be analyzed, interpreted, and delivered to clinicians and patients, thereby improving care delivery. In the field of pathology, the ready application of technology has become an industry norm, with fully automated workflows replacing manual processes in pre-analytical, analytical, and post-analytical phases in the laboratory cycle, generating enormous clinical data sets. This is largely due to the realization that the number of active laboratory professionals is on the decline, with most countries facing a shortage of pathologists. Data shows that 60% of active physicians in pathology are 55 years or older. There was a 10% decrease in pathologists from 2008 to 2013, and 20% of pathologists work overtime weekly or have to outsource their services.[1] This may also be due to the increasing workload, with a projected increase of 70% of new cancer cases within the next two decades.[2]

As necessity is often the mother of invention, it stands to reason that the application of methods or software that can reduce the work strain on lab professionals while still delivering timely and accurate reports will be readily implemented. Clinical decision making and the target towards personalized medicine with the help of investigations and genomics start with lab-processed data, which has led to the paradigm shifts in the implementation of AI-based software in pathology workflows to help develop new diagnostic and prognostic models. The segment that has shown significant advances is image analytics with the help of whole slide imaging and digital pathology software, integrated with robust AI algorithms to derive actionable diagnosis and prognosis of both oncology and inflammatory conditions in body tissues. Diagnostic precision is enhanced through deep machine learning and data integration that drives the field of *Computational Pathology* forward.

However, the applications of AI are spreading beyond the limits of image-based diagnosis in anatomical pathology and venturing into clinical pathology workflows as well. Considering the amount of data generated from a medical lab, these applications will significantly improve the interpretation and delivery of results to both referring physicians and patients. The various sections in laboratory medicine- hematology, bio-immunology, microbiology, histopathology, and blood banking – all require sample collection (***pre-analytical phase***), sample processing (*analytical phase*), and interpretation culminating in result delivery (***post-analytical phase***) as part of the workflow. Applications or platforms that have already been put into practical use, especially in hospital-based laboratory settings, have given rise to tangible benefits like early diagnosis of conditions, operational improvements like the reduction of wait times and turnaround times, thereby improving the provision of care with targeted therapeutics.

Pre-Analytical Phase and Point of Care Testing

Traditionally, in clinical pathology, blood or body fluid samples are collected manually, either by phlebotomy or fluid aspiration techniques, labeled, sorted, and sent for processing.

The past few years have seen a rise in remote patient monitoring through the use of wearables for temperature monitors, heart rate, respiratory rate, pulse oximetry, and ECG monitors to determine patient's physical well-being. Point of care testing devices used for routine monitoring like glucometers or coagulometers are also being used in conjunction with wearables to produce a holistic view of health status, which can be viewed by both the patient and his physician. When connected to and analyzed in real-time, this invaluable database can provide immediate care to patients by drastically reducing the turnaround time of lab reports. As an example of AI-enabled ambient computing, it demonstrates the deepening integration of computing platforms in routine living, assimilating into the background, and performing computations on autopilot without a direct command, through the Cognitive "Internet of Medical Things" (IoMT).[3] The AI-infused IoMT sensory data, if collated adequately, can be used effectively to help in modeling and forecasting disease progression or infections, ranging from localized tropical disease outbreaks like malaria or dengue to the recent COVID-19 pandemics.[4]

Arguably the most innovative application of AI in lab processes is the development of a robot by the researchers at *Rutgers University*, which uses artificial intelligence along with infra-red and ultrasound imaging to automatically perform phlebotomy or IV insertions for blood draws. If applied, it has the potential to drastically reduce the workload of bedside nursing staff or phlebotomists, as well as reduce the risk of disease transmission, due to reduced patient contact, especially in light of the recent COVID pandemic.[5]

Analytical Phase

At present, medical labs use advanced robotics to test minuscule volumes of blood, serum, and other body fluids from a number of different samples in a day and give highly accurate results on a large scale, one that is humanly impossible to duplicate. These analyzers function through conventional algorithmic programs that transform tedious manual processes into automated systems. Deep learning neural networks are not limited by human fatigue and are therefore able to process a multitude of information round the clock. Machine learning systems can be trained to take over a variety of repetitive tasks automatically, which can be applied readily in analytical systems of most clinical laboratories.

In microbiology, the seeds of AI were sown in the 1990s, with the introduction of *GIDEON (Global Infectious Disease and Epidemiology Network)*, a computer program that helped to diagnose infectious diseases, tropical diseases, and micro-organisms with antimicrobial sensitivity testing, globally, accounting for those more prevalent in certain countries.[6] Based on an extensive database of knowledge from peer-reviewed journals, electronic literature, drug reviews, and clinical trials, the system was able to generate a differential diagnosis based on signs, symptoms, laboratory tests, country of origin, and incubation period. It was used both for the diagnosis and simulation of all infectious diseases.[7]

In 2017, Harvard University's Beth Israel Deaconess Medical Centre used microscopes enhanced with artificial intelligence to help microbiologists diagnose blood infections faster to improve patient survival rates. The automated microscope collected high-resolution image data from microscopic slides from blood samples of patients with suspected bloodstream infections. A convolutional neural network (CNN) was trained to categorize bacteria by shape and size from large image data banks until it achieved nearly 95% accuracy in diagnosis.[8]

In histopathology, whole slide imaging, digital scanning, and AI-based analysis and interpretation have made considerable headway, alleviating pathologists' cognitive workload by streamlining routine slides while flagging complicated cases for an in-depth analysis, thereby saving time and expert resources. There are many companies that have developed neural network technologies to help with data analysis, some of which are *PathAI*[9] *and IntelliSite by Phillips*[10].

In hematology, companies like *Cellavision* provides an easy and fast option to automate manual differentials during microscopy of blood and body fluids, a task that is otherwise laborious and time-consuming, and is highly dependent on the availability of trained personnel. It uses digital imaging and artificial neural network technology to make the microscopic analysis more efficient.[11] More recently, *Athelas* released a compact personal patient monitoring machine for glucose, neutrophil, lymphocyte, platelets, and WBC (white blood cells) with morphologies, which uses deep learning and neural networks through computer vision to analyze blood samples, instead of traditional flow cytometry.[12]

In bio-immunology, molecular biology, and genome studies, the introduction of microfluidics has enabled the housing of multiple experiments on a single chip. *Microfluidics* allows the manipulation and analysis of very small fluid volumes within a multichannel system. This utilizes reduced amounts of samples and reagents when compared to large industrial analyzers. The reactions the sample undergoes to produce results are also faster, leading to rapid analysis. Appropriately called *"Lab on a Chip,"* microfluidic systems can be automated and standardized, reducing the chances of human error.

Thus, the results from the lab on a chip technology act as a data provider for AI systems, creating a synergy that can be leveraged for various applications in lab diagnostics. From the ability to perform tests on single analytes to multiple test parameters, covering various organs and functions in the body, lab on a chip is progressing to *Organ on a Chip and Human on a Chip* applications.

An example of a microfluidics system in immuno-assays is the FDA-approved *"Maverick Detection System" from Genalyte,* which uses resonance technology on a silicon chip, to perform multiple, simultaneous, rapid tests on a small volume of whole blood or serum. The system is cloud-connected for assay protocol retrieval and clinical oversight, delivering results in 20 minutes.[13] Similar devices have been produced to detect malaria, E. Coli, lactate and glucose levels, HIV, and Ebola, as well as drug levels in serum for levodopa, and in continuous monitoring of patients with Parkinsonism. Complementary technologies, like microfluidics, big data, and machine learning, may lead to exponential growth in e-health or digital health, catering to individuals for personalized diagnosis and therapy through rapid and cost-efficient means. In that process, a large biomedical database for targeted treatment depending on disease-specific symptoms or prognosis can be developed, serving as a more robust data set for further AI algorithms.[14]

The recent applications of AI in the analytical phase will result in *heuristic or self-learning systems* using numerous ways to arrive at the most opportune clinical decision, having been trained with exposure to holistic databases, data mining, pattern recognition, computer vision, natural language processing, and augmented reality, that will revolutionize the way labs generate and display results obtained from sample analysis.[15] In order to leverage *predictive analytics* to identify the likelihood of disease progression prior to the onset, AI-enabled systems use result databases and patient demographics as their training data banks. Through intelligent machine learning, patients prone to a certain illness can be flagged, bringing it to the attention of pathologists and treating physicians, who can offer preventive care instead of remedial care.

Post Analytical Phase

Report delivery and accessibility after data analysis and interpretation can be done in various ways so that both the pathologists and the treating clinicians are updated in a timely manner.

Integration of AI-based Software into Existing Systems

1. *Minimal or manual integration*: AI algorithms can be downloaded onto the computerized workstation where the pathologist authorizes reports so that it can run alongside the data retrieved from the LIS (laboratory information system) or the HIS (hospital information system) and deliver AI-augmented interpretations or results, which the pathologist then reviews and adds as required to the final report.

   This can be facilitated by a separate workstation or an extra computer dedicated to the AI software application.

2. *Fully automatic integration*: Results obtained from AI algorithms are automatically added to the reports authorized by the laboratory, in a standardized format, without a manual check or edit from the pathologist. This type of software needs to be extremely robust.

3. *Platform integration*: Instead of adding multiple software programs to the existing LIS, laboratories may decide to invest in third-party platforms, which integrate different AI algorithms onto one user interface, which is then connected to the LIS or HIS, in an approach similar to app stores for mobile devices. This is a boon for both AI providers and end-users like pathologists, who can benefit from the seamless integration of algorithms in their existing systems. An example of a connectivity platform is **Garuda,** which helps organizations connect and navigate through inter-operable machines and software, with a user-friendly dashboard and a gateway to a cloud-based repository.[16]

4. *Tag-along integration*: Laboratory systems have many existing software solutions, from quality management systems, lab and inventory management, internal and external quality control data, machine maintenance and error data in clinical pathology labs, to digital scanners

and storage systems, and automated tissue processors and stainers in anatomic pathology. Companies that provide AI algorithms or analysis can choose to integrate their software with existing programs to facilitate large-scale implementation. Although this is the most convenient way to access data from an end user's point of view, it may be tricky for AI developers to match their capabilities with those of the existing software.

5. *Multi department access with AI integration*: This type of integration can truly bring diagnostics to the final decision maker- the clinician. The integration of AI pathology software with systems that are accessed by referring physicians or administrators like patient EMR (Electronic Medical Records) and CIS (Clinical Information Systems) enables rapid communication of final reports for faster decision making. This has the advantage of filtering out normal results that do not require interpretation by pathologists to be accessed immediately, so that lab professionals can concentrate their time and energy on abnormal or complicated cases without cognitive or visual overload.

Challenges to Implementation

1. Even though state-of-the-art AI algorithms are released by researchers at a fast pace, adding another software extension to existing information systems in a multi-departmental laboratory can be cumbersome. Seamless integration of these algorithms into existing servers, incorporated as user-friendly software packages, may be required to improve buy-in by industry players.

2. Software implemented for medical use needs effective market checks and approvals from regulatory bodies like the FDA or the International Medical Device Regulators Forum (IMDRF). The FDA is therefore drafting a "Proposed Regulatory Framework for Modifications to Artificial Intelligence/Machine Learning (AI/ML) – Based Software as a Medical Device (SaMD)".[17,18]

3. Medical information obtained or analyzed by AI algorithms may be considered as Personal Health Information (PHI), and third-party software developers should be aware of complying with HIPAA

(Health Insurance Portability and Accountability Act) regulations when using this data for interpretation, as well as with data security.

4. Changes to workforce training requirements as well as clinical doctoral scientist mindsets will be necessary to fully participate in the growing revolution.

The application of AI solutions in the laboratory ecosystem will result in the prioritization of urgent cases, filtering out reports without abnormalities, and protocol adjustment based on AI interpretation of the data generated, thereby involving all levels of the current clinical and pathology workflows.

References/Further Reading

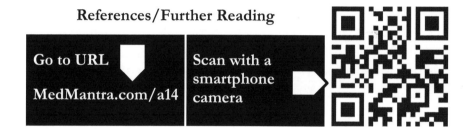

Go to URL
MedMantra.com/a14

Scan with a smartphone camera

"We've been seeing specialized AI in every aspect of our lives, from medicine and transportation to how electricity is distributed, and it promises to create a vastly more productive and efficient economy … But it also has some downsides that we're gonna have to figure out in terms of not eliminating jobs. It could increase inequality. It could suppress wages."

- Barack Obama

AI IN TELEHEALTH, COVID-19, DRUG DISCOVERY AND DEVELOPMENT, AND HEALTHCARE ROBOTICS

CHAPTER FIFTEEN

AI IN TELEHEALTH

Telehealth: The Basics

Telehealth involves facilitating healthcare and related services through telecommunication technology and electronic information.[1] Technologies used in telehealth include mobile health applications, video conferencing, remote patient monitoring, and much more.

In simple terms, you can receive all the benefits of medical care without visiting the hospital/doctor. Of course, AI is at the forefront of this field and is revolutionizing it in many ways.

Role of AI in Telehealth

1. Leveraging Innovations

With the help of AI, innovations are being leveraged in procedures and therapies through customization to match individual profiles and patient cohorts.[2] Such innovations are being used to enhance seamless communications across all aspects of healthcare delivery. If there is no communication or connection in this domain, healthcare quality will suffer, and so will patients.

Coordinated care is at the forefront of such innovations, as new technologies are needed to care for patients remotely. AI will help address this need and maintain a virtual knowledge base of a patient's disease and its management.

2. Quality Improvement

For the best patient care, healthcare quality and all its aspects must be improved. The field of telehealth is slowly noticing this improvement, as there is a movement toward the automated aggregation of patient information and universal EHR (electronic health record) systems. All of this is achieved by integrating AI with existing systems.[3]

The large data sets offer fantastic opportunities to extract new insights and improve health outcomes for patients. The data sets and information allow for improved clinical decision-making through automation. In the long run, telehealth will move toward smarter diagnosis and assistance.

3. New Models of Care

As the years pass, more people are affected by chronic diseases. When you combine this with the growing aged population, you can see that our current models of care are overburdened and unsustainable. On the other hand, the role of AI in telehealth offers a promising alternative for use in information and communications technology (ICT) to improve remote monitoring, diagnosis, and care delivery.[4]

Of course, to deliver new models of care, many challenges in telehealth must be overcome. To improve remote healthcare, there must be:

- Implementation of technological innovations

- Responsiveness and adaptability to the social and local healthcare system

- Support from front-line management and staff

Until these three points are exercised and there is a collaboration between management and staff, it will be difficult to get the most out of AI in telehealth.

Applications of AI in Telehealth

1. Monitoring Patients

Monitoring patients is the most common and basic application of AI in telehealth. The primary aim of this application is to create a cost-effective and quick way of offering consultations. This can be done through video conferencing and various other medical devices to record the patient's health data.[5]

This application aims to offer efficiency, ease, accessibility, and much more to patients. Researchers have recently designed telepresence robots to move in hallways and rooms and connect to the user through Wi-Fi. The most significant example of this is the Dr. Rho Medical Telepresence Robot.[6]

The robot consists of a screen for doctor-patient communication and a mobile body. The intuitive vision system of the robot follows the movements and gestures of the healthcare provider for procedures and examinations. Such robots have already been deployed in many hospitals.

2. Intelligent Diagnosis and Assistance

Diagnosis and assistance are other important aspects of telehealth. The aim of using AI for this purpose is to assist patients by analyzing evaluations to aid hospitals or by assisting patients physically. Tools for these aims are operated using machine learning (ML) algorithms.[7]

The self-diagnosis technology in telehealth is also expanding as mobile applications and software are released for self-diagnosis. These offer quick evaluations of vitals such as heart rate, pulse, breathing, and much more. One example of such technology is that of a start-up company known as Lemonaid Health. The company created an AI model for evaluating and screening patients through questionnaires and the fulfillment of several requirements.[8] After the screening, the patient is categorized depending on the clinical complexity. Then, a healthcare professional assesses the situation and conducts phone consultations to offer medical advice.

If such diagnosis and assistance are provided in emergencies, they can significantly improve telehealth in no time. Health centers can collaborate with ambulances and patients to offer quick and efficient healthcare services.

3. Collaboration and Information Analysis

Another application of AI in telehealth is collaboration and information analysis in consultations, medical research, and academic training. AI can connect medical professionals from various countries to collaborate and provide various perspectives and information on medical data for diagnosis.[9] This will revolutionize how healthcare professionals collaborate and consolidate clinical test results.

The aim of this application is essentially to detect patterns and analyze healthcare data. The use of AI analysis will eliminate bias and improve healthcare delivery to patients. Technology has a long way to go, and such collaboration is not being carried out right now. However, as AI is progressing rapidly in this field, we will see all of it soon.

4. Aiding Eldercare

Unfortunately, eldercare is a large field, as many people abandon their families in senior homes and other places. However, AI is developing smart machines that will decrease the cost of delivering healthcare to patients and improve their quality of life, especially seniors. For example, already, eldercare robots perform tasks and move semi-independently to assist elders.[10]

Stevie, a socially assistive robot, has been created to help seniors by engaging them physically and socially through activities and games. Stevie is equipped with autonomous navigation, which allows him to roam without assistance. However, there are still safety and insurance concerns when it comes to these types of robots, which is why Stevie never leaves his storage room without a handler.

As AI is implemented in the field of telehealth, we will soon see many robots assisting seniors and other people who need care. Stevie and other such robots are just the beginning of this journey.

Challenges With the Implementation of AI in Telehealth

1. Autonomous or Augmented AI

Autonomous AI is all about automating the healthcare workflow without the interference of doctors. The AI application solution design is critical to deciding whether the predictions served by ML models can be used to automate this workflow. It will also decide whether it can assist doctors in final decision-making (augmented AI).[11]

For example, let's say that a deep learning (DL) model is used to predict whether or not a person is suffering from an illness. Now, the solution design will need to include whether decision-making is automated or requires the assistance of doctors to have a say in the final decision based on the prediction. So, the question of autonomous or augmented AI must be answered before technologies in telehealth are created and implemented.

2. Ethical Challenges of AI

Ethical challenges involving AI exist in all fields of healthcare, including telehealth.[12] These challenges must be considered, and risks reduced, to create better AI. Here are the top three ethical challenges and risks that come with AI in telehealth:

Traceability

Who will be held accountable for incorrect predictions? Will it be doctors, hospitals, or the AI application? Incorrect predictions can lead to many conflicts, so the issue will have to be resolved by tracking who is responsible.

The AI application solution design will need to minimize this risk by incorporating accountability and who will be held responsible for these issues. Once that is done, this ethical challenge will be overcome.

Epistemic Risk

Creating an AI model for telemedicine is not an easy task. Researchers will have to come up with an optimal model that provides high performance.[13] Such a model will eliminate the risk of inconclusive outcomes and predictions.

Normative Risk

When the model makes incorrect predictions, the downstream applications will behave in a unique manner, which may lead to conflicts. In such a case, one must watch for related risks.

3. Governance Challenges of AI

The challenge of governance in AI is significant and exists in many fields. The telehealth domain will also face this issue, as the models require strong governance practices to reduce risks. Here are some of the practices to improve governance in AI:

Model Testing

Before the AI model is regularly used in telehealth, it must be tested with various data, including adversarial datasets. These will add to the performance of the AI model at frequent intervals. The dataset for which the AI model doesn't perform well will have to be included for purposes of retraining the prediction models.[14]

Model Retraining

After testing, one gets a better idea of the model performance. Based on this performance, the AI model will have to be retrained to include new features and models, tune hyper-parameters, and change the ML algorithms.[14] Of course, what must be done will depend on the performance results.

Model Monitoring

The performance of the AI model must be monitored at frequent intervals. Based on the inflow and distribution of data, the monitoring can be done daily, weekly, or even monthly.

4. Data Security

Security is one of the most fundamental challenges of AI. That is because building a telehealth AI model requires proper security to improve efficiency and model predictions.[15] Patients' data are highly sensitive and must be regulated or kept secure.

To overcome the challenge of data security, here are some of the practices that can be implemented in telehealth:

- Unless compliance requirements are met, the data shouldn't be accessed by external sources
- Access to data for internal stakeholders, even data scientists, should be controlled
- The requirements of data security must be met for data in transition or at rest

Conclusion

That was your complete guide to understanding AI in telehealth, including its role, its application, and all the challenges to be overcome. The field of telehealth is just beginning to transform, and there is a long way to go before any of this can happen on a large scale. Many hospitals and healthcare centers are employing this technology, but it remains in the building phase.[16]

As more technologies are implemented, we will have more data and insight on how to improve them. The field of healthcare is vast and expansive, which is why the trial and error phase will last throughout the coming years or decade. It will still be a while before we perfect these technologies and offer better healthcare to people.

However, you will soon witness remote AI and healthcare. Hospitals are already overburdened, and many researchers and entrepreneurs are working on these technologies for a better future.

References/Further Reading

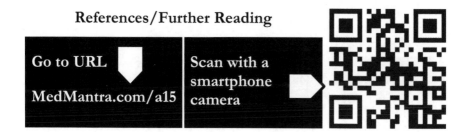

Go to URL
MedMantra.com/a15

Scan with a smartphone camera

CHAPTER SIXTEEN

AI IN THE FIGHT AGAINST COVID-19

The Coronavirus Disease 2019 (COVID-19) pandemic caused by Severe Acute Respiratory Syndrome Coronavirus 2 (SARS-CoV-2) has affected millions of people worldwide.

To limit the spread of infection, the main goal is to screen numerous suspected cases so that quarantine and treatment can be carried out swiftly. Although the gold standard is to carry out pathologic laboratory testing, it is time-consuming and has a risk of high false-negative results. There is an urgent need for alternative diagnostic techniques to fight the disease.

The contribution of artificial intelligence (AI) has been explored in this worldwide health crisis. Deep learning techniques which are part of AI have shown promising results in predicting, screening for, and treating COVID-19 cases in order to minimize the inception and spread of the infection as much as possible. AI algorithms have been found to have tremendous potential for saving time and critically controlling the spread and severity of the disease.

How does it work?

In March 2020, the White House put forth a call to action in collaboration with research centers and technology corporations. It prompted AI researchers to build innovative text and data-mining methods to support research related to COVID-19.[1] An initiative has been taken by the Allen Institute to provide the COVID-19 Open Research Dataset (CORD-19) in partnership with leading research groups. CORD-19 contains more than 280,000 scholarly articles, including more than 100,000 full-text articles about COVID-19, SARS-CoV-2, and other relevant coronaviruses. The data set is weekly updated and is free and open-source for the research community, in order to create new insights for ongoing research and innovation against COVID-19 through the application of advanced NLP and other AI technologies.[2,3]

Amazon recently developed an AI-powered technology, "Distance Assistant," to maintain social distancing measures for its employees. It works through a local computing device, depth sensors, a 50-inch monitor, and an AI-enabled camera for tracking and monitoring the real-time movements of employees. When the employees get closer than 6 feet from one another, highlighted red circles around their footsteps alert them to move to a safe distance.[4]

Philips IntelliSpace Portal 12 uses AI-powered quantitative assessment tools to detect pulmonary infiltrates in COVID-19 patients. It enables radiologists to differentiate COVID-19 pneumonia from other diagnoses based on ground glass opacities in lungs on chest CT scans.[5]

The extensive data about coronavirus-infected patients can be incorporated into and evaluated by highly developed machine learning algorithms. This paves the way for better appreciation of the trends in the spread of the virus, the progression of the diagnostic rate and precision, the development of new efficient remedial approaches, and the identification of the people at risk based on genetic and physiological attributes.

What can artificial intelligence do?

Viral infectious pandemics pose a grave danger to humanity. In the past, viruses have caused serious infectious pandemics, and COVID-19 will not be the last. We should be geared up for any such pandemics in the future. For this purpose, researchers are working hard to gather as much information as possible about the virus. Research institutions from various parts of the world are collaborating to accumulate data and develop solutions.

In light of this, machine learning has been remarkably meritorious in serving as a tool to perform the following tasks efficiently. It is also continuously evolving to be more advanced.

1. Identification of high-risk patients

2. Prompt diagnosis

3. Faster development of drugs

4. AI-based contact tracing

5. AI in patient care

6. Discovering the role of pre-existing drugs

7. Forecasting the spread of infection

8. Helping understand the virus

9. Facilitating mapping of where such diseases come from

10. Predicting the onset of upcoming pandemics

1. Identification of high-risk patients

AI has remarkable potential in the prediction of the risk of COVID-19 infection and its complications.

The risk factors:

- Any pre-existing health conditions

- Overall hygiene practices

- Social behavior

- Age

- Level of interaction with humans (including number and frequency)

- The area and climate of residence

- Socio-economic status

Predicting the possibility of infection

Machine learning (ML)-based research for the existing pandemic is still immature. A study has been carried out using ML to develop the initial vulnerability index for the disease.[6] Multiple other ongoing studies will hopefully improve the data quality and reliability over time as well as provide advanced AI applications in infection risk prediction.

Screening and triage of patients

Those who have been diagnosed with COVID-19 have different levels of urgency with regard to receiving medical care. The already burdened healthcare system would be unable to give immediate treatment to each and every patient regardless of the urgency of their need for treatment.

To relieve the pressure on hospitals, AI can help screen and triage such patients and identify those who need immediate treatment. For example,

Zhongnan Hospital in China employed machine learning-based software which detected signs of pneumonia in COVID-19 patients through CT scan images of lungs. This helps radiologists to mark the patients who need immediate treatment and further testing.[7]

In South Korea, the government released an AI-powered app for its citizens to self-report symptoms and to indicate whether these citizens leave their "quarantine zone" in order to prevent "superspreaders" from spreading COVID-19 infection in a large population.[8]

Predicting disease outcomes

After a person has been diagnosed with the infection, there is a need to identify the risk of the development of complications as well as for advanced medical care. Some people experience only mild symptoms, while others have the potential to develop serious respiratory conditions which can be life-threatening. Using machine learning, it is now possible to identify those who are at risk of developing serious conditions and providing immediate treatment to them.

Machine learning has been found to identify the risk of a patient developing acute respiratory distress syndrome and the risk of death simply by examining the initial symptoms.[9] Recently, a team of engineers from Rensselaer Polytechnic Institute developed a new algorithm to predict the need for ICU intervention in COVID-19 patients. The algorithm was built by combining CT images (which evaluate the severity of lung infection) with non-imaging data like vital signs, demographics, and lab test results to predict the disease outcomes.[10] This AI-based algorithm can define a valuable treatment approach for COVID-19 patients in terms of ICU bed allocation and hospitals' bed management systems.

Predicting treatment outcomes

Predicting treatment outcomes is an important tool for evaluating the results that will be produced through a specific treatment plan. This would be very useful for doctors in the prescription of medicines. Machine learning has already been used to predict the treatment outcomes for epileptic patients[11] as well as how cancer patients respond to immunotherapy.[12] There is also immense potential for AI-based algorithms to be applied to the prediction of treatment outcomes specific to COVID-19.

2. Screening and diagnosis

Face scans for patient screening

Artificial intelligence has also proved to be useful in screening people for fever using face scans. Hospitals in Florida and Israel have employed automatic face scans to screen hundreds of patients entering the hospital at a glance. These scans use machine learning to detect people with fever.[13]

Independently, the technology might not be very strong and useful. However, when thousands of people are involved, like in a pandemic such as this one, it acts as a very powerful tool to help screen and identify high-risk patients.

In Thailand, a team of researchers has developed an ML-based temperature screening system named μTherm-FaceSense. It can evaluate up to 9 people at a time based on increased temperature.[14,15] Baidu has built a "non-contact infrared-based sensor system" to screen individuals with fever in large crowds. It has already been deployed in major hospitals and railway stations and has replaced manual thermal scanning.[16]

Use of wearable technology

The Apple Watch has been very famous medically for its detection of heart rate and rhythm, helping to identify common heart problems. Ongoing research indicates that alterations in resting heart rate can facilitate the identification of influenza-like-illness (ILI).[17] This implies that AI algorithms can be used to predict more specific issues such as the diagnosis of COVID-19, although the research is at its early age. The recently launched Apple Watch has some new features to aid in diagnosing COVID-19 patients. Along with the remote ECG monitoring tool, it has a blood oxygen sensor, which is a cutting-edge addition from Apple due to the immense need in current times.[18]

Likewise, Oura-sponsored research at the University of California, San Francisco (UCSF) has collected profound physiological data.[19] This has been achieved by a sleep and activity tracking ring that makes use of body temperature, breathing rate, and heart rate. The research seeks to develop an algorithm to spot the inception, development, and recovery of COVID-19.

Researchers at Scripps Research Translational Institute recently launched the DETECT (digital engagement and tracking for early control and treatment) study to assess changes in heartbeat, activity, and sleep by using devices like Fitbit, Garmin, and Apple Watch for tracking potential cases of COVID-19. Initial results of the study have demonstrated that Fitbit can successfully predict 78% of patients with COVID-19.[20]

Employing chatbots

With an increasing number of queries and illnesses, doctors cannot respond to all patients, as they must attend to the more serious ones. Many countries have formulated self-triage systems to help patients evaluate their conditions. Patients fill out a questionnaire related to their symptoms and medical history and then are directed to either stay at home, consult a doctor, or visit a hospital.

Microsoft has developed chatbots to help direct people as to whether they should seek at-home treatment or visit a hospital, according to their symptoms.[21] IBM recently developed "Watson Assistant for Citizens," a new chatbot solution for updated information and guidance about COVID-19, recommended by the CDC. Watson Assistant for Citizens can answer common questions about symptoms, prevention, and protections against COVID-19.[22] Bespoke launched an AI-embedded chatbot, named "Bebot," that provides updated COVID-19 data and also helps patients check their symptoms.[23]

Role of AI in radiology

Recent studies have shown that radiology images contain information about the presence or absence of COVID-19 infection. Radiology combined with AI techniques can aid in the accurate detection of the infection and can also overcome a lack of expertise in remote areas. According to this study, a model for automatic COVID-19 detection with the help of chest x-rays is proposed. The DarkNet model was used to classify chest x-rays employing the "you only look once" (YOLO) detection system. This model can be utilized to help radiologists confirm the initial screening, as well as to immediately screen patients remotely via the cloud.[24]

Moreover, AI software is used to facilitate diagnosis using CT scans of the chest. This software is considered useful in classifying the infection into various severities. Thoracic VCAR software is a helpful tool for radiologists for the diagnosis of COVID-19, providing quantitative measurements of lung involvement. Thoracic VCAR enables the generation of a sound, prompt, and precise report to communicate important medical information to referring physicians. After evaluation, this software recognizes the natural parenchyma and differentiates it from surrounding consolidation, quantifying them as a percentage of the healthy parenchyma, thus allowing for estimation of the severity of lung involvement.[25]

Researchers have recently built a deep learning model named COVNet (COVID-19 detection neural network) to differentiate between community-acquired pneumonia and COVID-19 based on 2D and 3D visual features extracted from chest CT scans.[26] After the COVNet experience, researchers developed COVID-ResNet by using automatic and discriminative learning models. COVID-ResNet proved better than COVNet in terms of progressive image resizing in diagnosing COVID-19.[27]

3. Faster drug development

When a new pandemic hits, it's critical to have a quick provision of reliable diagnostic tools, drugs for treatment, and vaccines. As of now, this is a time-consuming process; it can take months to years to come up with an effective vaccine. Artificial intelligence can speed up this process without compromising quality.

As for the Ebola virus, researchers used Bayesian machine learning models to prioritize compounds for testing, in search of small molecule inhibitors of the Ebola virus (EBOV).[28] The results showed that data sets with fewer than a thousand molecules could create authenticated machine learning models which can be used to identify new EBOV inhibitors in the culture medium.

According to other research, a **virtual screening** approach was employed to identify influenza virus inhibitors with the help of molecular docking coupled with an AI-based scoring function. This led to considerable improvements in score accuracy.[29]

4. AI-based contact tracing

Contact tracing is a vital monitoring component for combating an infectious disease like COVID-19. It consists of three basic steps: contact identification, contact listing, and contact follow-up. TraceTogether is an AI-powered contact tracing app deployed in Singapore. If an individual is found to be COVID-19-positive, the TraceTogether app notifies every user of this app who was in contact with that infected individual within 2 meters for longer than 30 minutes.[30] Alipay Health Code, Immuni, COVID Near You, and CoronApp are other examples of AI-based contact tracing apps that are being used widely amidst the pandemic.

5. AI in patient care

Artificial intelligence is also playing a vital role in the area of COVID-19 patient care. Biofourmis created an RPM (remote patient monitoring) system with a biosensor and AI application to accelerate diagnosis and interventions for COVID-19 patients, which is part of the hospital-at-home solution.[31]

CLEW launched the AI-powered TeleICU, which uses clinical predictive analytics to predict respiratory deterioration in advance.[32]

6. Discovering pre-existing drugs

Drugs must be approved by a federal organization such as the FDA, and companies invest generously for that purpose. This is important to ensure that these drugs do not have untoward harmful effects. However, this process is time-consuming and would undermine the treatment procedure during a pandemic. One way to speed up the process is to repurpose already tested and used drugs. This is where machine learning comes into play. Several other projects, like Polypharm DB, are seeking to identify potential candidates against COVID-19.

Biomedical knowledge graphs

Many research articles contain knowledge about drugs, vir
behave. Natural language processing which involves ML a
be used for studying and evaluating a large number of Bene
knowledge graphs, a hefty storehouse of prearranged medical information. These include several associations extracted from systematic literature by artificial intelligence. They explore the potentially beneficial drugs that are approved and mark those which can inhibit the process of viral infection. Baricitinib is, thus, expected to decrease the ability of COVID-19 to infect the lungs.[33]

It has been found that coronavirus presumably makes use of the protein **ACE2** for gaining entry into the lung cells through a process referred to as **endocytosis**. This process is regulated by another protein, **AAK1**. The drug Baricitinib hinders AAK1, preventing the entry of SARS-CoV-2 into the lung cells.

Prediction of drug-target interaction

Ongoing research employs machine learning to predict interactions between the target drugs and the virus protein in order to identify the appropriate drug candidates. Scientists use neural networks to identify highly complex drug-target interactions (DTIs). These neural networks are specialized in huge DTI databases to extract lists of drugs that are most likely effective against the virus proteins.

Researchers have designed an end-to-end framework for processing knowledge graphs with the help of neural networks. This model is then advanced for the interpretation of knowledge graphs and precise prediction of DTIs. With the help of this technology, researchers are already exploring a potential drug candidate, which is presently under clinical trial.[34]

MT-DTI (Molecular transformer-drug target interaction) is an NLP-based tool that may be beneficial for assessing binding affinity values between antiviral drugs available on the market and target proteins on SARS-COV-2. It has been proved that Atazanavir is an effective agent against target proteins on SARS-COV-2.[35]

Forecasting the spread of infection

When a pandemic strikes, there is an urgent need for strategies to combat it. The government must answer several questions, obviously, with the help of the healthcare system. These include the number of people who acquired the infection, the location of the infected, etc.

With a pandemic, which evolves and spreads rapidly over time, it is difficult to keep up with the growing number of cases. New numbers of cases diagnosed with the infection are calculated and published by the corresponding agencies daily. However, one limitation is that there is a time-lapse between an individual acquiring the infection, the appearance of initial signs and symptoms, and the positive test. This can result in massive changes in the growth trend of the spread of infection.

Nevertheless, access to social media makes things favorable, thanks to the Internet of things (IoT) in this digital world. A local in a small town does not have immediate access to healthcare settings for checkups or screening but can leave indications of developing symptoms of the disease and the spread of infection, which can be taken up and processed at scale only by an artificial intelligence model.

This implies that interpretation of the public interaction content on social media can be carried out by a machine learning model to evaluate the risk of novel virus contraction. The model might not be able to categorize individuals independently, but it can use all the data to estimate the spread of infection in the pandemic. Also, it enables the ML model to predict the spread of the disease in the following days and weeks.[36]

BlueDot and Metabiodata are the companies that rely heavily on AI, ML, and NLP to predict infectious diseases, as in the current case of the COVID-19 pandemic, including severity, intervention, and spread of infection.[37] Applying NLP algorithms, BlueDot and Metabiodata collect a huge amount of data from biological, political, socioeconomic, and social media sources to accurately predict the severity and duration of outbreaks. Facebook is also currently using AI techniques to forecast the COVID-19 spread 14-days ahead in counties across the United States.[38]

Covid-19 case identification using a mobile app

A. Rao proposed that machine learning algorithms can be used to better identify COVID-19 cases quickly, employing a mobile phone-based web survey. With this technique, the spread of infection in high-risk populations under quarantine can be decreased.[39]

A mobile-based online survey is used to lessen the time required to mark a person under investigation (PUI) for COVID-19 and quickly isolate them. Basic travel history is obtained, including common signs and symptoms. This data can be used by most countries for contact tracing (using GPS) and warning users if an infected person has been nearby, as well as to screen and identify possible COVID-19 patients. They also have educational and informational uses. AI is used to process thousands of data points to evaluate and categorize patients into high-, minimal-, moderate-, and no-risk groups. This enables the earlier quarantine of the high-risk cases and reduces the chance of the spread of infection.

It is noteworthy that this information holds immense significance in the process of decision-making at the government level during the wildfire of a pandemic.

8. Understanding viruses

To fully know a virus, we must know its structural proteins. Whether an individual will get sick and how their body will react to it depends on the interaction between the virus and their body. Artificial intelligence makes it easy to obtain an in-depth understanding of the protein structure of a virus.

Prediction of interactions

The knowledge about the interaction of a virus with the human body holds great significance for the formulation of novel therapeutic programs as well as new drug breakthroughs. The human body reacts to an infection based on the interaction of body cells to the pathogens, referred to as protein-protein interactions (PPIs). This virus-host interactome is the complete interaction between the proteins of a virus and a host and acts as a blueprint showing the way the virus affects our bodies and reproduces in the body cells.

Multiple ongoing studies seek to decrease the array of probable interactions. Artificial intelligence models developed through protein data have already been employed to predict the likelihood of H1N1 and HIV virus-host PPIs.

Prediction of protein folding

It is an established finding that the structure of a protein is interrelated to its function. The unraveling of this structure is what makes its role inside a cell clear and paves the way for the development of drugs that are capable of affecting the distinctive shapes of the proteins.

On the other hand, it is not so simple to unravel the three-dimensional shape of a protein. This is because one protein is capable of forming a hoard of probable structures. For example, a protein that consists of 100 amino acids can conform to more than 3000 possible shapes/structures.

As of today, out of more than one billion protein sequences identified, less than 0.1% have been identified. Scientists have been successful in developing AI models that can envisage protein sequences with the help of neural networks. This makes it viable to recognize protein structures by means of computational techniques.

AlphaFold is an AI-based program developed by Google DeepMind for determining 3D shapes of proteins. It is designed by using deep learning models and helps to create an understanding of the proteins in the SARS-COV-2 viral genome, helping to explore the detailed structure and further mutation capacities of SARS-COV-2.[40]

9. How to target the virus

To fight the virus, it is imperative to figure out how to attack it. One way is to unravel and categorize its epitopes. An epitope is the cluster of amino acids located on the outer surface of the virus. Our immune system works to form antibodies that bind to these epitopes before eliminating the virus from our bodies. Thus, it is crucial to classify the epitopes in the development of vaccines.

In general, vaccines based on epitopes are safer than the conventional ones containing inactivated pathogens. Epitope-based vaccines are capable of preventing infection without the risk of side effects.

However, locating the correct epitope requires a lot of investment and time, which is not a suitable thing to do during a pandemic. Prompt recognition of the epitopes makes the vaccine development process faster. Artificial intelligence has a solution to this. Hidden Markov models, neural networks, particularly **deep learning** and support vector machines (SVM), have been found to be more precise and quicker at categorizing epitopes as compared to human scientists.

Baidu launched a webserver, "LinearDesign," in collaboration with the University of Rochester and Oregon State University. LinearDesign algorithms may greatly aid giant vaccine companies in optimizing their vaccine designs based on the most stable secondary structure of the viral mRNA genome.[41]

10. Identification of hosts

COVID-19 is a zoonotic pandemic, meaning that it is due to an infection stemming from a different species, like bats, and then spreads to humans. Such viruses—for example, Ebola, COVID-19, or HIV—can stay alive overlooked in the environment for a long time, with a high risk of mutation and spread of infection. These viruses hibernate in animals which are called reservoir hosts. This means that these animals only carry the virus silently, without suffering illness themselves, but have the potential to spread it.

Identifying the reservoir hosts is critical to combating a pandemic. After they are found, strategies can be developed to control the spread of infection, thereby preventing greater damage.

Unfortunately, the traditional method of discovering the reservoir hosts may take years of scientific research; still, many stray viruses have not been categorized as coming from an animal host. So, what can be done to overcome this issue? The answer to this comes from artificial intelligence.

The procedure of identifying the full DNA sequence of an organism, called Whole-Genome Sequencing (WGS), can now be carried out quickly and economically. Studies have found that machine learning models can make use of genome sequencing information coupled with specialist knowledge to mark the variety of animals that presumably played the role of host for the virus.[42]

By examining the small division of species, the course of identifying these pathogens in the wild can be sped up remarkably.

11. Prediction of upcoming pandemics

Precise prediction of the behavior of the influenza strain with regard to making a zoonotic transformation (i.e., to leap from one species to another) is important. This will enable doctors and other healthcare workers to foresee possible pandemics and, thus, plan and organize in accordance. For example, the Influenza A virus is found predominantly in the avian population. However, it has the potential to shift to human hosts. Scientists studying the influenza A virus isolated more than 67,000 protein sequences from the record. These protein sequences were filtered to include only the dataset record of the influenza virus, which contained the full sequences of 11 proteins of influenza.[43]

With the help of artificial intelligence, scientists have identified the zoonotic strains of the influenza virus with advanced levels of precision. However, there is a need for more effort to set up prediction models for direct transmission. The first thing to be equipped with to prepare for an upcoming pandemic is to know which strains of influenza virus are expected to make the leap to becoming zoonotic.[44]

12. Better resource management

As a result of the pandemic, there is a shortage of protective gear, medicines, ventilators, and hospital beds. ICUs are overburdened throughout the world. To better manage these resources, hospitals can make use of the forecasting tools driven by artificial intelligence.

For this purpose, Qventus has designed software that aims to support hospitals during the pandemic. This model considers the number of new cases and the associated deaths related to COVID-19. It also forecasts the effects of the pandemic on the capacity of the hospitals, such as the availability of beds, ICUs, and ventilators.[45]

Published research states that with the help of collected data, an artificial intelligence framework can be used to predict the clinical severity of COVID-19 patients. This will also assist in clinical decision-making. As per this predictive model, real patient data is used to foresee those who will develop acute respiratory distress syndrome (ARDS), which is a serious complication caused by coronavirus infection. According to the study, these models have been successful in achieving 70 to 80 percent precision in predicting the clinical severity of cases. This enables them to identify patients for advanced support.

Methods and techniques like these help to better categorize and prioritize patients and dispatch resources accordingly in due time. This will ultimately reduce the burden on healthcare organizations.

Pitfalls of using AI for COVID-19

Despite all the merits of artificial intelligence tools, it is vital to note that machine learning alone cannot provide a complete solution. Rather, these algorithms should be taken as support for healthcare professionals. For example, BlueDot employed an algorithm that identified trends with the help of colossal data, which would otherwise require a lot of time by a human. After these trends had been identified, doctors and epidemiologists were the ones who evaluated them to reach a final conclusion and judgment.

The developments and progression put forth by the ongoing maneuvers made by artificial intelligence and deep learning pave the way for a bright future in the field of medicine. It is emerging as an asset for the healthcare system, tremendously facilitating the practitioners, and will continue to do so even after the pandemic is over.

As the virus moves from the environment to humans, it also undergoes mutations. These mutations are critical because they alter the genome sequence of the virus. It is the genome sequence on which the diagnostics, treatment, and vaccines are based. Alterations in this sequence would cause alterations in the therapy and its outcomes. Although artificial intelligence algorithms are successful in screening and diagnosing patients, they are currently not very strong in terms of detecting mutations. Hence, there is a need for the development of algorithms that not only perform screening and diagnosis but also are robust in detecting mutations.

Full-potential AI has still not been utilized against COVID-19. Its application is hindered by either lack of data or too much data. There is a need for vigilant balancing between data security and public health, as well as meticulous human-AI interaction to surmount the constraints. However, it is implausible to address them in short enough time to be helpful during the current pandemic. Meanwhile, it is vital to gather extensive diagnostic data, have specialized AI tools, and minimize economic injury.[46]

Another example of how artificial intelligence can be good and bad simultaneously is as follows. As NLP algorithms may alert against any possible outbreak by mining data from different sources, a recent study found that running a standard NLP model emits 626,155 pounds of CO_2 while it is trained; this is over five times the CO_2 an average car emits in its lifetime.[47]

Concerns related to the efficacy and privacy of machine learning models are valid and require a determined effort on the part of the authorities to ensure the safe and effective use of artificial intelligence. Yet, there is no doubt that the upcoming pandemic cannot be tackled without the execution of intelligent tools far before it strikes.

Conclusion

Artificial intelligence is a significant way to combat the present pandemic. If it is employed efficiently and coupled with the expertise of healthcare professionals, it can save a lot of time, money, and energy.

Despite its many uses and support for the healthcare system, machine learning also has some limitations and is not very robust against mutations. Thus, it is reasonable to be cautious and aware of the likely privacy concerns and risks associated with the use of such novel technology in unexpected circumstances. However, with constant research and the combined efforts of scientists and engineers, these developments will gradually evolve and enable us to better prepare for future outbreaks.

References/Further Reading

Go to URL ⬇	Scan with a smartphone camera ➡
MedMantra.com/a16	

CHAPTER SEVENTEEN
AI IN DRUG DISCOVERY AND DEVELOPMENT

Artificial intelligence (AI) in drug discovery:

Though traditional methods of drug discovery are risky, expensive, and time-consuming, they can bring extensive benefits with high returns if successful. Research shows that since 2016, companies spend an average of around ten years and $2.6 billion on developing a single new drug.[1]

Therefore, in the expansive field of new drug discovery, companies in the pharmaceutical industry pursue strategies that increase the possibility of success while reducing the risk of failure. AI shows the potential to reduce costs as well as save time during the production of drugs, thereby gaining significant attention in recent times.[2]

Drug discovery is a lengthy and complicated process that can be broadly categorized into four major stages:

1. Target selection and validation

2. Compound screening and lead optimization

3. Preclinical studies

4. Clinical trials

The first step is to identify the target related to a specific disease after evaluation of cellular and genetic components, genomic and proteomic analysis, and bioinformatic predictions.[3] This is followed by hit identification, using methods such as combinatorial chemistry, high-throughput screening, and virtual screening to recognize compounds from molecular libraries.[3]

To improve the functional properties of newly synthesized drug candidates, cellular functional tests along with structure-activity and in silico studies are used in an iterative cycle. Then, animal models are used for in vivo studies like pharmacokinetic investigations and toxicity tests. In the last stage, the drug candidate has successfully passed all preclinical tests and can be administered to patients in a clinical trial.[3]

The drug must then go through the following three clinical stages in order to confirm the efficacy and safety of the compound:

- Phase I: **testing drug safety** using a small number of human subjects

- Phase II: drug **efficacy testing** with **a small number** of patients affected by the targeted disease

- Phase III: **efficacy testing** with **a larger number** of patients

The drug can then be reviewed by regulatory agencies like the FDA for subsequent approval, distribution, and commercialization.

Artificial intelligence (AI) in drug screening:

Searching for active compounds through traditional means is a tedious process in the discovery of new drugs, as it is time-consuming and tends to drain resources during the screening stage. However, modern rational methods of drug discovery make use of core techniques like **molecular docking** to **virtually screen** potential compounds. This enables the computational selection of effective compounds from large compound libraries.[2]

Computer-aided drug design (CADD) is based largely on virtual screening technology. To select compounds that meet the expected criteria from known databases of small molecules, theoretical knowledge of molecular biology and computer science are required to analyze the target biomacromolecules' three-dimensional (3D) structure as well as their quantitative structure-activity relationship model. Subsequently, various experimental methods are chosen for the targeted drug screening to aid in the treatment of specific diseases.[4]

In the pharmaceutical industry, virtual screening is considered to be a leading CADD tool used to effectively screen large chemical structural libraries. It then condenses this data into a set of potential candidate compounds that are related to specific protein targets.[5] Its value lies in its efficacy in searching for lead compounds and the enhancement of compound activity.[6]

Though many algorithms have been programmed for docking in virtual drug screening using the in-silico method, the discovery of lead compounds or "perfect hits" is rare. To maximize the potential of the screening process, many companies are investing in AI methods like machine learning (ML) and its application to the present procedure of molecular docking with a focus on the scoring function. This may also lead to more effective drug repurposing.[2]

Algorithms, such as nearest-neighbor classifiers, random forests (RF), extreme learning machines, support vector machines (SVMs), and deep neural networks (DNNs), are used for virtual screening (VS) based on synthesis feasibility and can also predict in vivo activity and toxicity.[7,8]

Prediction of physical properties:

It is important to select drug candidates that exhibit desired properties with respect to bioavailability, bioactivity, and toxicity. The melting point of a drug compound identifies the ease with which the drug will dissolve in an aqueous medium. To determine cellular drug absorption, the calculated logP that measures relative solubility between water and oil is useful. These physical properties are, therefore, important factors that influence the bioavailability of a drug molecule and should be taken into account in the design of a new drug.[9,10]

Considering the importance of the physical and structural properties of drug molecules, recent AI drug design algorithms include molecular representations like:

- Simplified molecular input line-entry system (SMILES) string or molecular fingerprints

- Ab initio calculations and other similar measurements for potential energy

- Atoms or bonds with differing weights for molecular graphs

- Coulomb matrices

- Fragments or bonds in molecules

- 3D coordinates for atoms

- The electron density around the molecule[11]

Kumar et al. developed six predictive models utilizing 745 compounds for training, which included: SVMs, artificial neural networks (ANNs), k-nearest neighbor algorithms, linear discriminant analysis (LDA), probabilistic neural network algorithms, and partial least square (PLS). To predict and analyze intestinal absorption activity, these were later used on 497 compounds employing parameters like molecular surface area, molecular mass, total hydrogen count, molecular refractivity, molecular volume, logP, total polar surface area, the sum of E-states indices, solubility index (logS), and rotatable bonds.[12] Along similar lines, RF and DNN-based in silico models were developed to determine the human intestinal absorption of a variety of chemical compounds.[13]

Prediction of bioactivity:

To investigate a single localized change to a drug candidate as well as the impact on its bioactivity and molecular properties, Matched Molecular Pair (MMP) analysis[14] has been used with a focus on quantitative structure-activity relationship (QSAR) studies.[15] MMPs are generated through retrosynthesis rules for *de novo* design tasks in typical studies.

A static core, along with two fragments describing the transformation, is used to chemically define a candidate molecule.[15] After the core and these fragments are encoded, three machine learning (ML) methods—random forest (RF)[16], gradient boosting machines (GBMs)[17], and DNNs[18]—are used. These were previously applied without MMP and are now used to analyze and present new fragments due to static core transformations or modifications. These models were used on the IC_{50} data to derive five different kinases and a protein-containing bromodomain.[19]

It has been observed that DNN has a better overall performance than RF or GBM in predicting compound activity.[19] Because of the exponential growth of ChEMBL and PubChem, which are public databases that contain numerous structure-activity relationship (SAR) analyses, MMP with ML may predict many bioactivity properties. These include oral exposure[20], distribution coefficient (logD)[21,22], intrinsic clearance[23], distribution, absorption, excretion, metabolism[24,25], and mode of action[26].

In attempts to further predict the bioactivity of drug candidates, other methods have recently been developed. A drug target site signature was extracted by Tristan and colleagues using a graph convolutional network. This was done by encoding distinct chemicals into a seamless latent vector space (LVS).[27] Gradient-based optimization in molecular space is permitted due to LVS, which, in turn, allows for predictions based on different binding affinity models as well as other properties.[27]

Prediction of toxicity:

In drug development, the toxicology profile of a compound is an important parameter. Hence, toxicity *optimization* during the preclinical stage is arguably the most time-consuming and resource-draining task involved in a drug discovery project.[28,29] This makes accurate predictions of the toxicity of compounds extremely valuable for drug development.

An ML algorithm called the *DeepTox* gave remarkable results in the Tox21 Data Challenge.[30,31] This was a contest in which participating groups competed to computationally predict, through specifically designed assays, a range of 12,000 environmental chemicals and drugs for 12 different toxic effects. Initially, the chemical representations of the compounds are normalized by the algorithm. Then, numerous chemical descriptors are categorized as static or dynamic and are computed as inputs for ML methods.

Static descriptors include factors like atom counts, surface area, the predefined substructure in a compound[32], 2500 pre-defined toxicophoric features[32], as well as additional chemical features extrapolated from molecular fingerprint descriptors, which are also taken into account.

Dynamic descriptors are calculated in a pre-specified way, keeping the dataset within manageable limits despite the possibility of an infinite number of dynamic features.[33] The DeepTox algorithm has shown accuracy while predicting the toxicity of compounds in typical trials.[34]

To evaluate the safety target prediction of 656 marketed drugs with respect to 73 unintended targets that may produce adverse effects[35], the *Similarity Ensemble Approach (SEA)* was used to develop an ML approach. The resulting program, eToxPred, was then applied to the dataset to analyze the toxicity and synthesis feasibility of small organic molecules, for which it demonstrated 72% accuracy.[36]

Similarly, open-source tools, like *TargeTox* and *PrOCTOR* are also used in the prediction of toxicity. TargeTox uses the guilty-by-association principle to identify target-based drug toxicity and predict risk based on a biological network. This demonstrates that entities with similar functional properties share common biological networks.[37] It can produce protein network data and unite pharmacological and functional properties in an ML classifier to predict drug toxicity.[38]

AI in designing drug molecules:

Prediction of the target 3D protein structure:

During the development of a drug, evaluating a drug compound that binds only selectively to a potential target is both challenging and expensive. Very few chemical molecules of candidate formulas have received approvals, while several drug compounds still may have unknown interactions or reactions with proteins.[39-41]

For successful treatment, it is important to assign the correct target while developing a drug molecule. Numerous proteins are responsible for the manifestation of a disease, and sometimes they are overexpressed. Hence, for selective targeting of a disease, it is vital to predict the target protein's structure in order to design the drug molecule.[42] By predicting the 3D protein structure, AI can help with structure-based drug discovery. The design is usually in accordance with the target protein site's chemical environment, thereby helping to predict the effect of a compound on the target along with safety considerations before their synthesis or production.[43]

Recently, a competitive event—the Critical Assessment of Protein Structure Prediction Contest—witnessed the launch of an AI tool: *Alpha Fold*. This performed well while predicting the 3D structure of a target protein using primary sequences and was still able to correctly predict 25 out of 43 structures. Its performance was better than that of the second-place contestant, which could correctly identify only 3 out of 43 test sequences.

It relies on trained DNNs to predict protein properties based on its primary sequence, providing both the distances between pairs of amino acids and the φ–ψ angles between neighboring peptide bonds. These probabilities are combined to give a score that determines the accuracy of the proposed 3D protein structure model. With these scoring functions, Alpha Fold evaluates the landscape of the protein structure to find similarities with predictions.[3]

Several VS experiments have found success with Naive Bayesian (NB) classifiers. Yu and colleagues used one in conjunction with 3D quantitative structure-activity relationship (QSAR) pharmacophore hypothesis modeling to find prospective inhibitors of PI3Kα, a key target protein for many cancers; in vitro assays confirmed the discovery of some novel inhibitors.[44]

To produce new and structurally diverse hits for mGlu1 receptor inhibitors[45], Jang and colleagues used an NB classifier as an indispensable step in their workflow for drug delivery. In addition, Lian and colleagues combined Support Vector Machines with their NB models to create an enhanced ensemble model capable of producing nine potent Influenza A neuraminidase inhibitors.[46]

Predicting drug-protein interactions:

It is imperative to identify drug-target interactions (DTIs) in the case of new drugs because this helps to narrow down the number of prospective candidates by detecting side effects early in the process.[47] It also enables insights into the experimental designs needed for drug discovery through the evaluations of reactions that take place between drug and target molecules.[48]

DTIs are predicted using significant computational methods that are mainly divided into three strategies:

- Ligand-based approaches[49]

- Docking approaches[50,51]

- Chemogenomic approaches

Ligand-based methods are unreliable when target proteins have insufficient known binding ligands. Docking methods require the 3D structures of proteins or drugs.[52] Therefore, research efforts have focused mainly on chemogenomic-based methods, which may give successful extrapolations of DTIs based on widely available biological data.

A large proportion of these methods are based on the assumption that similar drugs tend to bind to similar targets and vice versa.[53] To demonstrate this, Chen and colleagues[54] proposed a system that predicted ligand binding sites for proteins in DTI. In addition, Yamanishi and colleagues[55] developed a unified novel framework that was integrated with genomic, chemical, and pharmacological inputs to enhance research productivity aimed at genomic drug discovery.

It was postulated that similarity in pharmacological effect is more valued than similarity in chemical structures while predicting unknown DTIs. Keiser and colleagues[56] used a method based on chemical similarity, with the assumption that in cases of drug-protein connections, similar drugs will usually react with similar target proteins.

To calculate the relative potential energies as well as molecular structures of an atom arrangement or conformations of a molecule, molecular mechanics (MM) is usually applied in large systems.[57-59] While the electrons in the system evaluated are not considered individually, the atomic nucleus with its associated electrons is taken as a single particle.

The Born-Oppenheimer approximation has been used to justify the exclusion of electrons in the MM.[60] This allows for the uncoupling of electronic and nuclear motions so that they can be considered separately.

The differences in energy between the conformations are more significant in these calculations than the absolute values of potential energies.

The quantum mechanics (QM) principle considers molecules to be collections of nuclei and electrons without considering "chemical bonds." Therefore, QM is important for understanding the systemic behavior at the atomic level and the approximation of the wave function and for solving Schrödinger's equation.[57,61]

QM—or, alternatively, QM/MM hybrid—methods have shown remarkable potential in drug discovery due to their ability to predict protein-ligand (drug molecule) interactions.[62,63] Taking into consideration the quantum effects for the simulated system (or the region of interest, in the case of QM/MM) at the atomic level, these methods, therefore, offer better accuracy as compared to classical MM methods.

When evaluated alongside MM methods, the time-cost for QM methods is greater because MM methods tend to apply atomic coordinate-based simple energy functions.[64,65]

Therefore, when applying AI to QM methods, there is a trade-off; one must consider the accuracy of QM on the one hand as compared to the favorable time-cost of MM models.[48] AI models can match the speed at which MM methods calculate, as they have been instructed to replicate QM energies from the atom coordinates.

The study performed by Zang and colleagues suggests that ML-based computations have several advantages for applications in MM or QM calculations. The ability of the ML-based and QM calculator while predicting the potential energy co-incidence provides these advantages, which include:

- the avoidance of artificial distortions

- the elimination of a buffer zone in adaptable MM/QM applications

- accounting for the coupling period through the development of simpler methods

- the provision of a singular surface of potential energy for kinetic sampling and thermodynamic approaches[66]

When DNNs are trained for big datasets, the potential energies for quantum chemistry-derived density functional theory (DFT) should be calculated.

Artificial intelligence (AI) in advancing pharmaceutical product development:

Commercial product development, ranging from a fairly simple formulation (e.g., oral liquid, capsule, or tablet) to a formulation with a controlled release (e.g., an implant), is inherently a complex, time-consuming process.

In most cases, a primary formula of the constituent drugs is mixed with a variety of ingredients (excipients). As development and experimentation continue, the process of choosing the types and amounts of these ingredients and their manufacturing processes is optimized. These modifications then result in the build-up of large datasets that are difficult to analyze and understand.[67]

One of the earliest studies in this field was reported by Turkoglu and colleagues[68], who modeled a hydrochlorothiazide-containing direct compression tablet in order to improve the tablet strength and select the best lubricant.

In another study, Kesavan and Peck[69] modeled caffeine in a tablet formula to relate both formulation variables (like diluent types and binder concentrations) and processing variables (a type of granulator, method of addition of binder) as well as granule and tablet properties (friability, hardness, and disintegration time).

Both these investigations showed that neural networks performed better than conventional statistical methods. Subsequently, the data produced during this study were reanalyzed using a combination of genetic algorithms and neural networks.[70]

Similarly, Rocksloh and colleagues[71] used neural networks to successfully optimize the disintegration time and crushing strength of a tablet with a high dose of plant extract. In another study, Do, and colleagues[72] showed the advantages of leveraging both neural networks and genetic algorithms in the formulation of antacid tablets.

Chen and colleagues[73] used neural networks to predict the concentration of the drug in addition to the hardness of the intact tablets of ophylline when mixed with microcrystalline cellulose with the aid of their near-infrared spectra. The model performed better than a statistical model generated with the same data. Sathe and Venitz[74] also discovered the superiority of neural network models over statistical models when they predicted the dissolution of 28 diltiazem tablet formulations developed for immediate release.

Neural networks have been applied to modeling immediate-release tablet and capsule formulations, rapidly disintegrating or dissolving tablets[75], as well as a new oral microemulsion combination of rifamycin and isoniazid formulated for the treatment of tuberculosis in children.[76]

While designing controlled-release formulations, Chen and colleagues[77] used pharmacokinetic simulations and an ANN, or artificial neural network. Seven formula variables, in addition to three tablet variables, such as the size of particles, moisture content, and hardness, evaluated for 22 formulations of a chosen primary drug tablet were used as model inputs for the neural network.

A similar model was developed by Zupancic Bozic and colleagues[78] to optimize diclofenac sodium sustained-release matrix tablets. Variables like the concentration of cetyl alcohol, polyvinylpyrrolidone/K30, and magnesium stearate in addition to sampling time were chosen as inputs. Twelve nodes were included in the hidden layer. The amount of the drug released at each sampling time point (calculated as percentages) was used as the output. A trained ANN model was applied to predict the drug release profile and optimize the composition based on the percentage of compound released.[78]

Various mathematical tools, such as computational fluid dynamics (CFD), discrete element modeling (DEM), and the finite element method, have been used to evaluate the effect of the flow property of the powder on the die-filling and process of tablet compression.[79,80] CFD can also be utilized to study the impact of tablet geometry on its dissolution profile.[81] The combination of AI with these mathematical models could aid immensely in the production of pharmaceutical products.

AI in quality control and quality assurance:

In addition to its successful implementation in the performance of clinical trials, there is tremendous potential for the use of AI in manufacturing and the approval of licensing steps that must be taken when a new drug is introduced to the market.[2]

Drug candidates that are similar to the new drug will eventually progress to clinical trials, which are arguably the most cumbersome obstacles in drug development, as they are stringently controlled and require the cooperation of administrative bodies like the FDA, CMC (Chemistry, Manufacturing, and Control), etc., to obtain commercial drug licensing.

The use of AI to select subjects and optimize the trial design with appropriate screening can increase both the efficacy and the reliability of clinical trials. Although still in its infancy, efficient processes that use data similar to smart factories with good manufacturing practice (GMP)-based drug manufacturing are needed for effective AI utilization in drug production.[2]

AI can also be implemented in the regulation of in-line manufacturing processes to achieve the desired standard of the product [82]. Using ANN-based monitoring of the freeze-drying process, a combination of self-adaptive evolution along with local search and backpropagation algorithms is applied. This may be utilized to predict the temperature and desiccated-cake thickness at a future time point $(t + Dt)$ for a particular set of operating conditions, eventually helping to keep a check on the final product quality.[83]

AI in clinical trial design:

Improper patient cohort selection and recruiting mechanisms fail to bring the best-suited patients to a trial in time. Technical infrastructure is required to cope with the complexity of running a trial, especially in its later phases.

Without reliable and efficient patient monitoring, adherence control, and detection systems for clinical endpoints, a clinical trial can come up short. AI can be used as an effective tool for combating these deficiencies in design.[84]

By using a profile analysis based on the patient-specific genome–exposome, AI can assist in selecting a target population for recruitment in Phases II and III of clinical trials. This, in turn, helps in the early prediction of available drug targets in these patients.[85,86]

The preclinical discovery of molecules along with the early prediction of lead compounds before the commencement of clinical trials, while leveraging the use of ML or similar techniques for reasoning, leads to the discovery of potential drug molecules that could pass clinical trials with consideration of the selected patient population.[86]

Artificial intelligence in pharmaceutical product management:

Business to business (B2B) companies also increasingly use AI technologies to help in sales negotiations and closing. Specifically, based on several customer characteristics such as industry, size, and prior relationship, AI algorithms compute a buyer's reservation price, which can be a useful benchmark for salespeople. To strengthen customer relationships, B2B companies use AI technologies to predict a buyer's churn probability from recent purchase behaviors. Salespeople can then initiate retention measures, drawing inspiration from this guidance from the AI-generated analysis. Furthermore, companies are increasingly using AI-powered chatbots to provide quick customer service.[87]

Market prediction is essential for different distribution companies, as they implement AI in the field, such as "Business Intelligent Smart Sales Prediction Analysis," which uses a combination of time series forecasting and real-time application. This helps pharmaceutical companies to predict the sale of products in advance to prevent costs of excess stock or prevent customer loss because of shortages.[88]

A company determines its product's final price based on market analysis and cost incurred during development. When AI is applied to determine this price, the main aim is to harness its ability to mimic the thinking process of a human expert in order to assess the factors that control the pricing of a manufactured product.[89]

Pharmaceutical market of AI:

Robotics is a field within the realm of artificial intelligence. A
of systems that combine sophisticated hardware and responsive software
with detailed datasets and knowledge-based processing tools to enable
effective human-like decision-making. It enables mechanical computer-
controlled devices to perform precise, tedious tasks that may be considered
hazardous if performed by human beings. Traditional robotics applies
artificial intelligence techniques to program robot behaviors.[89]

Implantable nanorobots have been developed for the controlled delivery of
drugs and genes that require considerations such as dose adjustment,
sustained release, and controlled release. The release of the drug requires
automation controlled by AI tools, such as ANNs, fuzzy logic, and
integrators.[90] Microchip implants can be used for programmed release while
detecting the location of the implant in the body.

In 2019, Pfizer announced a partnership with *Concreto HealthAI* to help
patients suffering from solid tumors and hematologic malignancies, with
early diagnosis. Applying AI tools to Pfizer's real-world data, the company
aims to identify novel, precise treatment options and completely restructure
study designs to improve the completion time of the outcome study.

In January 2020, *Bayer* partnered with a UK-based AI-driven drug
discovery company to work on early research projects using the AI platform
and Bayer's large database. They are striving to identify and optimize new
lead structures for potential drug candidates to treat cardiovascular and
oncological diseases.

Leading organizations in the industry, also called "Big Pharma" companies
(namely, Merck, AstraZeneca, GlaxoSmithKline, Novartis, Roche, Pfizer,
Sanofi, AbbVie, Johnson & Johnson, and Bristol-Myers Squibb), have
either acquired artificial intelligence technologies or entered into mutually
beneficial collaborationism with third-party technology providers to take
advantage of the undeniable opportunities that AI brings to the table.

Several biopharmaceutical companies, such as Bayer, Roche, and Pfizer,
have teamed up with IT companies to develop platforms for the discovery
of therapies in immuno-oncology and cardiology.[85]

References/Further Reading

Go to URL

MedMantra.com/a17

Scan with a smartphone camera

CHAPTER EIGHTEEN
AI IN HEALTHCARE ROBOTICS

Robots are making their way into healthcare and transforming many aspects of this industry. By 2025, global medical robot expenditures are expected to reach over $24 billion.[1] Keep in mind that robots can't replace many aspects, such as creativity, which is why they will be integrated into some aspects of the existing healthcare system.

History of Healthcare Robotics

Robots in healthcare are not new. They emerged in the 80s, and the first robots offered surgical assistance. However, with time, AI has been integrated into the system, which has allowed for wider applications of healthcare robotics.[2] For example, medical robots can now be categorized into:

- Surgical assistance

- Service assistance

- Social assistance

- Modular assistance

- Mobile assistance

- Autonomous robotics

Robots are used in operating rooms and clinical settings to improve patient care and support healthcare professionals. The spread of COVID-19 has led to the higher deployment of robots for many tasks. The operational capabilities of these robots are limitless.

In the pandemic era, robots can reduce person-to-person contact in infectious disease wards, clean patient rooms, prepare patient rooms, and much more. The best part is that they take less time to complete these tasks and thereby enhance efficiency.

Applications of AI in Healthcare Robotics

1. Improved Diagnoses

AI is powerful when it comes to detecting patterns in healthcare data and records. AI can scan thousands of cases simultaneously and look at the different patterns and correlations between them. It is so accurate and precise that you will not find these correlations and patterns in current medical work.

Tests done to understand healthcare robotics have concluded that these robots can compete with the best doctors and surpass their abilities in no time.[3] For example, IBM Watson provides cancer diagnoses with an accuracy rate of 99%. Also, an endoscopic system from Japan that detects colon cancer in real-time has an accuracy rate of 86%.

2. Improved Performance Accuracy

We humans have limitations because we get tired and have emotions and short attention spans. AI and robots don't face these problems, which is why they can quickly improve accuracy. Thus, many hospitals worldwide are now employing robots.

Such robots can bridge the gap between technology and humans, performing tasks with improved strength, high precision, and no tremors (while performing surgery). The only thing needed is the correct software setting for the procedure being performed. The doctor can take a supervisory role. The most exciting element is micro-robots, which can go anywhere inside the body and perform micro-surgery in sensitive areas.[4]

3. Supporting Daily Tasks and Mental Health

Hospitals worldwide are opting for service robots that perform daily tasks such as routine checkups. These robots are used in conjunction with healthcare professionals, and they aim to assist. Many of these robots are utilized in eldercare and similar fields.

Companion and conversational robots make senior patients feel less lonely and remind them to stay positive. The robots also remind patients to take medicines, and perform routine daily tasks for them.[5] Think of these robots as personal assistants for seniors and other such people.

The robots come with built-in personalities and the capability of sentiment analysis. These qualities are helpful for depressed patients, as they improve the patients' quality of life. More such robots will be deployed in the future.

4. Remote Treatment

While it might seem like remote treatment was developed during the pandemic, the idea first arose in the 90s from Defense Advanced Research Projects Agency (DARPA).[6] However, at that time, we didn't have strong communication networks to offer necessary support to soldiers on the battlefield. Current 4G, 5G, and satellite communication technologies have made this problem irrelevant.

DARPA continues to fund efforts to promote remote treatment. Keep in mind that robots still require human assistance and supervision for hygiene purposes and many other tasks. That is why the concept of remote treatment is still more complex and is not currently cost-effective.

As healthcare robotics improve and new remote treatment methods are discovered, we will see a boom in remote medical and surgical management.[7,8]

Top Medical Robots That Are Transforming Healthcare

1. Endoscopy Bot

Endoscopy is a checkup procedure in which a tiny camera on a long tube is inserted into the body through a natural opening to search for disease, foreign objects, or damage. The procedure is delicate and uncomfortable for patients.[9] However, medical companies such as Medineering have improved the process with robots.

These robots are flexible and slender and can be driven like remote-controlled (RC) cars to the precise location that the healthcare professional requires. These bots can stay there and perform any endoscopic procedure without hassle.

Another fantastic invention in this department is capsule endoscopies. In the capsule procedure, a pill-sized robot is swallowed. It then travels along the digestive tract, where it takes pictures and gathers data to be evaluated for diagnosis.[10] Gone are the days when endoscopy was a painful and delicate procedure for the patient.

2. DaVinci

DaVinci is the standard for robot-assisted surgery and one of the best medical robots out there.[11]

The surgeon always maintains full control of the machine, but the strides it has made are nothing short of brilliant. Healthcare professionals use the DaVinci system for many operations that can be done with a few incisions and precision. This lowers the risk of infection and promotes fast healing and less bleeding.

The most shocking part is that DaVinci has been in the healthcare game for over eighteen years and is further advancing as time passes. However, many big tech companies have developed similar systems with more autonomy, which is why we might soon be seeing updated and more autonomous DaVincis.

3. Disinfectant Bot

While hospitals look clean, they are some of the dirtiest places out there. With the pandemic and COVID-19 on the rise, they are now hotbeds of many viruses and infectious diseases. You could go to a hospital for treatment and come out with a new illness.

That is why hospital rooms must stay clean and germ-free at all times. Of course, when it comes to such a vast space, the cleaning staff can do only so much. That is where modern disinfectant robots come into play, as they can easily clean the entire hospital without errors.

These robots autonomously move from one room to another. Once they enter the room, they use high-powered UV rays for a few minutes.[12] They emit these rays until no harmful microorganisms are left in the hospital room or area.

4. Companion Bots

Not all medical robots are used for high-risk procedures and treatments. Some are used to provide company and to help people feel mentally better.

Millions of people are disabled or elder or suffer from chronic illnesses. To function well, such people need regular checkups and companionship. In many areas, there are shortages of professional caretakers, which is why a companion robot is needed. These robots improve the quality of life and provide care to many people.

For example, they can make conversations, carry out routine checkups, and ensure that the patients feel less lonely. BUDDY is a new robot in this arena, and it interacts with patients on a unique emotional level.[13] Due to these advancements, it won the Innovation Award in 2018.

5. Nurse Robots

While many people praise doctors, nurses go underappreciated. They are the backbone of any medical setting. Without nurses, a medical setting will not work optimally, and there will be many issues. Globally, there is a nurse shortage, which is why researchers have introduced nurse robots into the mix.

These robots can fill out digital paperwork, monitor patient conditions, measure vital signs, and much more. Some of the most recent nurse robots can also perform tasks like moving gurneys and drawing blood. We can only wait and see what else these nurse robots have to offer in the future.

Nurse robots are critical for any hospital because they make processes more efficient, reduce cost, and save the time of many people. In the long run, they will allow the hospital to take care of patients in a much better way.[14]

Top Three Ways Robots Can Improve Healthcare

1. Slashing Rates of Hospital-Acquired Infections

Whenever you visit a hospital, you are at risk of contracting an infection. According to the CDC, one out of thirty-one patients has an infection associated with hospitals. UV disinfectant robots can significantly slash the rate of these infections.[15]

In the long run, hospitals will be less burdened and people will feel more safe entering medical settings. Many recent studies have shown that UV can decrease the amount of live coronavirus on surfaces by 99% and airborne coronavirus by 99.9%. Several companies are creating robots to battle the virus in hospitals and reduce infection rates.

2. Offering Contactless Access to Healthcare

The best part about medical robots is that they can easily assist in monitoring patients. These robots are typically equipped with a screen, a keyboard, a camera, and medical tools. Such devices allow doctors to communicate with their patients and provide care remotely.[16]

As COVID-19 keeps increasing, many people are isolating and going into quarantine. During such times, contactless access to healthcare is the best option because it reduces the risk of doctors contracting the virus. It also allows patients to quickly receive healthcare. Even after COVID-19 is gone, we will see these robots in hospitals and other medical facilities.

3. Ensuring Safe Lifting of Patients

Did you know that nurses need to lift their patients more than forty times on a regular day? Such heavy physical activity is a big part of the job, and it can put both the nurse and the patient at risk of injury. Robots designed for this purpose can ease the burden on nurses and easily lift patients a hundred times a day.

To that end, the Riken-SRK Collaboration Centre created Robear in Japan. The robot is bear-shaped, weighs forty kilograms, and can easily lift and move patients.[17] It moves the patients onto wheelchairs, helps them stand, and turns them frequently to prevent bedsores.

The Robear is still in its experimental phase, but it shows great promise for the future of nursing and patient care. In the long run, it will relieve the staff from burdensome and physically straining tasks.

Conclusion

That is everything you need to know about AI in healthcare robotics. Soon, we will witness more robots being employed in hospitals and other medical settings.

Robots will never replace humans, but they will make the healthcare system more efficient. The primary aim of such technologies is to improve processes without burdening human staff and personnel. We can't wait to see more of such technologies and how they revolutionize the healthcare industry in the coming years.

References/Further Reading

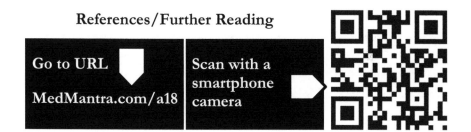

Go to URL

MedMantra.com/a18

Scan with a smartphone camera

"By far the greatest danger of Artificial Intelligence is that people conclude too early that they understand it."

- Eliezer Yudkowsky

AI IN ELECTRONIC HEALTH RECORDS, HEALTH INSURANCE, AND MEDICAL EDUCATION

CHAPTER NINETEEN
AI IN ELECTRONIC HEALTH RECORDS

Brief history

Medical records were always kept and documented on papers, filing systems, lab reports, and prescription notes up until the 1960s. Such records were labeled with the patient's name or the clinical number for identification and were kept in long vertical shelves for storage purposes. A man named Lockheed developed a clinical information system during the mid-1960s; it was on this basis that the electronic health record system began to evolve. Other companies had begun improving this technology, and by 1980 the use of the electronic health record (EHR) for medical purposes had increased. By 2004, medical records had been converted into electronic health records and also adopted into the healthcare industry.

What is an electronic health record (EHR)?

An EHR is a compilation of all medical records and personal health records of the patients. An EHR provides an in-depth view of patients' health by assembling demographics, a wide range of test results, immunization documents, past and present prescriptions, medical history, family history, and history of present illness so as to increase treatment productivity. An EHR is designed to store data and record the status of a patient's health over time. Using an EHR defeats the purpose of keeping medical paper records in ensuring accurate data representation of health. In essence, an EHR is an electronic detailed health record that provides a wider scope of patients' health.

Is an EMR (electronic medical record) the same as an EHR (electronic health record)?

Though EMRs and EHRs are both non-analog documentation of a patient's health information and the terms can be used interchangeably, or sometimes referred to as the electronic patient record, they serve different purposes. An EMR is an electronic medical record, which is a digital representation of a patient's one-time chart. More often than not, an EMR stays within the confines of a doctor's office or a hospital. An EHR, however, contains multiple EMRs and provides a broader view of the patient's medical history. Most people like to think of EHRs as a compilation of all EMRs. This may be true because EHRs cover the general health status of a patient, while EMRs are brief medical records. Both EMRs and EHRs may be seen to perform the same function on the outside, but when looked at in detail, an EHR focuses on the overall health of the patient.

Overview

The principal aim of using EHRs is to provide easy access to patients' medical data to both medical providers and the patients themselves. A standard EHR should be able to provide secure transferrable medical data in the event that a patient changes doctors or hospitals. The EHR is very instrumental in preserving the patient's records and offering accurate medical solutions. The EHR was originally designed to be very effective and cause a major breakthrough in the healthcare industry, but along the line, it developed functional problems, which, in turn, reduced the efficiency of the EHR. This caused a reduced efficiency in the healthcare delivered by medical providers. The dysfunction of the EHR has been known to cause major burnout among medical providers, thus reducing their overall productivity. Taking all these problems into consideration, it was later concluded that technological advancement would be the best option for harnessing all the benefits of the EHR.[1]

After the HITECH (Health Information Technology for Economic and Clinical Health) act was passed in 2009, EHRs were brought into the healthcare industry to improve the use of data among medical practitioners. At the time EHRs were introduced into the system, about 48% of medical providers were using them. Later on, the percentage increased to 85%. This system was designed to work and completely transform the method of operation of the healthcare sector, but it had begun developing problems. Research was conducted, and the results concluded that EHRs did more harm than good because they took more time to respond and provided less accurate information. Moreover, EHRs encountered difficulties in sharing data between medical providers and, hence, resulted in medical providers diverting their attention away from patients. Most people perceived that EHRs were still capable of causing transformation, but there had to be another way to limit drawbacks and increase efficiency. Fortunately, the incorporation of artificial intelligence (AI) into EHRs seems to hold a promising future for the healthcare industry once again. EHR/EMR vendors are beginning to adapt by incorporating AI into their products.

EHRs with artificial intelligence

Artificial intelligence is one of those technologies that evolved over time to imitate human reasoning in computerized systems. With relevance to artificial intelligence, John McCarthy said, "Every aspect of learning or any other feature of intelligence can in principle be so precisely described that a machine can be made to simulate it. An attempt will be made to find how to make machines use language, form abstractions and concepts, solve [the] kinds of problems now reserved for humans, and improve themselves."

The incorporation of artificial intelligence into electronic health records has produced better and more effective results. Not only that, but it has also made data widely available. With machine learning tools, EHRs can perform advanced functions like ambient learning and predictive analytics. Putting together AI and EHRs will properly structure the amassed data and interpret such data in a less complex way, which will, in turn, make it easier to proffer solutions.

The merging of the healthcare industry with data science can facilitate an increase in the efficiency of healthcare operations. Artificial intelligence through EHRs can provide quality medical data and analysis, which, in turn, can help the healthcare industry provide better management. Over the years, the use of artificial intelligence or machine learning has proven to be effective in many fields. Out of the many applications of AI, it was found to be very useful in the medical sector and can enhance the productivity of healthcare providers through the use of augmented EHRs.

More discoveries have been made with regard to the effects of using machine learning-augmented EHRs to strengthen hospital management systems. Apart from providing accurate and complete personal health information, EHRs grant quick and secure access to healthcare providers by sharing the electronic records in the event that the clinicians or allied health professionals are changed. They also enable well-structured medical care with reduced risks and errors, facilitating reliable drug prescriptions. Overall, they constitute a safe and cost-effective method for storing and managing health data.

AI with relevance to EHRs

Artificial intelligence (AI) is considered one possible way to limit the problems associated with using EHRs. The director of MedStar Health's National Center for Human Factors in Healthcare noticed that the introduction of artificial intelligence into EHRs produced far more efficient results. More AI-augmented EHR models were created, and an increase in efficiency and functionality was recorded. The more the machine-learning models were fed the right data through algorithms, the higher their productivity was. Later discoveries further proved that if the data was properly grouped according to type, it produced more refined and useful results. The healthcare industry is data-bound, which means that most of its work is data-based, and its response varies according to the data received.

With the inclusion of AI, the EHR can process data more efficiently, principally through data mining and data extraction.

- *Data Mining*: Through data mining, the EHR can intelligently trace patterns in large data sets and transform such data into an understandable structure fit for use. Data mining in itself is the extraction of knowledge from the discovery of patterns in the database. Data mining is achieved through the analysis of large-quantity data into groups of data records ranging from cluster analysis to sequential pattern mining. The patterns formed are the summarized input data that is further used in predictive analysis through a decision support system. This machine learning technique will enable the EHR to bring together relevant information from medical history and treatment records to further assist in decision-making. In the case of patients, data mining will make available different treatment types and outcomes for similar cases.

- *Data Extraction*: Through data extraction, the EHR can recollect ungrouped data from data input and further process it to get an understandable data output. EHRs that use this machine learning technique are most suitable for medical research and storing data related to public health. This AI technique will group data based on specific terms and results across the EHR's database.

- *Predictive Analytics*: EHR with incorporated AI simplifies data processing and identifies the pattern of grouped data to predict occurring propensities across various health records. With a reference database, a machine learning EHR can foretell likely outcomes based on the reference. Predictive analytics is a machine learning technique that provides a wide range of possibilities for medical practitioners to look into and make accurate decisions from.

- *Natural Language Processing*: This AI tool is used to program computers to know how to analyze natural language data. Basically, natural language processing is the interaction between computers and human language. Former EHR models were known to cause physician burnout during "check-in" sessions because they had to manually input the patient's complaints, the analysis, and the recommendations themselves. This is not to say that the former EHR models could not document it; rather, the amount of time they took in documenting it made the machine a primary focus of the physicians. EHRs with AI can document conversations between patients and doctors and simplify them to properly fill out the EHR. As a result, burnout will be reduced, and there will be more of a focus on the interaction between a doctor and a patient. This machine learning tool is very flexible and is used not only for verbal transcription but also in data finding (a portion of data mining) by context, terms, and phrases. In 2017, an iOS app was launched using this machine learning tool. This app, named Kara, could listen to conversations between the patient and doctor and then process them into orders, clinical notes, and diagnoses.[2]

EHRs are capable of so much more with artificial intelligence (AI).[3] Here's why:

- *Data Visualization*: This AI method is responsible for providing readable information to medical providers. Data visualization utilizes statistical graphs, charts, and information graphics to communicate information. Visualization is key in effectively accessing data from the EHR. Visualization represents the data in the electronic health record well so that it can be easily understood. However, the visualization template must be customized within the framework to make the patients' data comprehensible. In general, this machine learning technique provides easy access to data when needed.

- *Privacy, Compliance, and Confidentiality*: Any type of data can be sensitive depending on its content. We know that an EHR carries sensitive content of more than just one person. For this reason, an EHR is more susceptible to breach and data loss. Machine learning tools can protect your privacy no matter what. The only time your privacy might be breached is when your health records are transferred to another doctor.

- *Predictive Algorithms*: AI has proven useful in predicting medical outcomes via data analysis. The predictive algorithms will provide information and possible implications of the patient's health to the medical provider. It is on this basis that the medical provider will take action accordingly.

- *Decisiveness*: Determining an underlying condition or the most suitable prescription for a patient is one of the most critical decisions a medical provider has to make. It is critical because any mistake in diagnosis or drug prescription can cost the patient his or her life. Machine learning-augmented EHRs have a higher percentage of accurate diagnosis and, as a result, can positively increase the decisiveness of the medical providers.

- *Data Availability*: Artificially intelligent EHRs have granted the healthcare industry and medical providers access to a large amount of data that can influence problem-solving strategies in the healthcare system of a healthcare organization and the nation at large. The more accurate the accessed data, the more problems would be solved in healthcare.

- **_Sharing Data_**: The lack of adequate data increases the risks taken by medical providers. If a patient's EHR record cannot be accessed by the right people, it means that the EHR is experiencing disruption of workflow. Consequently, medical providers will not be able to work with any available data to provide quality healthcare for patients. However, machine learning EHRs can improve data interoperability within a healthcare organization and the healthcare industry at large.

- **_Artificial Documentation_**: Before the incorporation of AI into EHRs, medical providers took it upon themselves to manually input and correct data saved by the EHRs. During this time, medical providers would pay more attention to the machine than to patients. Because of the natural language processing (NLP) machine learning tool, EHRs can now accurately document clinic notes needed for making the correct diagnosis.

- **_Listening EHRs_**: Normally, medical providers listen to their patients' complaints and draw a list of possible conclusions. Most of the time, before a final result is obtained, the medical provider will have exhausted almost all the options through trial and error. Listening EHRs, however, will help the medical provider give full attention to patients while they document patients' complaints and predict a more accurate list of outcomes.

Will EHRs be better in the future?

Just like no one would have thought it possible to create an electronic health record, the extent to which EHRs will advance cannot be definitively predicted. However, we can guess that in a few years, EHRs will be capable of securely and efficiently transferring patient's data over a long distance to medical providers. Also, clinicians can provide medical care and prescriptions without physically meeting with the patient.

One way or another, with one technique or another, AI plays a very important role in the operation of EHR. It provides new levels of accessibility to data and a framework for data, which, in turn, makes the merging of AI with EHRs one of the biggest breakthroughs in healthcare operations. As things evolve, there will be newer models of machine learning EHRs, thus leading to better and more cost-effective healthcare.

Four vendors and their role in merging AI with EHRs/EMRs

EHR vendors and the healthcare industry noticed increased effectiveness of EHRs when merged with artificial intelligence. Four of these healthcare software companies have developed four models of EHRs that are being used by thousands of hospitals worldwide to hold their patients' health/medical records.[4]

Epic Systems Corporation

Epic is one of the most renowned healthcare software companies. It develops and manages its EHR with health information exchange software (initially between Epic software only). Later on, Epic and all other major healthcare software companies set a common Interoperability software standard as a requirement for electronic health records. Along the line, the software started developing problems that caused major physician burnout, especially among Danish healthcare professionals. The system remained unstable and slow during this period. As a result, many medical practitioners began losing hope in it. In 2015, however, Epic had begun developing EHR models with artificial intelligence by using algorithms to determine the outcomes of real-life situations. The company began selling these models and developing newer and more advanced ones, leading to more sales. Epic is one of the companies to provide solutions in the healthcare industry by taking advantage of artificial intelligence for clinical decision-making and population health management. Epic uses AI's predictive analysis method to predict patient risk levels, mortality, sepsis, hospital-acquired infections, hospital readmissions, the utilization of emergency departments, and more. With AI, EHR customers can easily access their records. Epic is currently in the process of developing virtual computerized scribes. The company now has many models of machine learning EHRs, with each model being targeted at a specific purpose.

Cerner Corporation

Cerner, previously known as PGI & Associates, is a US-based company that offers health information technology services. By 1990, Cerner had begun developing an IT system, called HNA (Health Network Architecture), to automate healthcare processes. Four years later, Cerner had sold about 30 full HNA systems. As time passed, Cerner kept expanding and upgrading its HNA systems. From 2002 to 2014, there was documentation of failures of the computerized health system until it merged with Amazon Web Services. Recently, Cerner has taken to machine learning initiatives to enhance the operational effectiveness of the health systems. Like Epic, Cerner is taking advantage of artificial intelligence for clinical decision support and population health management. Specifically, Cerner is utilizing AI to predict heart failure and hospital readmission. Other AI applications of Cerner include Charge Assist (coding support), Chart Assist (documentation support), Chart Search (NLP-driven search engine), Virtual Scribe (conversation transcription), and Voice Assist (use of voice commands to complete certain tasks). It is the only vendor at the time of this writing that offers coding and documentation support.

Meditech

Medical Information Technology, otherwise known as MEDITECH, is a software and services company that sells healthcare information systems. The company initially began by developing the MIIS programming language, an implementation of MUMPS. Later, it adopted the MAGIC programming language for healthcare information systems and another software platform known as client/server. While the MAGIC programming language runs the code, the client/server executes it. On January 29, 2020, MEDITECH announced the launch of a mobile application software called Expanse Patient Care. This software allows nurses and therapists to conduct administrative tasks. MEDITECH aims to enable voice navigation within patient charts and ambient listening to further promote virtual assistance. For this reason, MEDITECH's main focus is on artificial intelligence beyond its existing machine learning models.

Allscripts Healthcare Solutions, Inc.

This is a US-based vendor that provides electronic health records and practice management systems to physicians, hospitals, and other healthcare providers. Allscripts had already merged with about two of its competitors at the end of 2010, and by 2012 its small practice software was discontinued because it did not meet the EHR standards. In March 2013, however, Allscripts bought a developer of system interfaces and data analytics tools and a developer of personal health records, namely, dbMotion, Ltd. and Jardogs, LLC, respectively. By 2020, Allscripts had been named best in the category of Global Acute Care EMR, according to KLAS (Kumon Leysin Academy of Switzerland), and had formed a merger with Israel's Sheba Medical Center. As a result of this merger, this vendor has been working on a model to predict acute kidney injury via machine learning to reduce clinicians' workload.

Future of machine learning-augmented electronic health records

The history of EHR is a long one and is still being written. With the constant evolution of technology and artificial intelligence, the future of EHRs is, without a doubt, very bright. Some medical practitioners suggest the integration of telemedicine—an access to virtual healthcare. Also, EHRs by then would have mastered the machine learning technique of predictive analytics. This means that EHRs will be able to accurately predict and avoid negative outcomes in real-time.

Summary

In this text, we discussed the brief history of EHRs, how they came about, and how they evolved every step of the way. Upon reviewing the similarities and differences between the EMR and EHR, we were able to decide which was best for handling large data over a long period. Principally, we looked at the effect of artificial intelligence through machine learning on EHRs and how it was able to transform the failing system into something it was originally designed to be. Furthermore, we acquainted ourselves with the four vendors of EHR, their histories, and how they incorporated artificial intelligence into their EHR systems. Finally, we concluded that EHR with artificial intelligence would only get better in the future.

Conclusion

The transformation of the healthcare industry began when artificial intelligence was brought into electronic health records. It was after this that EHRs began to gain more recognition. The roles each machine learning technique played in the EHR go on to prove that the EHR is capable of much more than thought. AI-integrated EHR systems were, and will be, able to achieve more feats through data analytics, such as data mining, data extraction, and data visualization. They could, and will, also predict outcomes in real-time through natural language processing and predictive analytics. Overall, the utilization of artificial intelligence with electronic health records will store large and grouped sets of data, enhance predictive outcomes, narrow the endless options through document searching, secure patients' health data, and, above all, prevent clinician burnout.

References/Further Reading

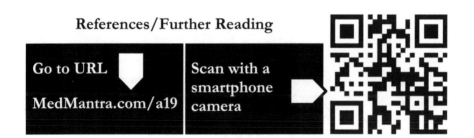

Go to URL
MedMantra.com/a19

Scan with a smartphone camera

CHAPTER TWENTY

HEALTH AND MEDICAL DATA OWNERSHIP

Patients' medical records and health data lay open to the healthcare system and the pertinent medical professionals. The medical data is currently owned and stored by the hospitals, corporations, or doctors; although, it is the patient who pays to generate this data. Many situations have arisen that sometimes have called into question the credibility of the data in the doctor's hands.[1]

Doctors, at times, are prone to overlook the prevailing health conditions of the patients. Patients, on the other hand, shower their faith blindly upon doctors. This works in many scenarios, but it has its own drawbacks. In the forthcoming discussion points, we will look upon the importance of patients owning their own data. Everyone must understand how the healthcare industry works in general and how it can potentially benefit or harm us.

Using EHR for Patient Data

There has been a consensus on the use of electronic health records (EHR) to understand the disease state of a person. EHR is an efficient way of tracking disease susceptibility in a personalized manner.[2] However, much research says otherwise. EHR in itself does not hold all the health records of a person and, therefore, cannot be reliably used to predict disease susceptibility, outcome, and prognosis.[3]

While EHR is widely used to outline the disease state and medical condition, it cannot be confidently labeled as being the best method. Patients must own their medical and health-related data to better understand what they specifically seek from a doctor. This allows patients to explore the physiology of their bodies, thereby allowing for a proper doctor-patient relationship.

Controlling Your Data

A significant concern being raised today is that we are not in complete charge of our data. Instead, the healthcare system has sole ownership of our medical data.[4] This raises a big question: Is our data secure with healthcare institutions? The confidentiality of our bodies and health must be well-secured for obvious reasons.

Having access to our health data allows us to better understand our body physiology, enabling us to communicate with doctors better during healthcare checkups.

Essentially, the law itself should address this fallacy in the system. Every patient has the right to confidentiality and information. Every patient should be given the right to access their medical data because the healthcare system itself has many flaws which, if breached, allow for enormous mishaps, physical and otherwise. The possibility of the data security breach and the misuse of our data in an already flawed healthcare system cannot be ignored.

Data Sharing with Third Parties

One of the most significant concerns about letting the healthcare system control our data is the potential risk of data sharing with third parties. Our data can easily be misused by third parties such as insurance companies[5], which can mold the data to avail financial advantages from our medical records for their companies.

More often than not, our data can be sold or hacked into without our informed consent. This allows for undue situations that can take place. We have no idea when or how our data can be misused.

There have been reports of hacking and selling of healthcare data. Our data can be transmitted across several industries in no time, and the consequences are dreadful to imagine. Therefore, having control of our data ensures safety and security to stop our data from being misused. By securing it in a central server accessible to only us, we can better protect our data.

Why Should You Own Your Data?

There are several reasons why we should be given sole ownership of our data. The primary reason why we should own our data is to prevent data breaches. Further, the following are the reasons why we should be allowed to own our data.

- *You are Paying for this Data*

  We must all know that every time we get any biochemical or microbiological tests done or even visit our doctors, we give our information to them. We pay for all of these tests, yet we do not receive access to everything. We spend an exorbitant amount of money on our data throughout our lives, yet we do not obtain the accessibility that we should be given.

- *Your Medical Data has Value*

  Rarely is any data more valuable than our medical records. They contain everything about us: our anatomy, physiology, and biochemistry. Having access to this data is vital to understanding our bodies.

- *Privacy is Essential*

  We have discussed how third parties can easily use our data for their financial and other benefits.[6] Data hacking and theft can also be a consequence. Having ownership of our data ensures privacy and gives us adequate control over ourselves.

- *You get to Share it*

  Finally, we must have sole control over our data and be given the right to share our data with whoever we deem necessary.

References/Further Reading

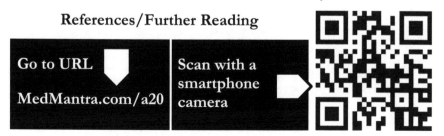

Go to URL
MedMantra.com/a20

Scan with a smartphone camera

CHAPTER TWENTY-ONE
AI IN HEALTH INSURANCE

The insurance industry is the central pillar of the economy by virtue of the magnitude of its investment, the scale of premiums plans it collects, and, more importantly, the essential role it plays by covering the personal health and business risks. The majority of the healthcare spending comes from health insurance, with the private healthcare insurance expenses crossing $1.1 billion in 2017, according to Centers for Medicare and Medicaid Services. This corresponds to a 4.2% rise from last year and constitutes around 34% of the total National Health Expenditure.[1]

As the world population is aging, the current health insurance system is being cut off at the knees with the increasing workload and complexity of claims processing. According to OECD predictions, the current insurance system is incapable of hosting future advances and is in dire need of major reforms. With the new diseases being diagnosed and the long-term treatment of chronic diseases, the insurers will need to invest in ways to handle claims more proactively—a process that is mostly manual and takes anywhere from weeks to months.

Artificial intelligence has been adopted by many health insurance companies to take advantage of this revolutionizing technology in claims processing, insurance package selection, improving cost efficiency, minimizing waste of health resources, and detecting fraudulent claims.

Application of AI in health insurance

Artificial intelligence has the potential to revolutionize all the industries on the face of this planet and is thus known as the 'Fourth Industrial Revolution.' The health insurance industry is no different in this regard. The lack of flexibility in the health insurance industry can be eliminated with the use of intelligent algorithms. For example, an AI system can help in coining customized insurance plans for patients suffering from chronic diseases. The extent of potential gains is beyond the horizon.

Artificial intelligence is capable of contributing more to the healthcare and insurance industry. Machine learning algorithms can augment the expertise of case managers in processing claims. This hybrid scheme will increase the efficiency of workers in the screening of claims and will help them make better-informed decisions. Intelligent algorithms continuously evolve with the increasing flow of data—making their own ever-changing rules and revamping the conventional inflexible methods of claims management. A system operating on such algorithms can precisely flag the errors in claims applications while decreasing the human effort in scratching around for possible discrepancies.

Now, we will discuss how machine learning can help fasten claims processing, detect frauds in insurance claims, the role it can play in minimizing the healthcare expense burden, and how it can be of value in predicting investment outcomes.

Revolutionizing claims processing

A glimpse at the process will help understand the complexity of insurance claims processing and the probability of mismanagement. A mid-sized insurer with around 1.5 million customers gets to deal with 0.7 million claims per year in the name of cost refunds. These claims go through a screening process that requires several hundred workers to check if the claim is valid and make interventions where required.

The whole process drains the human resources of a company only to find the majority of claims incorrect. The workers can decide on the basis of available patient history from hospital forms to accept or decline the claim request—an intervention linked to a specific rule book of the company. The correct interventions are important, as the claims audit procedures absorb precious time, manpower, and resources. However, with this current sluggish system, the health insurers can cut the amount to be paid by merely 3%. It's becoming ever challenging to correctly identify fraudulent claims and is costing both health insurers and providers a fortune.

Machine learning algorithms enable prompt and accurate identification of false claims in a really short amount of time, i.e., in a matter of seconds. The algorithms are trained on already processed claims data of millions of cases. It can efficiently tag only those cases that need human intervention and defer acceptable cases to automatic processing—that, too, at superhuman speed. The system also comments the reason for rejecting the claim, resulting in a quicker, simpler claims management process.

This way, the auditor can focus on cases that are unusual from 'correct' claims determined by AI. This self-learning system only gets better and better as it learns the results of human intervention in cases it was unable to resolve.

On the client's end, this system requires the least amount of effort to submit claim forms. They simply need to take photos of their hospital bill and submit it from the smartphone app and, within few seconds, receive the transaction slip for the amount credited to their account—simple and insanely fast!

Detect fraudulent claims

Fraud detection in hospital claims can also be empowered with AI. For example, the general cost of hospital treatment in Germany amounts to around €73 billion, which accounts for 30-40 percent of the expenses in insurers' budget. However, the ratio of false claims received is as high as 10%. Identifying these false claims with certainty would benefit both health insurers and providers—a win-win deal.

A software company based in New Jersey is using machine learning algorithms to detect and notify insurers of fraud on its custom insurance platform. The name of the company is 'Azati' and was founded in 2001. The company's AI system is trained on huge data of previously processed claims. Fraudulent claims can be identified by detecting connections between data submitted to the platform and revealed to the health insurance company through digital notifications. If the system detects a potential fraudulent case when parsing new applications, it notifies professionals at the insurance company so that an investigation and possible intervention can be done. The software platform also provides details for flagged claims, describing the points used in making that determination. Azati claims that it has helped an unnamed company detect fraudulent claims with three times more accuracy than before—owing to its AI algorithms, and the amount of precious human time saved is another pearl of it.

Cut the health costs

According to OECD, an estimated 20% of healthcare spending is wasted globally.[2] The Institute of Medicine (IOM) reckons this figure to be around 30%. In light of both estimates, the top 15 healthcare budget countries waste an average of 1,100 to 1,700 USD per person in a year, whereas the bottom 50 countries spend around 120 USD per person in a year. In other words, the average per-person waste of money in the top 15 countries is 10 to 15 times more than the average amount spent on healthcare by the bottom 50 countries. Digging deeper into statistics showed that the factors causing this waste include over-treatment, failure of healthcare delivery, and inappropriate care delivery, which are preventable system inefficiencies.

The human experts working in the health insurance industry are prone to make mistakes, not due to lack of expertise but because human nature is fallible. This preventable human error is a huge burden on the insurance system. AI can change the fundamental way a health insurance system works by suggesting accurate diagnoses and predicting the cost of treatments across different hospitals in a state.

Temple University Health System (TUHS), based in Pennsylvania, has benefitted from AI implementation in this regard. Its employees working on the TUHS health plan were infrequently scheduling for medical appointments that increase the insurance expenses. This was estimated to be causing four percent revenue loss per year.

After working in collaboration with Accolade, an AI-powered platform, TUHS was able to dramatically reduce its healthcare costs. The company official said that they achieved around 50 percent more employee engagement and saved more than two million dollars in one year after using AI. In the next year, those cost savings in health care claims have more than quadrupled—amounting to 9.8 million dollars.

Personalized packages

In countries with private health insurance, like the USA, certain treatments such as cancer care are so expensive that only the privileged with premium insurance plans can afford it. Whereas in countries with socialized medicine, where everyone has access to basic health care, new medical interventions are hard to roll out on a nationwide scale, as the system cannot afford it, decreasing the overall standard of health.

Helping clients decide the insurance plan according to their health status is an arduous process with current rule books. It is nearly impossible to list all the rules that go into policy-making, and it gets more and more challenging with new diseases being diagnosed and newer treatments coming out all the time. This is further crippled by the U.S. law that only permits consideration of a mere five factors for calculating premiums. These factors include age, tobacco addiction, location, the applicant (individual vs. family), and plan category. Analyzing the needs of the client based on this limited data is a shot in the dark.

The health insurers must be able to assess the risk flawlessly in order to offer the right premium. If they offer low price packages, it can cost them a fortune. But, if they go a little above the expected cost, they might lose that client next year. Owing to this, the value of their investment always remains questionable.

Prognos is an example of a platform for health insurance companies that are using AI algorithms to accurately assess the level of risk involved in a particular case. They run predictive analysis on each of the new clients to determine which of the members will cost them more in the long term and which ones won't, so the insurers can disburse their resources accordingly. They have trained their algorithms on a large dataset comprising clinical diagnostics data, with 20 billion records of 200 million patients. It is capable of early prediction of the incidence of disease, need for treatment, hospital readmission rates, clinical trial opportunity, and level of risk involved by running algorithms on more than 30 diseases. This provided us with insight into already existing data that was unseen to human workers and help tune the premiums in favor of benefitting both parties.

Interactive Bots

Gone are the days when customers needed to visit health insurance offices or the insurers needed to send workers to inquire about insurance policies or sign clients, respectively. The ambiguity of health premiums had the clients confused about what treatments are covered by their insurance plans and what is the status of their claim processing request. Above that, the stubborn insurance industry, with its tedious workers and long queues, made it really hard to inquire and extract information regarding insurance status.

AI-powered bots promise a solution to the above-mentioned drawbacks of red tape in health insurance. Chatbots can play a crucial role in the efforts to scale for client's needs. That's not to say that health insurers plan on having a monopoly on chatbots and other AI-augmented fronts. What is surprising here is that the insurance industry, with long hold perception of being inflexible, is investing a fortune in getting their hands-on AI bots. According to the survey by Global Trends Study, there is an average investment of 124 million USD per company in this technology. That's 54 million USD more than the average investment across all other industries listed in the 2017 survey.[3]

Trying to comprehend the differences between term-life versus whole-life insurance can be confusing if you're unfamiliar with the field. A chatbot can help reduce this confusion or even eliminate it by using natural language processing algorithms, thus reducing confusion jargon and increasing the chances of a customer opting for an insurance plan. Also, chatbots are available all the time every day and are not limited to business hours only. No one knows when a calamity will happen—road traffic accidents and life-threatening events can and do occur at all times of the day, requiring an insurance claim. People often find themselves restrained to call within working hours if they need help in filing a claim. A chatbot is online at all times, even during holidays and at night. Also, its performance remains unparalleled with high call volume, so customers don't have to wait for hours before their request is answered.

According to a McKinsey report[4], "Chatbots will be the key source of communication for the insurance customers by 2030, and the human personnel engaging will drop by more than 70 percent compared to 2018. China is already leading in this technology by using chatbots in its largest insurance company, ZhongAn Tech. Around 97% of the time its customers interact with AI bots when they reach out to check the benefits, subscribe for coverage, or submit a medical claim; the remaining 3% of the requests are directed to human representatives."

The AI-driven chatbots are being used by 68% of the insurers, as pointed by an Accenture survey[5], to reach out to their customers. And there are reports that more than 2 billion USD can be saved by health insurance companies by using this technology for interacting with customers.

Conclusion

Up until now, the health insurance industry was not doing enough to serve the clients because of routine stuff burdening the stakeholders. Machine learning is capable of handling the massive datasets that need to be analyzed and processed to streamline health insurance workflows. Artificial intelligence is tantalizing the insurance industry with its promising potential to revolutionize the way claims management works these days.

It goes without saying that AI technologies will play a major role in healthcare management. But looking at the future, the solutions to the challenges faced by health care may not be as easy as we would like to believe. They will require careful planning and participation of governments, the private sector, and the citizens. In anticipation of these future trends, we can expect to see an increased implementation of AI-augmented projects in the health insurance industry among major stakeholders endeavoring to decrease costs and scale-up performance.

References/Further Reading

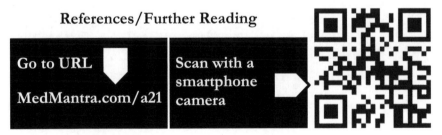

Go to URL
MedMantra.com/a21

Scan with a smartphone camera

CHAPTER TWENTY-TWO
AI IN MEDICAL EDUCATION

Artificial intelligence (AI) is an emerging technology that is quickly overtaking not just simple, manual tasks but also more complex, decision-based tasks as well. Some may view AI as a threat to their jobs and professions. However, the better way to view it is as a tool. Within the medical profession, AI has the potential to substantially affect future medical practice. Although many doctors are already using new health AI technologies in clinical practice, it is only a matter of time before every doctor is expected to incorporate these new technologies.

Current medical education does not fully prepare future doctors for the impending AI revolution in their medical practices.[1] The medical curriculum should be transformed in a way that can improve future healthcare providers' capacity to practice in a big data environment, supported by AI.[2] Medical students need to have a clear knowledge of the volume, velocity, veracity, and variety of big data. They must be familiar with how AI and big data are analyzed, aggregated, and personalized in the context of clinical decision-making.[3] While in school, medical students should acquire solid knowledge and understanding of the practical applications of AI in healthcare in order to apply these technologies to patients in their future medical practices. The role of medical students as future health professionals is gigantic; thus, AI tools must be incorporated into their curriculum.[4]

As the interest of current and future healthcare providers in using advanced technologies grows, a standard framework is essential to ensure equal ability across the medical field. The goal is to update the existing medical educational framework with modern technologies. To understand how the current curriculum can be updated effectively, physicians must first understand what AI can offer to healthcare.

Examples of AI Applications in Healthcare

- **Diagnosing Diseases with Deep Learning:** Thinking of symptoms like data points, a doctor can input a patient's symptoms into an AI model that has been trained with volumes of diagnostic data to output a list of possible diseases. This method drastically reduces the time to diagnose a patient, which can minimize the diagnosis-treatment-recovery cycle for many patients.

- **Radiology and Machine Learning:** A team of researchers out of Osaka University developed a deep learning algorithm that reliably diagnoses neurological diseases. Instead of using symptom inputs like above, this method uses patient scans from MRI (Magnetic Resonance Imaging) results and compares them against the images of tens of thousands of other scans from healthy patients.

- **Reduction in Operational Costs:** A different approach to looking at the benefits is in terms of the healthcare business itself. One of the main benefits of AI applications is time. A lot of costs are involved in running a healthcare organization. AI has allowed these organizations to cut costs and let providers extend their budgets at every level. These increases in budgets lead to more resources for practice, more time for patients, and many more positive outcomes. One example is the use of AI in the field of joint replacement surgery. A program known as *PeerWell* helps patients prep for surgery by guiding them through a course pre-operatively. Patients saw a reduction in surgery costs of about $1200 when using the AI program.

Each of the above examples shows the use of AI in practice and the benefits it brings to the medical profession. Notice how, in each example, AI application was in the form of a program or tool that the physician would use to improve their work and results. If a doctor understands how to use AI to their advantage, the effect is not only improved work but also improved patient health. Artificial intelligence isn't about replacing people; it's about making better use of resources and focusing on what matters most.

Artificial Intelligence in Context

Because AI is built on the backbone of data, context is very important. Updating the medical curriculum requires students to understand AI in two settings: clinical and professional.

- **The Clinical Context:** doctors must understand AI in practice the same way they understand any other technology they use. They must know how to use it, interpret it, and explain it. These three requirements allow the physician to be comfortable with the technology and provide the patient with peace of mind when interacting with these tools.

  - To use AI technologies is the simplest way out of the three above-mentioned issues, as machine learning and deep learning methods have transformed the procedure into an easy process of input and output.

  - Interpreting AI means understanding both the data input and the makeup and structure of the model being used. This includes the variables involved, the relationships between the attributes, and the assumptions the model makes, if any. For interpreting AI, students must learn the basics of data structures and how they're used and arranged to build out these models.

  - To explain AI is to help the patient understand the results by effectively communicating the output in a way they can understand. The problem with current AI models is that we don't understand exactly how the model is achieving its results. A fair degree of understanding of the algorithms involved would alleviate some concerns regarding this. However, forcing students to understand the algorithms is too complex, as each can be different. A better approach toward making them understandable is to communicate the nature, origin, and rationalization of an algorithm's results. It is better to understand the data instead of the algorithm, which is what students already learn in the traditional curriculum.

- **The Professional Context:** This context is broader, as it extends past the clinical setting and toward leadership and health advocacy. Due to the simplification that AI imposes upon some of the manual processes that physicians perform, there is a tendency for complacency. This, of course, presents a risk in practice, as doctors may trust the results of an algorithm even if they can't seem to understand why. That's why it is necessary to understand that a model is just like the data it's presented with. There's a term used within AI literature, known as "Garbage in Garbage out (GIGO)"; it is essentially the "Do No Harm" of the data world. Users must be attentive to the data feeding the model, as it directly impacts the results provided.

Another issue accompanies the topic of health equity. A bias issue arises from building and training an AI model. The model can be just like the person building it; if the individual holds certain biases, whether apparent or not, those biases may be built into the algorithm and the mindset of the model. Studies have shown that factors like utilization of those datasets that lack minority population representation or gender discrepancies lead to biased, wrong results.

Privacy and data security are the other issues that must be considered. Physicians should be aware of all the risks involved with AI in order to conduct themselves in the appropriate, professional manner. The risks described above should be incorporated into the ethical portion of the medical curriculum so that students can learn about the risks of AI in addition to the benefits.

Incorporating AI into the Medical Curriculum

Any update of the current medical curriculum must incorporate the knowledge gaps addressed above. There must be a baseline for teaching students about data structures and how models are built. Then, students must understand and learn to deal with the risks involved with AI. Finally, students must practice with AI tools to become comfortable with the technology, as well as practice interpreting and communicating the results. Implementing these three points into the medical educational framework can ensure that future physicians are ready to use these new technologies to improve their practice.

The Readiness of Medical Education to Meet the 21st Century's Healthcare Demands

Is medical education ready for transformation to meet the 21st century's healthcare needs? Well, it might not be totally ready; however, with the recent rapid advancements in different AI tools, medical education will tremendously improve the outcomes of patient-centered care. The rise of artificial intelligence systems is promoting healthcare's digitalization in medical education by creating a major paradigm shift in teaching and learning methodologies.[5] Current reforms and modifications in medical education are necessary; however, these may not be sufficient to meet the 21st century's digital healthcare delivery needs.[6]

The acquisition of AI-based skills for advanced medical practice requires a more comprehensive and radical transformation in medical education. It is clear that AI should be incorporated into the medical curriculum at all training levels and should provide the opportunity for learners to compare their performance based on different AI algorithms.[7] Various challenges such as enhanced quality/continuity of care, sustainable cost, and agile teaching, and educated guesswork about the effectiveness of treatments are provoking physicians to consider new AI-based technologies in order to meet these challenges.[8] Medical educationists are also making efforts to update existing educational frameworks according to the 21st century's digital healthcare realities.

Medical Education and the Characteristics of Future Medical Practice

How can medical education be transformed from the dominant 20th-century model into the 21st century, especially with the application of AI and big data in professional practice? Medical educationists are incorporating AI in medical education on the basis of the idea that future medical practice will be based on a partnership among physicians, healthcare professionals, machines, and patients.[9] AI may transform medical education and future medical practice in the following four dimensions:

- Due to large data storage and processing infrastructures, care will be provided in multiple locations simultaneously.

- One-to-one doctor-patient care may be replaced by patient-to-multiple healthcare providers (e.g., nurses, home health aides, care managers, social workers, physical and occupational therapists, etc.).

- Physicians will practice in an environment in which clinical decisions will be made by a combination of machines, patients and their families, and expanding varieties of healthcare providers. Care will be provided with artificial intelligence and a growing array of accessible, large data sets collected from multiple sources. Machine-based analysis of large data sets will be the standard for patient care, leading to patients' continuous monitoring and valid assessment.

- There will be an interface between machines and medicine by using different AI tools. Machines may know more and perform more tasks in many areas.

Using AI to Transform Medical Education

Not only can students learn about AI and be ready to encounter these technologies in practice, but medical professionals and faculty leaders can use AI to improve the curriculum itself.

AI can be incorporated into medical education through curriculum analysis, learning, and assessment. Through analysis, the adoption of AI can help students in their reviews, automating time-consuming tasks, and creating curriculum maps. A major barrier to the use of AI in this area is the lack of digitalization in the AI-based learning management system (LMS), which greatly impacts the ability to meet the data pool requirements to develop AI-based systems. This lack of digitalization is more pronounced in medical institutions, where non-digital tools are used for different domains such as assessment, teaching, and evaluation.[10] Medical institutes can utilize AI-based technologies to create curriculum maps and assessment tasks by overcoming this barrier effectively.

Another application is providing students with instant, personalized feedback as they complete assignments. This can be done by assigning the grading to an AI model that can receive the work as input, and that can output not just a grade but also personalized feedback. This learning improvement can be expanded to provide students with pathways to improvement and less supervision. Therefore, AI-based personalized and adaptive feedback models may provide additional insight for students to fill their knowledge gaps effectively.

Major parts of the radiology and pathology specialty examinations can be automated using AI. Image analysis components of other medical specialty examinations can similarly be automated.

Other applications include the use of virtual patients (VP) and virtual reality (VR). This allows the students to practice a wide array of tasks over and over again without putting any patients at risk or potentially damaging instruments. Other VR simulations include performing a physical examination and making therapeutic and diagnostic decisions. The implication of VPs and VR for medical students has been widely accepted. A VR-based education system can be used anywhere and anytime, with an internet connection. VR training material can be accessed and shared with educational institutions online, with quick delivery of the latest updates to medical scenarios. It has the potential to take medical learning beyond the traditional classroom experience. VR has multiple benefits in medical education, such as enhanced student engagement, improved knowledge retention, and experiential learning. This simulation-based technology has much potential to revolutionize our medical education system according to the 21st century's healthcare demands.[11] VR has made it possible for medical students to experience their medical learning in more immersive and engaging ways than textbook learning. VR has provided the new concept of "digitalized classroom sessions," in which both teachers and students can gain classroom insights by recreating and recording real classroom sessions. If a student misses a class, he/she can use VR recordings to learn the missed lesson as in real-time.[11]

Chatbots, also known as virtual humans or virtual assistants, are AI-based programs designed to simulate human conversation via speech or text.[12,13] Will AI-based medical chatbots cause a major paradigm shift in future medical education? Yes. *PatientX* is an example of a chatbot that allows medical students to exercise their clinical knowledge and receive feedback in order to enhance their diagnostic skills. In medical education and training, chatbots can be used for two basic high-level functions: "understanding" and "answering." No matter the type of chatbot, they are all built for a similar purpose, i.e., to understand regular human language inputs and then provide relevant answers. Chatbots are everywhere, and we are expecting to experience more of them for the health sector as educational assistants, virtual nurses, and more.

Lastly, AI can improve the knowledge and retention of medical students through performance assessment. The Journal of the American Medical Association published a study in which an AI model was tested to distinguish surgeon trainees based on their stage of practice in simulated situations. The study tested 50 students in 250 simulated cases of tumor resection and showed that the ML algorithm classified the students with 90% precision across six metrics. The model was able to classify hand movements corresponding to each surgical device, the tissue removed or bleeding caused, and other metrics. The AI can be applied to the assessment of surgeon trainees along with surgeons in top certification evaluations, thereby saving both money and time.

Expanding the Reach of Medical Education

The implementation of artificial intelligence into the curriculum for students to learn, as well as applying it to the learning itself, will lower the barriers to education.

Medical students learning how to use and understand AI models in practice will create a net benefit to society, as physicians can work faster and have more time to focus on the patient instead of the data entry or results. Hours of tests will be cut down to minutes of runtime as the model works to solve the inputs of data. Physicians will be able to use, interpret, and explain AI applications to focus more on the care of the patient and, thus, bettering their work.

Transforming the curriculum with AI will lead to the ability of medical education to increase its reach. As AI evaluators and virtual environments improve, students will not be held back by the size of the class, the number of available professors, or even world-class facilities. Improving the learning experience will allow more students to practice and perfect the basics with more time using fewer resources, thus effectively lowering the cost of medical education over time.

The Learning Environment and Beyond

As more technologies, and not just AI, are adopted into the medical field, it is crucial for medical professionals to foster an effective culture of learning at every level. This would enable both students and the current workforce to reframe their knowledge within an increasingly technology-driven world.

To foster a culture of learning, the medical profession must encourage lifelong learning, have an openness to collaboration, and understand human intelligence. The first two incorporate the idea that as new technologies emerge, medical professionals must be open to learning new ideas and looking for applications in their everyday work. The latter is specific to artificial intelligence in that, to be able to understand the data, the models, and the algorithms, one must understand the nature of intelligence itself. It's a way of acknowledging that the machines are just like the people who program them. This realization will prevent physicians from becoming complacent and unquestionably trusting the model. It is a risk that comes with the adoption of AI in any field, but a risk that is amplified in medical practice due to consequences involving the health of patients.

Furthermore, collaborating with data scientists and AI programmers will allow medical professionals to be involved in the development of these new technologies, ensuring their effectiveness. If the medical field fosters an environment of continuous learning, it may be possible to work hand in hand with technology experts to bring forth the future of healthcare together.

In conclusion, the fast growth of AI in healthcare around the globe is a glimpse into a shining future, where artificial intelligence-driven tools are likely to define new methods of medical practice. Although no one can predict exactly how AI will transform medical education in the future, the main focus of AI in medical practice will be the development of tools such as robotic surgery, e-Patient, etc., to deliver patient-centered care.[14] We can assess that the development of future medical education will be based on a partnership among physicians, machines, and patients. Thus, health professionals must be ready for their new roles with transformation in medical education.

References/Further Reading

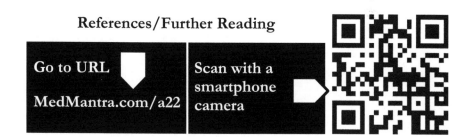

Go to URL
MedMantra.com/a22

Scan with a smartphone camera

"People worry that computers will get too smart and take over the world, but the real problem is that they're too stupid and they've already taken over the world."

- Pedro Domingos

AI IN GENOMIC AND PRECISION MEDICINE AND VIRTUAL ASSISTANTS AND HOSPITALS

CHAPTER TWENTY-THREE
AI IN GENOMIC MEDICINE

Outline:

A. Introduction

B. Application and Growth of AI in GM (Genomic Medicine)

- Pre-sequencing

- Sequencing

- Data processing

- Analysis and interpretation

    i.   Clinical interpretation

    ii. Research reporting

C. Stepping into the Future: Existing and Emerging Uses of AI in GM

- Cancers

- DNA sequencing

- Genomic sequence data processing

    i.   Variant identification or variant calling

    ii. Genome annotation

- Analysis and Interpretation of data reports

- Venturing outside the DNA helix: Integrated multi-omics and multi-modal data analysis

- Other research efforts toward complex genomic data analysis

    i.   Population genetics

    ii. Polygenic scores

Introduction

The application of artificial intelligence (AI) into the field of genetics is not surprising. After all, genomics is largely data-driven and requires the integration of large amounts of information derived from sequencing technologies with relevant biological, molecular, and clinical data. AI makes it possible to rapidly analyze large data sets to derive new conclusions and insights that pave the way forward in the fields of genetic research and personalized medicine.

AI techniques like deep learning (DL) offer advanced computational abilities needed to streamline and organize genomic and biomedical datasets. Interest in the rise of AI is clear, as major corporations—like Facebook, Google, Baidu, Tencent, Microsoft, Apple, and Amazon—are investing heavily in AI expertise in healthcare, where genomic analysis in addition to health monitoring and the diagnosis of medical conditions through digital devices and apps and virtual health assistants have made considerable headway.

The availability of raw materials or resources (hardware, software, and datasets) needed for the building of machine learning models has grown and led to a wide spectrum of analytics based on genomic data from single cells to studies of large populations

Application and Growth of AI in GM

With the study of genomics in humans, an individual's genetic information can be utilized to navigate their clinical care through the help of personalized diagnostics or therapeutics.

The large data pool that is required to link genomic data to other contributing factors that determine disease onset or progression and the responses of genetic variants to different therapeutic models is challenging for researchers to analyze and compute. They must also account for and integrate phenotypic information (physiological measurements and organ assessments), clinical records (family history, pathology of diseases, imaging records), and multi-omics datasets like proteomics, metabolomics, and transcriptomics.

Due to this, there exists a growing requirement for computational-based solutions to simplify the classification of heterogeneous, diverse, and high-dimensional data groups. Machine learning (ML) and DL seem to be an optimum solution to this need, as they can predict outcomes and facilitate the discovery of previously unknown or unrecognized patterns within complex data sets.

ML can be used to augment the various stages of the genomic data processing sequence:

a. ***Pre-sequencing*** – collection and preparation of the genetic sample for sequencing. This could be a blood sample, tissue or tumors, and even groups of cells or pathogens.

b. ***Sequencing*** – the genetic material is transformed into its raw sequence data, which is millions of fragments of DNA, called sequence "reads." The timeline for this is generally in hours.

c. ***Data Processing*** – a genome sequence is generated from the sequence reads or raw data. This is then compared to a genome in a reference database to detect point-based or region-based variants, which usually takes hours to complete.

d. ***Analysis and interpretation*** – this is the most intensive phase and can take a long time to complete, ranging from days to months. The processed data undergoes analysis to generate outputs that could lead to:

- **Clinical interpretation** and clinical reporting used for diagnostic, therapeutic, or reproductive decision-making.

- **Research reporting**, adding to the genomics knowledge base, such as molecular functions at cellular levels, like learning how ,cancers evolve and examining microbiomes.

By enabling ML and DL in genomics, algorithms are being trained to discover relationships between genetic variants and the manifestation of a disease, identify new disease biomarkers, and predict response to individualized, targeted treatment.

Stepping into the Future: Existing and Emerging Uses of AI in GM

1. Cancers

Histology or tissue-level analysis of cancers is used for both diagnosis and prognostication of tumors. Beginning with AI's potential to augment workflows in digital histopathology, various ML projects have been initiated that demonstrate its potential further. To deal with the computational demands of large high-dimensional and multi-attribute datasets, GPUs and DL neural networks are also being introduced to gain new insights.

The application of DL in medical imaging data has revealed that AI can outperform radiologists, pathologists, and dermatologists in the diagnosis of metastatic breast cancer, melanoma, and several eye diseases. It has aided in pharmacogenomics, which can enhance cancer screening and monitoring, to increase the prediction of adverse events and patient outcomes.[1] US-based company Freenome uses ML on its multi-omics platform to identify cancer risk signatures from blood samples, thereby decoding cell-free DNA (cfDNA) as biomarker patterns, leading to a low invasive screening test for multiple cancers.[2]

Research has shown that deep convolutional neural networks (DCNN) have emerged as an important image analysis tool, which is being used to predict outcomes in disease progressions from histology images integrated with genomic marker analysis. This has seen remarkable results in the diagnosis and classification of brain tumors, where overall survival in gliomas could be predicted using data from *The Cancer Genome Atlas (TCGA) Low-Grade Glioma (LGG) and Glioblastoma (GBM)* projects.[3]

US-based healthcare company *Proscia developed Concentriq,* an AI-based software platform for digital and computational pathology, which helps anatomical labs use ML in image analysis. This aids in cancer discovery and treatment by connecting relevant data points.[4]

However, there are restrictions to the widespread implementation of imaging based on digital pathology with genomics data due to the reluctance with which whole slide imaging is adopted, which is necessary to capture digital images to create a database. The standardization and aggregation of data also differ across research centers, which makes the data incongruous for analysis.

2. DNA sequencing

Any relevant technology used to sequence genetic data may be prone to errors or noise. To avoid these errors, complementary DNA probes must be designed so that the DNA target regions can be captured and bound efficiently during sequencing. Using the sequence data, DNA binding rates can be determined with ML with greater accuracy.

3. Data processing of genomic sequences

Identification of variants (variant calling) is a process by which the differences of an individual genome, as compared to genomic information in a reference data set, are picked up and analyzed. ML tools are being developed to improve the accuracy of this analysis. The DCNN can assimilate information from observational training data to differentiate true variances from artifacts due to cross-contamination or sequencing errors.

Google's Deep Variant tackles variant calling as a problem solved by image classification. Its method constructs multi-channel images or tensors, in which one aspect of the sequence is represented by a single channel. These images are then used to train a DCNN model, which is used to call single nucleotide polymorphisms (SNPs). Though it has been trained without specialized knowledge about genomics, this tool has performed well, as its strength lies in image analysis.[5]

Another challenge for identifying disruptions in sequencing is somatic variants. Although they are not inherited into progeny cells, they do arise in cell subsets and must be analyzed for potential uses in cancer treatment. Copy number variants (CNVs) are parts of the DNA strands that are either duplicated or deleted and which need to be accurately identified, as they contribute to approximately 4.8-9.5% of the genome.[6] Some of them have no effect on health and disease occurrence, while others have been identified as the causes of genetic disorders, both inherited and sporadic.

Genome Annotation: ML methods are used to identify specific elements and patterns in the genome, like splice sites, transcription start sites, promoters, and enhancers, to predict what effects they may have on disease risk.

4. Analysis and interpretation

After the identification of variants, it is important to prioritize and classify these variants based on the likelihood that they will cause disease or gauge whether they would respond to a personalized treatment modality. This functional analysis can be done by various algorithmic tools like *CADD* (combined annotation-dependent depletion), which combines predictive features in a different variation with respect to ML, and **DANN**, which combines CDNNs to demonstrate improved performance using the same set of input features. Illumina Inc. also released open-source novel AI software called **Primate AI**, which could distinguish between potential disease-causing mutations and benign genetic variants in individuals by using training data from nearly 120,000 human samples.[7]

5. Venturing outside the DNA helix: Integrated multi-omics and multi-modal data analysis

Due to the still-undiscovered knowledge about DNA sequences and their interpretation, researchers are also looking at the molecular components of the cells, taking into account changes in cellular processes, the dynamics of the surrounding environment, and disease variants that are acquired, not inherited, all of which may affect the molecular genotype and phenotype interactions.

That is why an integrative "omics" approach is better suited to fully understand the biological complexity of disease pathology. The combination of multiple "omics" technologies with health records and environmental monitors can provide machine learning software with high-dimensional data sets to analyze and discover patterns. The application of this strategy is used to examine the proliferation and spread of infectious diseases, especially in the diagnosis, etiology, transmission, clinical management, and response to treatment, along with potential resistance.

6. Other research efforts toward complex genomic data analysis

Population genetics

While dealing with the study and collection of genetic differences within and between populations, as a part of evolutionary biology, researchers are faced with the daunting task of making sense of the overwhelming amount of information. Supervised ML can certainly help with faster and unbiased accumulation and segregation of data sets

Polygenic scores

Polygenic scores are allotted after the analysis of the effects that single nucleotide polymorphisms (SNPs) or variants have on genetic traits. Multiple SNPs influence the genetic base of complex traits and are important to predicting diseases and potential actionable outcomes. Polygenic models and machine learning could improve the predictive value of these models because they can recognize more intricate patterns in correlated data.

Microbiome studies

All genetic material present in microbiological organisms in the human body, like the intestines or skin, can be sequenced and analyzed to investigate links between hosts and disease progression. *DeepMicro* is AI-based software that offers DL techniques that can be applied to high-dimensional microbiome data to obtain similar data clusters. Predictive problems that may be analyzed with microbiome data are drug response prediction, forensic human identification, and food allergy prediction.[8]

Single-cell analysis

Omics technology can be applied to individual cells to demonstrate the diversity in different cell populations while providing information about the disease's molecular characteristics.

Cancer evolution modeling

As cancers evolve and change, they do so in a temporal order, which, if tracked and analyzed, could provide early strategies for disease detection and progression. Several research groups are developing machine learning tools to track the evolution of cancer and determine the factors that drive cancer proliferation.

7. Clinical decision support

Time-sensitive analysis and periodic re-analysis

The successful application of AI algorithms would result in a significant increase in speed and accuracy by providing immediate provisional diagnosis, independent re-evaluation in cases in which a manual interpretation of data has failed, and the automated re-evaluation of clinically unsolved cases. This is particularly useful in time-sensitive cases like critical pediatric and newborn diseases.

Researchers at San Diego's *Rady Children's Institute for Genomic Medicine* (RCIGM) utilized clinical natural language processing (CNLP) and ML to diagnose fairly rare genetic diseases with the help of an algorithm, which extracted the phenotype data of children from electronic health records. The process was 80% precise and demonstrated a recall result of 93%. The system correctly diagnosed ICU infants while saving time (a mean of around 22 hours), which, in turn, affected the kind of treatment they received. This demonstrated the implementation of precise treatments due to genome sequencing augmented by automated phenotyping and interpretation.[9]

US-based company *BostonGene*[10] has curated an expansive updated AI-driven database of cancer research and clinical information, along with a cloud-native software that delivers a patient-centric list of the best treatment options based on its data analysis of the tumor as well as patients' clinical and environmental factors. Similarly, *Cambridge Cancer Genomics*[11] enables data-driven precision oncology to develop biomarkers that indicate treatment response and helps with clinical decision-making. *Perthera's Precision Oncology Platform*[12] aims to help by providing therapeutic intelligence to generate a comprehensive clinical and prognostic report based on multi-omics, showing improved treatment plans for patients.

With the genomic database rapidly expanding, it is only a matter of time before machine learning methods in the future could lead to systematic variant re-analysis to determine any changes in the reporting and analysis of existing results. This may, in turn, result in breakthrough treatment modalities.

Genetic counseling: Result feedback to patients and physicians

It would be difficult for genetic specialists or counselors to communicate test results or key findings to both mainstream physicians and patients, especially with the increase in genetic testing at present. To deal with this challenge and scale-up means for genetic counseling, companies have developed AI chatbots that can communicate with end-users about the results and interpretations of tests or analyses.

Geisinger and Clear Genetics, Inc. have introduced chatbots to improve communication with patients who received clinical information about actionable genetic variants from the **MyCode® Community Health Initiative**. The chatbot tells patients about key topics like goals, benefits, and risks before testing. They also suggest and remind patients about appropriate actions to take after the results are obtained. They can prompt cascade testing for relatives who may also be at risk. This provides an acceptable, user-friendly, scalable approach to manage ancillary genetic counseling tasks, thereby reducing the burden on human counterparts.[13]

8. Drug delivery and therapeutics

Drug discovery

ML is being applied to pharmaceutical and prescription databases to define disease subtypes, biomarkers, target discovery, drug repurposing, and prediction of drug responses.

The platform of Canadian-based company **Deep Genomics**[14] helps in the development of drugs used for neuromuscular and neurodegenerative disorders. Its new software, "Project Saturn," analyses 69 billion varying cell components and provides researchers with actionable feedback.

San Francisco-based **Atomwise**[15] developed its neural network, Atom Net, to predict drug activity in the body and identify characteristics required for volunteers in clinical trials. It screens 10 to 20 million genetic variants each day and can supposedly deliver results much faster than traditional Big Pharma companies. The company is currently working on new drugs for the treatment of drug-resistant malaria and tuberculosis. By 2026, **Astra Zeneca**[16] pharmaceuticals are planning to analyze up to two million genomes and study huge amounts of patient data points from their drug clinical trials.

Genome editing

Genome editing processes have widespread use in therapeutics by replacing or altering a defective or disrupted gene in patients' DNA sequences. Currently, the most cost-effective tool and versatile tool is **CRISPR (Clustered Regularly Interspaced Short Palindromic Repeats)**, which makes use of algorithmic networks backed by machine learning to predict and guide the moves made by the editing system, including intended and unintended or off-target gene edits and their consequences. *Editas Medicine*[17] focuses on CRISPR technology to target mutations that cause serious genetic diseases. In April 2020, the FDA approved the trial for *EDIT 101*, a CRISPR-based gene editing medicine administered via subretinal injection that is being investigated for the treatment of Leber congenital amaurosis type 10 (LCA10), which causes congenital blindness.

9. Rare diseases

Diseases with low rates of incidence in patient populations are difficult to trace and monitor. Large-scale investment in new pharmaceutical treatments is difficult and expensive. The application of AI in drug research for these diseases has reaped benefits.

Heal X[18] has introduced its Rare Treatment accelerator program, which connects the efforts of academic groups, patient groups, and early-stage biotechnology with its AI software to analyze the possibility of re-purposing its available drugs to aid in the treatment of rare diseases in order to benefit patients suffering from these illnesses.

AI-based technology like Disease-Gene Expression Matching (DGEM) allows for the identification of viable candidates in the study of drug repurposing for the treatment of Fragile X syndrome, which is a rare neurodevelopmental disorder. The study revealed the potential for Sulindac and nutraceuticals as treatment options.[19]

10. Research tools for literature mining

The application of AI tools worldwide has led to the publication of a large amount of scientific literature that provides an abundant data set for AI algorithms to mine and extract relevant information. The rising volume of scientific publications indicates that multiple theories are being tested at the same time, which makes it harder for researchers to keep up with relevant advances in their field without the help of automation. This, in turn, impacts their ability to arrive at coherent conclusions in their studies, which is necessary for evidence-based recommendations in precision medicine.

The application of Literome, an automated system for curation, used to extract genomic information from PubMed articles to facilitate browsing, searching, and reasoning, has greatly benefited research efforts. Another tool, *Phillip's IntelliSearch*[20] Discovery, provides AI solutions for medical research as well.

Applications During the COVID-19 Pandemic

- *Building data sets: Analysis of the viral genetic code*

  The COVID-19 pandemic caused global disruptions of economies and healthcare systems, infecting and killing millions of people worldwide. In a bid to understand more about the virus, its first genome sequence was identified. Since then, there have been large, concerted efforts to analyze the virus' genetic code as well as that of its most affected hosts or patients in a bid to arrive at a vaccine or effective cure to the disease at the earliest possible time. Leveraging the power of genomic AI, the Cog *UK Research Consortium*[21], in the United Kingdom, consolidated resources from the Sanger Institute, the NHS, and other research institutes, and then sequenced more than 16,000 viral samples from patients who were diagnosed with COVID-19. *Nextstrain*[22] is an open-source coronavirus project that delivers publicly accessible sequencing data along with analytic and visualization tools. Around 20,000 sequences were uploaded to the Global Initiative on Sharing All Influenza Data (GISAID), which acts as a dataset that researchers can use to illustrate a family tree demonstrating the spread of the virus. Similarly, *23andMe*[23], which is a consumer genetics testing and analysis company, has enrolled its willing customers into a study to find potential associations between the severity of coronavirus symptoms and genomic structures. These research efforts aim to examine the evolution and origins of the virus as well as the host cellular response to infection.

- *Exploring novel drug treatments*

  UK-based *Benevolent AI*[24] is working with major pharmaceutical companies to use its AI platform to identify existing drugs that could be used to treat the novel coronavirus. Their research led to a clinical trial with Eli Lilly and the US National Institute for Allergies and Infectious Diseases, which validated the AI's hypothesis for the use of Baricitinib as a possible therapeutic drug.

Policy and Regulations

When considering the road ahead for the application of AI in GM, it may seem paved with difficulties due to its inherent complexity. This may result in roadblocks to progress, which must be overcome.

The dark side: Limitations and challenges

Various ethical and legal challenges can hinder the development of safe, clinically validated, and beneficial algorithms.

1. Though the FDA has approved many AI algorithms, a few ethical concerns and regulatory gaps raise concerns due to the **sourcing and privacy** of the data that is used to train the systems. There are also concerns about **data security** and the hacking of algorithms to disrupt patient health care plans as part of cyberattacks, as well as problems raised regarding **informed consent** when using AI tech or chatbots for personal patient information.

2. There is **regulatory ambiguity** in terms of liability in the event of prediction errors. This may be addressed by the open sharing of AI models, codes, meta graphs, etc., with the entire scientific community to improve transparency.

3. **Bias in datasets** occurs due to the imbalance of genomic data sampling and available information about some populations, which may lead to misdiagnosis and uneven success rates when the AI-analyzed outcomes are put into practice. Faulty input will lead to the faulty output. The results of the analysis could be skewed to under-represent a community considering that the input data was inherently lacking in diversity. For example, **Deep Gestalt**, an AI system for the analysis of facial morphology, demonstrated poor accuracy in identifying Down's syndrome in patients of African versus European descent (36.8% versus 80%, respectively).[25] To counteract this, the NIH and the US Department of Health and Human Services established the *All of Us*

Research Program, which aims to build a diverse health database with participants of all backgrounds, races, and ethnicities.[26]

4. **Lack of reproducibility** is a challenge due to inaccessible exact research methods or codes or incomplete training data. These data silos make it difficult to integrate data for analysis effectively.

5. **Adequate computing, data mining, and storage infrastructure** is also a requirement that may be difficult for some organizations to achieve. Cloud computing services may be a solution to this issue, but specialist intervention is required to manage the interface and configure the AI models for the cloud service and research organization. **Building domain knowledge** that covers an understanding of the healthcare ecosystem, genomics, multi-omics, and the necessary technical skills to collaborate on research projects are also required.

6. The application of AI in GM and human health requires safeguards, oversight, validation, concentrated ethical appraisals, and public engagement. The **validity and clinical utility** of the technology must be demonstrated by promoting explainable AI and algorithmic interpretability.

These concerns will need to be dealt with rapidly if the advantages of this technology for the field of genetics are to be effectively utilized for the safe deployment of healthcare solutions.

Current policy changes that have taken place toward the advancement and adoption of AI applications are:

1. The US government published draft guidance for the regulation of AI applications with ten core principles. This was followed by an Executive Order that launched a coordinated government strategy, "The American AI initiative." It also launched a new website, AI.gov, to make information about AI more available to the public.

2. In 2019, the Organization for Economic Co-operation and Development (OECD)[27] drafted its "Principles of AI," which was signed by more than 40 participating countries to promote ethical AI initiatives. The G20[28] released its AI principles based on those specified by OCED later that year.

3. In 2018, the European Commission adopted its AI strategy by creating the European AI Alliance and developing AI ethics guidelines, which promotes the slogan "Trustworthy AI." EU member states like the UK and Germany have also released their national strategies for the ethical application of AI.

These guidelines addressed common principles[29] like:

- Investing in AI research and development and unleashing AI resources with a cost and benefits analysis.

- Setting up AI governance standards with human agency and oversight to ensure transparency and accountability.

- Establishing standards for risk assessments and technical robustness.

- Building the AI workforce with expansive training.

- Fostering interagency coordination and international engagement.

- Building up public trust in AI, thereby encouraging public participation.

- Maintaining scientific integrity and information quality, with guidelines for disclosure and transparency.

- Encouraging fairness and non-discrimination in the collection of data.

- Ensuring the safety and security of health data through effective data governance.

The bright side: Imagine the possibilities

To address the challenges encountered in the collection and sharing of genomic data, like inferior data quality, isolated information islands or silos, tampered-with or distorted data, incomplete records, gray data transactions, or even the leakage of personal data, there has been a concerted effort to apply new blockchain technology to protect sensitive personal genomic data because of its inherent ability to decentralize information while providing encryption algorithms, antitampering features, and traceability.

One such blockchain-based big data platform, *LifeCODE.ai*[30], manages data ownership, sharing, and security. Blockchains are publicly distributed ledgers that seal blocks of information or data with timestamps and encrypted hash links, enabling users to encrypt data with their own individualized and personalized keys. It has an open-source sharing protocol that enables data logging and storage by all participants simultaneously. This ensures that the details of the transactions recorded cannot be changed after input, without the approval of the network, thereby adding to data security. Due to the blockchain's decentralized architecture and governance, it is fairly safe from attacks or collusions.

Conclusion

The applications of AI in the field of GM are far-reaching, with encouraging results opening up possibilities for further advancement in the future. Steps are already being taken to regulate the industry and implement policy changes to fully reap the benefits of this technology, with positive impacts on healthcare delivery in the future.

References/Further Reading

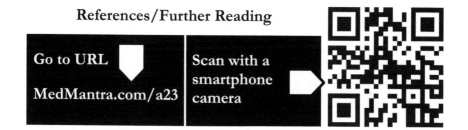

Go to URL

MedMantra.com/a23

Scan with a smartphone camera

CHAPTER TWENTY-FOUR
AI IN PRECISION MEDICINE

Introduction

Precision medicine is the branch of medicine that utilizes information from an individual's genes, variability in environment, and lifestyle to find the most appropriate, most cost-effective, and best preventive measure against the development of disease or infirmity. It considers various individual factors such as personal characteristics, environmental exposures, genotypic details, immunization history, and clinical and biological data[1] to best tailor to a definite subgroup of patients rather than taking a one-drug-fits-all approach. The terms "precision medicine" and "personalized medicine" are sometimes used interchangeably. Personalized medicine is sometimes misinterpreted as medical care specific to an individual; however, according to the National Research Council, personalized medicine is an older term for precision medicine[2], both of which significantly overlap in their meaning and are used synonymously. The Swiss Personalized Health Network (SPHN) is an initiative of the Swiss government that offers several programs focused on personalized medicine. The main goal of this initiative is to bring Switzerland to the forefront of personalized health research by establishing an extensive nationwide network of biomedical information. This network promotes research related to personalized medicine among multiple disciplines such as clinical medicine, engineering, and health care. It attempts to further dig into the complexities of precision medicine and to explore its endless possibilities.[3]

Use of AI

To make healthcare precise or personalized, as mentioned before, a large quantity of data must be stored and analyzed. Correlations must be made between various parameters related to health and disease. That is where Artificial Intelligence (AI) comes into play. The use of artificial intelligence has revolutionized all the branches of medicine and healthcare. The immense computational power, high-performance abilities, specific decision-making skills, and machine learning capabilities of AI are changing the future of healthcare, and precision medicine is no exception.[4] Machine learning algorithms such as Support Vector Machines (SVM), logistic regression, random forest, Naïve Bayes, K-nearest neighbor (KNN), hidden Markov model (HMM), etc., are frequently applied in medicine.[5] Precision medicine requires a gigantic volume of data processing power using various phenotypic and genotypic details of an individual.

AI systems can store and analyze massive volumes of data related to genetic variants and their phenotypic expressions and, hence, can help establish previously unknown gene-protein and protein-drug interactions.[6] This can unravel a multitude of possibilities for manipulating those interactions to get the desired output, like preventing or treating a specific disease. Hence, AI can significantly aid this field of medicine by precisely identifying the risk patterns and diagnostic, therapeutic, preventive, and prognostic modalities of various diseases.

Use of AI in precision medicine

Breast cancer

Although at a very initial stage of development, the application of AI has proven revolutionary in multiple fields of medicine, from neurology to critical medicine to oncology. In an international AI competition organized by the Symposium of Biomedical Imaging, AI could diagnose malignant breast carcinoma from the available images of lymph node biopsies with 92.5% accuracy. An experienced oncologist takes the accuracy to about 96.6%. This also demonstrated that the combination of AI with human diagnostic abilities can significantly increase the diagnostic success rate to 99.5%.[7]

Cardiovascular disease

Conventionally, statistical data based on prevalence and correlation studies have been used to detect individuals at risk of certain diseases. AI systems can store a considerable quantity of genomic data and predict disease risk better than conventional statistical methods. An AI system developed by Intel has been able to predict disease risk with an accuracy of up to 85%.[8] It could predict cardiovascular disease risk in 23 individuals who would not have been considered at risk by traditional statistical methods.

Radiology and Cardiology

Medical Sieve is a program launched by IBM that assists in clinical decision-making in radiology and cardiology by analyzing radiology images quickly and more reliably.[9] An intelligent, cognitive, and analytical clinical assistant with clinical knowledge and reasoning skills is a possibility for the near future. In China, AI systems running on Intel Xeon processors have been deployed in multiple health facilities to detect abnormal thyroid nodules. This has decreased the workload of health workers and increased the diagnosis rate of abnormal cases. The average accuracy of clinicians' diagnosis is around 75%, while that of AI systems is around 95%.[8] The health workers can now focus on more challenging cases requiring human knowledge, which has led to increased job satisfaction.

A Dutch company, Zorgprisma Publiek, analyzes data from various hospitals and insurance companies and generates information about the mistakes made by clinicians and hospitals in the diagnosis of a particular illness.[8] This can help improve treatment in specific disease conditions and avoid unnecessary hospitalization of patients.

Pediatrics

Precision medicine is also being used in the field of pediatrics. AI is being used in patient selection for clinical trials to identify a specific subpopulation in whom the therapy of interest may be trialed. In the last two years, multiple clinical sequencing studies in pediatric oncology have been reported. These studies have shown several actionable genetic variants and the feasibility of sequencing in clinics.[10]

Some centers have recently started using precision medicine tools to manage pediatric sepsis. Bioinformatics tools that use the multi biomarker-based approach are being used to identify patients at risk of poor outcomes so that they are managed appropriately.[11]

Neuro-Developmental Disorders (NDD)

AI has also been used in neurodevelopmental disorders (NDD) such as autism spectrum disorder, epileptic encephalopathy, intellectual disability, and other rare diseases. Machine learning algorithms can help identify the exact loci of the affected genes and mutations in the disease processes. AI-based solutions have offered a reasonable degree of success in diagnosing congenital and neurodevelopmental disorders.

Conclusion

Precision medicine is still in its infancy, although the future use cases are endless. Possibly, in the not-so-distant future, precision medicine and AI will revolutionize healthcare and enable people to live longer and much healthier lives. The application of precision medicine does have some downsides. AI replacing humans in specific jobs is seen as a challenge, although an equally large number of the workforce would be required for handling the AI machines and technologies. It involves that a myriad of expertise is operated correctly, and it also can make the cost of healthcare unaffordable for many. Questions of ethics and safety can be raised and quite reasonably. Errors might arise when adequate data is not available for the statistics to build upon, especially in never-before-seen cases and in novel drugs and interventions. These factors may form a barrier against precision medicine implementation, and they must be dealt with tactfully. AI should not be thought of as something that will replace humans but, rather, as a tool that will go hand in hand with human expertise and knowledge. Adequate safety protocols and ethical guidelines must be developed, and it should be obligatory to put them into practice. Precision medicine can be the Holy Grail for modern medicine if handled rationally.

References/Further Reading

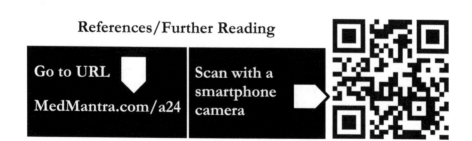

Go to URL
MedMantra.com/a24

Scan with a smartphone camera

CHAPTER TWENTY-FIVE

VIRTUAL HEALTH AND MEDICAL ASSISTANTS AND VIRTUAL HOSPITALS

There has been much talk on how AI can help revolutionize the face of the healthcare industry. One of the many possibilities is the introduction of virtual assistants into the healthcare system. With the introduction of virtual assistants and virtual hospitals, AI can steadily and massively change how the healthcare system works.[1]

While much remains to be done in this vast field, there is no denying the fact that the possibility of this happening is quite large. More than that, the effectiveness of AI has already been observed in many healthcare settings. With the development of virtual assistants and hospitals, individuals can be provided with more focused advice and measures to take care of their health.

How Can AI Impact Various Parts of the Healthcare Sector?

Through AI, various aspects of the healthcare industry can evolve. It can not only benefit individuals by the creation of virtual assistants but, if properly implemented, also transform the entire healthcare sector. Let us take a look at how AI can impact and massively change the different sectors of the healthcare industry.

- **Use of Voice-Controlled Devices for Virtual Medical Assistants**

  One of the biggest utilities of AI in healthcare is the idea of voice recognition. Currently, there are many applications of voice recognition around the world.[2] However, their use is minimal. The most dominating voice recognition application used across the globe is Alexa.[3] Is it possible to incorporate the use of voice recognition in the healthcare sector? Many possibilities exist, but various challenges prevail alongside it.

  Voice-controlled devices are being heavily assessed as to whether they can be implemented in the healthcare sector. This is because they could prove to be the most effective way of offering service to patients. The hands-free, inexpensive, and quick nature of the assistants highly increases their convenience for day-to-day use.[2] Once they are properly set up, there will certainly be many virtual health and medical assistant users. However, for now, there seem to be various issues that must be addressed before this possibility is introduced.

A few observations have been made to figure out whether voice-controlled devices are useful for the healthcare sector. With thorough investigations taking place, one prominent issue is that these voice-controlled devices and AI apps are perhaps too narrow when it comes to their capabilities to assess various kinds of diseases.[4] There may not currently be any effective solution to help in evaluating various diseases in one-go. A lot of work and the creation of many prototypes are required to come up with an AI device that might have more to offer. At this stage, no inventions can solve the issue of limited capability.

Another significant observation is that there have been mainly studies in which AI apps have been useful. These studies are conducted on a relatively small scale, and the subjects are situation-based instead of random trials. This means that there is no clear evidence that this might work out on a larger scale. Because most of the tests and trials are run on studies that happen to be of a smaller scale, there are yet-to-be-successful tests and trials done on larger, more randomized bodies. Even those that have been conducted on a larger scale and randomized have not shown any outstanding results. Essentially, this denotes that much must be done to ensure the effectiveness of virtual assistants with voice-controlled apps or devices. This makes us believe that the actualization of virtual medical and health assistants still has a long way to go.

- **The Workforce and the Workflow**

One must also consider the workforce of the healthcare industry. There are current tasks that one worker in the healthcare sector must accomplish. Redundancy, exploitation, and many other forms of issues are present in the industry.[5] AI can help diminish these issues and streamline things. When it comes to the large number of tasks associated with every member of the healthcare industry, things will be much less burdensome with AI applications.

There is bound to be more ease of access to faster work because AI will take over and control most of the redundant and mundane work that an employee has to do. Not only will this make things more effective, but it will also allow for the possibility of lower costs. The problem of over-burdened doctors and nurses will decrease as most of the documentation and paperwork will be handled through AI mechanisms. It is practical and highly possible for the workforce and the workflow of the entire healthcare system to be much more effective by implementing AI.

Another thing that AI promises to ensure is the safety of the patients who come for their checkups.[6] Often, doctors prescribe tests and exposure to radiation that can be harmful. Through AI implementation, this exposure can easily be minimized, leading to a more effective and streamlined way of assessing who requires what kind of treatments. AI will take over more work, allowing doctors to evaluate patients accurately.

- **Hospital Rooms will Become Obsolete**

There is a lot of talk about trying to implement AI to create a virtual hospital that has more to offer patients than ever before. While space will always be available in hospitals, many patients will be staying in their homes, being taken care of properly through the right AI mechanisms. All of this might seem absurd, but it is in the process of being implemented in the distant future. AI is here to change the way hospitals work. One such way is to make hospital rooms obsolete.

AI devices come in many forms and shapes. Incorporating such devices for use in virtual hospitals is a possibility that many can see coming. There will be fewer people in the hospitals for treatments, and there will be more people in the comfort of their homes getting treatments from their doctors.[6] While you might think that this is something you cannot see at this particular time, there will be a time when this will become the norm. Using robust sensors and AI can ensure that industry professionals help patients in the most effective ways. More than that, there is a high possibility that AI will diagnose patients much better. So, even if someone showcases no symptoms, AI mechanisms will assess whether there is a possibility of the onset of disease.

There is a massive possibility of virtual hospitals becoming a norm in the future. With the right kind of research applied in this situation, there are bound to be more and more changes in the way that hospitals work. More emphasis will be placed on making use of virtual hospitals as opposed to anything else.

Benefits of Implementing AI for Virtual Medical Assistants and Hospitals

Many benefits arise with the implementation of AI for use with virtual medical assistants and hospitals.

- ### Cutting Costs and Improved Maintenance

  On a different note, the implementation of AI creates many possibilities regarding how the healthcare industry is run. For instance, with the reduction of people working in the industry and with AI covering many operational activities, there are bound to be many cost reductions everywhere.[7] This is a motive that every business owner has, including people who are running hospitals, clinics, and similar healthcare platforms. There is a need to minimize costs everywhere. The use of effective AI systems can ensure that these costs are reduced drastically.

  More than that, the use of AI can help people maintain their health better. For instance, they have better access to information about patients. This will ensure that the patients know how to take care of themselves. With virtual medical assistants' presence, patients will be able to learn various tips to ensure that they maintain their health in the best possible ways as opposed to other options.

- ### Running Medical AI at a Larger Scale

  With AI's introduction into individual and industry-wide applications, there are bound to be national benefits of taking on this possibility.[8] For instance, with AI's help, there will be a better doctor-to-patient ratio in the long run. Plus, doctors will be able to help their patients get better in the best ways. With AI's introduction into the healthcare sector, there is a high chance of getting more information about patients and learning more efficient prevention and treatment paths.

Building a Virtual Medical Assistant

We have discussed the various observations of the use of AI and voice-controlled devices in the healthcare sector; there is a significant possibility of this happening in the distant future. We mean that perhaps these observations might get trumped once the right kind of technology is used to create an effective system using different types of resources. With a more thorough and compelling look into what is doable with this, there are sure to be many possibilities in the distant future. Currently, much work is required to ensure that this is a possibility. This mostly involves the fact that many challenges are present in this context.

Challenges of Building a Virtual Medical Assistant

Many challenges make it challenging to create virtual medical assistants [9]. Let us take a look at some of the prominent issues that arise when one is building a virtual medical assistant or hospital.

- **Low-Quality Input**

  One of the more prominent issues is that while there are many ways to access information, there are lower possibilities of getting high-quality input. There is currently a high placement of various AI devices, AI algorithms, smartphones, and much more, through which data comes in. However, all this information is not necessarily of excellent quality.

  While the possibility of collecting data has increased, multiple issues persist. For instance, the inflow of significant data does not mean that all of this data offers valuable information. Work must be done to ensure that low-quality input is limited.

- **Difficulty of Nailing Down the Right Data**

  Another challenge is the fact that there is a significant issue with finding the right data to use amid the plethora of information coming in. While there are many ways in which data comes, the assessment of which data might be right, and which is irrelevant, is not entirely clear.[10] For instance, there is no clear identification of what kind of information should be covered when it comes to one person and how often this information should be covered.

A lot of confusion exists when it comes to getting a holistic view of an individual. While plenty of data is available, cutting it down to the right kind of information is essential for developing a virtual medical assistant or an entire hospital. There is also a significant possibility of coming across incidental findings that alter the whole process. Now, there will be more confusion about how to go about processing the right information for an individual.

- **Ineffective EHR Data**

We have discussed how the data collected through EHR is not entirely correct. Relying on information available in these records will not make the system more effective. Instead, there is a possibility that it will derail the planning of the entire system. EHR is an ineffective method through which data is collected and stored. Its use will prove to be counterproductive, as deep learning requires a more thorough understanding and detailed information.[11] With the widespread use of EHR, there is no denying that it will make things more complicated for virtual medical assistants.

It is essential to ensure that a different way of collecting data is present because EHR is incomplete and full of errors. It also does not adequately represent a person's health. Therefore, it restricts the possibility of understanding the person's health entirely. Moreover, deep learning requires clean data, and EHR does not provide this in any form.

- **Privacy and Protection**

A core challenge stemming from the possibility of creating a virtual assistant is that an individual does not have the right to their data. So, if patients have no rights, how will this system work? Will the virtual medical assistants have all the relevant information about their health and wellbeing? If that is the case, what will the process be? Because individuals do not have access to their data, people cannot use these virtual medical assistants effectively.

Another issue prevails, revolving around the fact that there is no privacy or protection of an individual's information. For instance, data theft is widespread across different channels. What is to say that the presence of virtual assistants in healthcare leads to the same thing? More than that, because patients do not have control over their data, they have no idea how to most effectively make decisions about their health. The privacy of information is a big issue that prevails politically when it comes to virtual medical assistants.

- **Information Blocking**

Another issue that is prevalent in the healthcare sector is information blocking. Access to patients' medical data is withheld from them even though they are the ones who pay for it. Doctors are concerned about losing control of their patients if they are given access to all of their data.[12] How will this be overcome if work is underway to develop virtual assistants? There is no standardized idea regarding what kind of information blocking will prevail across different states and countries. So, how can the application of a virtual medical assistant take place?

Will doctors start giving the full information to their patients over time? Or will this be an issue that persists for the long run? If the latter is the case, the possibility of introducing virtual medical assistants is challenged mainly because there is little access to data for patients. With limited access to medical data, how can patients optimize their virtual assistants' use?

- **The Form of the Virtual Assistant**

One thing that seems highly challenging to cover is the form that the virtual assistant might take. There are many issues regarding the way that virtual assistants will present themselves to individuals. There is no clear identification of what they might look like, as many prototypes must be made to get the perfect option. The only clear thing is the fact that the virtual assistant must be convenient to use. That means anything bulky is out of the question.

More than that, there are many things to consider in creating a virtual medical assistant. It must be in a form that anyone can use to avail themselves of the maximum benefit that it has to offer. Other than that, there is the pressing issue of how to make sure that people find a sense of ease in using it. For instance, currently, the self-driving car is one of AI's most distinguished forms. There must be something that will be easy to use and offer maximum benefits to users of the entire AI virtual assistant system.

Can the Health System Change with AI?

When it comes to figuring out whether the health system can change with AI, there is a clear indication that a significant change is possible. However, this requires a lot of work. With the implementation of AI into healthcare, there can be ease of work for many people in the system. One of the biggest ways that AI promises change is in the form of individual experience.[13] However, it is here to offer more than that. If given enough time and resources, AI can change the entire healthcare system. There is bound to be a series of massive changes once the adoption of advanced AI mechanisms makes its way into healthcare processes.

Can AI and Other Technologies Successfully Create Virtual Medical Assistants and Hospitals?

When it comes to this question, clearly, AI can transform how the entire medical system works. Whether it involves implementing the possibility of virtual medical and health assistants or large-scale conversion to virtual hospitals, there is no denying that AI, along with other relevant technologies, can make this possible. Much research and development are underway to make this possible on a large scale. You will certainly be seeing these features soon in the healthcare industry.

References/Further Reading

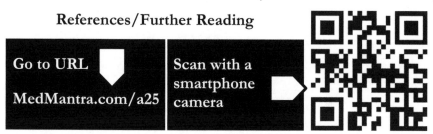

Go to URL
MedMantra.com/a25

Scan with a smartphone camera

"As more and more artificial intelligence is entering into the world, more and more emotional intelligence must enter into leadership."

- Amit Ray

PRESENT STATE & FUTURE OF AI IN MAJOR HEALTHCARE SPECIALTIES

CHAPTER TWENTY-SIX
PREVENTIVE HEALTHCARE

In the early 2000s, Google co-founder Larry Page[1] made an interesting prediction:

"Artificial intelligence would be the ultimate version of Google. The ultimate search engine that would understand everything on the Web. It would understand exactly what you wanted, and it would give you the right thing."

Twenty years later, the latest buzzwords in healthcare are Big Data and Artificial Intelligence (AI). Research shows that the field will see the growth of CAGR[2], which may reach 40% by 2024, giving rise to a 10-billion-dollar market focused on the different routes through which AI can impact healthcare delivery. These include broad-ranging fields, from medical imaging and radiology to lab medicine, diagnostics, genomics, personalized drug delivery, and even robotic AI assistants, through advanced Machine Learning, Deep Learning, and cognitive computing.

When Larry Page said that AI was the "ultimate search engine," he was referring to the fact that AI algorithms can process large amounts of data, analyzing them to give smart, actionable solutions. This has proved highly effective in the healthcare space. The 2020 pandemic has shown the global dearth of qualified and skilled healthcare personnel. The goal of using AI-based tools is to alleviate the cognitive burden of repetitive mundane tasks in order to free up healthcare workers so that they can focus on patient care, using their manual dexterity and skills. However, researchers soon discovered the untapped potential that AI offers, with solutions that can transform healthcare from a reactionary service to a preventive service.

All too often, patients are diagnosed with chronic conditions like endocrine issues or neoplasms simply because they missed symptoms or a diagnosis was delayed. This could be due to various reasons, but most research has delved into the ways in which patients can be diagnosed for health conditions at the earliest so that both curative and preventive measures can be taken to prevent mortality and morbidity, which may result from debilitative and costly late treatment measures. Studies have demonstrated that if patients have access to their own health data and if they are able to receive insights and feedback into their own health conditions, they are more willing to actively track their status and make lifestyle choices that are better for their health conditions. This concept ranges from routine monitoring of health parameters to active diagnosis and post-treatment evaluations.

The idea of remote patient monitoring seemed especially attractive in light of social distancing measures imposed by the 2020 pandemic. Patients were unable to visit treating physicians and depended on telehealth consultations, which, again, relied on health data collected by the patient himself through remote and user-friendly "wearable" devices. This large data set could reach treating physicians with the help of integrated smartphone applications, making it possible for real-time diagnosis and interventions. The large amount of data that was generated with remote monitoring devices were optimal for the application and training of AI-based algorithms. This could lead to machine-derived, predictive inferences, which in turn, would lead to personalized and preventive care for patients, catching disease symptoms earlier and more accurately.

If one plays devil's advocate, it is natural to ask: Can machines genuinely learn to think like doctors and surgeons? The multitude of research-based experimentation has answered that question with a resounding "yes." AI-based tools have already enhanced many healthcare branches by enabling doctors to make educated decisions, consultations, and interventions.

How AI is Revolutionizing Preventive Healthcare Now

Preventive healthcare has come into the limelight this past couple of years, especially as more people have called for an end to curative care. Stopping diseases and ailments before they have a chance to progress is critical to maintaining the health and well-being of any community. Thus, as healthcare is being reformed throughout the world, AI is offering modalities to get the job done. Thousands of startups working out AI for healthcare have popped up. These applications range from productivity in the office to enhancing the visuals of MRI scans and beyond. The best part is that both healthcare professionals and patients will have access to the data that AI will use, considering that the availability of knowledge is one of the most integral points of preventive care. Several healthcare IT applications are powered by AI, seeking to enhance patient care by reducing delays in treatment and highlighting risk factors within patients.

IBM Watson

Watson is famous for a number of interactions with humans, but its applications in healthcare are truly revolutionary. IBM created a special version of the *AI for oncologists*[3] to analyze and diagnose cancer states. It was found to be "concordant with the tumor board recommendations in 90 percent of breast cancer cases." With the multidisciplinary tumor board from India, Watson was concordant 96 percent for lung cancer, 81 percent for colon cancer, and 93 percent for rectal cancer. Now, Watson has become a reliable companion for oncologists throughout the world.

IBM Watson has also been used to power *Medtronic's IQ cast software*[4], which used the AI technology to train the application's *Sugar.IQ virtual* bot assistant to predict a patient's sugar level forecast, giving warnings for expected or sudden fluctuations in blood sugar levels and giving patients and physicians time to take interventions.

Healint

The main focus of the *Healint technology is* the *"Migraine Buddy" function*[5] that tracks migraines and keeps a diary. This data is analyzed using deep analytics and Machine Learning to give alerts on patient symptoms as well as medication results. The user can record the symptoms they get from their medication, which are sent to their treating physicians, who can then proactively adapt the treatment for such ailments.

What Can We Expect in the Future?

Every day, a discovery is made that will contribute to the healthcare of tomorrow. Aside from the benefits that are already obvious within the aforementioned examples, the advantages of incorporating AI into preventive healthcare are numerous. Here are just a few ways that AI is boosting the efficiency of the medical world for the present and future.

More Efficient Research Tools

Google and its parent company, Alphabet, are investing heavily in AI-based technology with a special focus on healthcare. Their subsidiary Verily is spearheading these attempts with data collecting research and analytics tools. Verily has focused its efforts on collaborating with medical research institutions around the world to find areas where they can apply AI-based solutions to capture biometric or health sensory data. Its wearable patient monitoring device, *the Study Watch*[6], is currently being used in clinical research programs as a prescription-only device to monitor patient conditions remotely for use in large population-based health trials as an easy way to accumulate data. They also introduced the *Verily Patch*[7], which is a novel sensor-based adhesive patch that can measure body temperature over long periods of time. It can be worn comfortably on the body continuously for up to 3 months. Another Alphabet subsidiary, Calico, is focusing on research into age-related diseases. It applies its algorithm to analyze large data sets and automate lab processes for faster diagnosis.

Better Data Management

AI can do something that humans can't—sift rapidly through data without getting distracted. In other words, AI will have access to billions of electronic medical records, scientific data, and other databases and will be able to find patterns and connections that humans may overlook.

Waqaas Al-Siddiq, founder and CEO of **Biotricity**, *states that AI's learning algorithms can "be deployed to traverse massive amounts of data and detect a few variables across hundreds of thousands of data points that are specific to certain conditions and diseases."*

Furthermore, fusing AI with blockchain technologies could enhance data management. An example would be **DeepMind Health**, another Google or Alphabet-owned enterprise that is leveraging AI for better health outcomes. Their algorithm mines data from medical records and expedites the treatment process. Most recently, through their **Alpha Fold** system, they have made computational-based predictions of the protein structures belonging to the COVID-19 virus, which will help in drug discovery research.[8]

Another system, called **Doc.ai**[9], uses blockchain to "collect masses of medical data globally" to generate individualized insights to patients for personalized medical aid.

Faster Online Consultations

The greatest asset AI brings to preventive healthcare is providing people with medical aid anywhere, anytime. As long as one has access to a cell phone connection or Wi-Fi, AI makes it possible to get consultations. An example of this is **Babylon**[10], an application that offers online consultations based on patients' individual medical records and medical databases. Users can input their data, report their illnesses, and receive feedback from the algorithm. The app also has functions like medication reminders and follow-ups that ask how you are feeling.

Similarly, **Engagely.ai**[11] provides personalized and accurate patient engagement by enabling physicians to diagnose with informed judgments. It also offers patients the right tools to make knowledge and evidence-based decisions about their health.

In the future, we can expect AI to grow more helpful with how it scans patients and gathers information. For example, a system called **AiCure**[12] is being developed by the National Institute of Health to use a smartphone's webcam to check up on patients, ensure that they are taking their prescriptions properly, and monitor a patient's overall condition, thereby helping doctors keep in touch with those who are having life-threatening conditions.

Conclusion

Artificial intelligence might seem like a futuristic concept, but it is here now, currently being used in wide-scale applications that most of us would be unaware of. With a number of algorithms being developed that learn how to think like a doctor, as well as with the automation of workflow, the creation of new medications, direct medical consultations, and better treatments, AI is fine-tuning healthcare daily. AI and medical professionals can now work together to create a more efficient system that stops ailments before they begin and treats patients quickly and more effectively than ever before. An exciting future with AI awaits.

References/Further Reading

Go to URL

MedMantra.com/a26

Scan with a smartphone camera

CHAPTER TWENTY-SEVEN

NUTRITION

In the modern world, diet is important. People are becoming much concerned about their health and wish to maintain a nutritious diet that helps them sustain their wellbeing. But the question arises: what is 'healthy'?

On some days, the Paleo diet is proclaimed as the best thing for your body. On others, there is the Ketogenic diet that has become a trend rather quickly.

While some diets are said to be beneficial on a day – eventually, they may be declared detrimental. Not only does this variation exist between specific diets, but it also exists in essential everyday foods that we consume regularly. Foods like eggs and coffee may be considered healthy today, but you could be reading a headline tomorrow that tells you to avoid them at all costs.

At this stage, consumers are confused. People find themselves in a dilemma regarding which diet to follow or who to listen to. But here is the unfortunate truth: each body is unique. The idea that a specified diet would be healthy for every human is biologically impossible[1] – mainly since the way our food affects us differs on an individual level.

To break free of this struggle to determine the best diet for ourselves, we turn towards technology. More specifically, we look towards artificial intelligence.

Artificial Intelligence

Technology has become an integral part of our survival as human beings. We are beginning to rely more on technological advancements to aid our existence with each passing day. As a result, societies are also evolving.

The latest type of modern technology that has integrated itself into human lives is artificial intelligence. With the widespread launch of smartphone applications such as Siri or Cortana, there is increased access towards the world of artificial intelligence.[2]

But how does that impact or benefit us?

Well, with AI voice assistants around your home and your phones, there is so much that you can achieve. Most importantly, you could ask them a simple question: What should I eat?

AI and the Food Industry

Food is essential for human survival, and now, so is technology. The importance of AI in the food industry dates back to a few years ago when multinational companies such as IBM invested in using AI to create practical solutions for food-related problems.[3]

For instance, IBM is actively involved in research that includes the use of AI to pair various ingredients to develop new flavors and recipes for people. This research could prove to be a significant breakthrough for the food industry – since creating an entirely new flavor can be considered both scientific and artistic.[3] Since the process was too lengthy and too complicated for humans, IBM decided to leave all the work to artificial intelligence.[3]

AI in the food industry has proven to be quite efficient. It can make quick calculations and analyses based on the data collected and make corresponding changes immediately.

By using AI to develop new flavors by identifying patterns and considering alternatives, there are many new avenues now ready to be explored. Lucky for us, that includes an individualized diet-plan or the AI diet.

The AI Diet

Artificial intelligence can be used to create a perfect algorithm that tells you what to eat.[4] Since all of AI's suggestions are based on research and calculations, there is no doubt in believing that an AI diet could help people become healthier and significantly reduce their risk of getting a disease.

But why do we need an AI diet? Don't we already know the difference between healthy and unhealthy eating habits?

The truth is, we don't.

Dr. Eric Topol, a renowned cardiologist, participated in a 14-day experiment that involved tracking his dietary consumption, sleeping habits, and physical exercise. A sensor that tracked blood-glucose levels was provided, and a stool sample was also taken to assess his gut microbiome. After comparing his data with more than 1000 other participants' input, AI was able to create a personalized healthy/unhealthy grading scale for him.[5]

The results were anything but ordinary. The cheesecake was allocated an A grade in the sweets section, but whole-wheat fig bars were given a C. In fruits, strawberries were given an A+, while grapefruit was an unhealthy C. Apart from that, assorted nuts were given an A+ grade, but vegetable burgers had a C.[5]

Despite being a health practitioner, the results contradicted his existing beliefs regarding healthy eating. While his current diet was somewhat healthy, according to him, consisting of veggie burgers and whole-wheat fig bars, his nutritional intake wasn't actually healthy at all.[5]

As a result of this research, he realized that he had been eating unhealthy for the majority of his life. To avoid glucose spikes in the future, he was required to make significant changes to his diet – including integrating cheesecake and strawberries.

The main takeaway from this research was that humans are vastly unaware of what is healthy or unhealthy for their bodies. However, AI can help you determine a diet plan that is individualized and suited to your own biology – something that differs significantly from popular beliefs regarding healthy eating.

AI and Dietary Habits: Initial Developments

To successfully program AI to determine our individualized diet plans, we must first know why such variance exists in the first place. In simpler terms, why is something healthy for me but unhealthy for you?

The first significant development regarding this area of research was made a few years ago at the Weizmann Institute of Science. A journal article titled "Personalized Nutrition by Prediction of Glycemic Responses" was published, including the research that the spike in blood glucose levels as a response to consuming certain foods is only one aspect of our individualized responses towards nutrition.[6]

During this research, scientists made use of machine learning – a specialized branch of artificial intelligence that focuses on patterns. The goal was to determine the critical factor that drove the blood-glucose response towards food for each individual.

After analyzing billions of possible factors, the research was concluded with about a hundred factors that were actively involved in this glycemic response in humans. Instead of the key factor being food itself, it was actually concluded to be the gut bacteria – or microbiome.

As a result of this research, two conclusions were made. One that our microbiome is mainly responsible for our spike in blood glucose levels, and two, that this groundbreaking discovery was only made using AI.[6]

For continued development, more research is underway to determine the different biological responses our bodies have towards the same kinds and amounts of food.[7,8] The fascinating part, however, that all of these researches now include AI to analyze the large amount of data being collected and to reach evidence-based results.

The Importance of Biotechnology

In order to successfully generate all of these personalized AI diets we keep referring to, there needs to be a method of handling big data. This process requires many different technologies to be combined into one major development – something that is beyond the expertise of nutritionists or the food industry.

This brings us to the need for development in biotechnology – or the application of modern technology in the creation of individualized diets. AI diets require chunks of data on both life and diet habits, which comes together under the branch of biotechnology[9] due to its close relationship with life sciences.

In simpler terms, the future of an AI diet could stand on the foundations of modern biotechnology. Since an effective AI mechanism to generate customized diet plans requires the filtering of fake data as well as the simultaneous processing of different information, biotechnology is the only branch of science that would be able to aid the process seamlessly.

The Problem with Fake Data

On the topic of how biotechnology aids the process of having an AI diet, it is also vital to understand what nutritional science lacks at the moment. While many people believe that our diet and health are interconnected, the connection is overly complicated.

Without using modern biotechnology or AI, it is nearly impossible to conduct randomized trials at large scales. Observing the effects of a specific diet may span for many years before any conclusion can be drawn – and such close adherence to a diet and tracking of behavior is rarely ever controlled.

As a result of these imperfect researches, there is a great deal of fake data available regarding dietary habits and nutrition.[10] For instance, if you look at the oxalate quantities in different foods, the values you find will vary significantly from one source to another.[11] The difference could be so vast that while one article would suggest a particular food to be great for your health, another would advise you to remove it from your diet altogether.

Our Diets Are Flawed: The Evidence

Before resorting to AI for customized diets, it is important to consider the various researches that have already concluded that our diets are extremely flawed. The main reason for the flaw, however, is the amount of fake data available to us regarding 'healthy' and 'unhealthy' eating habits.

Depending on which source we choose to follow, we could have a completely different belief system regarding the contents of certain foods. Consequently, we could be eating less or more of a certain food without having any concrete evidence regarding its effect on our body.

A 2017 study conducted in the US investigated the consumption of 10 specific foods in more than half a million people who died from heart disease.[12] In the research, diets that consisted of salty foods and processed meats were considered to have adverse outcomes. A similar strategy was used for other kinds of foods as well.

With "convincing" evidence, the study concluded that 45% of the deaths were due to the ten dietary factors being researched.[12] In simpler words, it was concluded that half of all deaths from heart disease are caused by a poor or unbalanced diet.

Similar studies related to diet and fatality have made conclusions such as that plant-based diets can lessen the chance of developing type 2 diabetes[13] and that regular consumption of whole-grain foods can result in lower cases of heart disease or cancer.[14]

However, there is a major flaw in all of these studies: the dependency on self-reporting. Participants may not have accurately reported their dietary and other habits, resulting in an influx of false information. Additionally, these researches also do not have any controls and fail to eliminate confounding factors such as socioeconomic environments or literacy rates.

Consequently, such researches that are low in reliability still make their way to the public in the form of media headlines or journal articles – thus impacting the kinds of diet, we consume. Depending upon the day, every type of food ends up labeled both helpful and harmful.

The Problem with a Fixed Diet

As a result of fake news that circulates based on flawed research, many problems arise with our typical fixed diet. The idea of collectively following a specific nutritional guideline is both biologically and physiologically flawed, especially since it fails to consider the individuality of each human body.

In all individuals, there are varying metabolisms, microbiome, and external environments that contribute towards their physiological reaction towards food.[15] Despite consuming the same amount of the same food at the same time, it is possible and highly likely for two people to have varying biological reactions.

This can be attributed to many factors, including how our unique DNA can react to foods in varying manners.

Solving the Problem with Modern Biotechnology

Since our bodies react to foods in different ways, it can be useful to understand what aspects of our DNA differ and how the use of biotechnology with AI can help us find a solution to the problem.

1. Whole Genome Sequence Analysis

With modern biotechnology, science can analyze a person's entire genome and further understand how specific genes are related to certain diseases.[16] By analyzing the genetic compound of a person, it is possible to create a customized nutrition plan that is in accordance with their bodily functions and helps them avoid the instance of illness.

2. Nutrigenetics

Contrary to popular belief that the only way food impacts our bodies is through the nutrients it contains, modern biotechnology has now proven that food has a significant influence on DNA expressions that impact an individual's health.[17] With these technologies, it is possible to understand the varying health effects of consuming certain foods with relevance to genetic expressions – thus allowing AI to gather data and create customized dietary plans.

3. Proteomics

The tRNA signal transduction system in our body is greatly affected by the food we eat[18], which could result in certain proteomes being synthesized. Since these proteomes are essential for bodily functions such as growth and balance, the data collected through DNA expression can be used to determine healthier food choices.

4. Nutrigenomics

The genetic structure of each individual is different. While food impacts our genetic expression, our varying genetic structures also lead to different metabolomic reactions within the body. This nutrigenomic data is, therefore, necessary during the creation of smart, AI diets.[19]

5. Metabolomics

While not causally related to food consumption, metabolomic data is still essential for the creation of AI diets since it allows for a deeper understanding of how overall lifestyle (sleep, exercise) impacts the health of an individual.[19]

6. Microbiome

Multiple studies have concluded that the food we consume affects not only our gene expression but also the gut bacteria that live inside our bodies.[20] While food does not change the DNA of gut bacteria, it does cause significant changes in the microbiome. This microbiome is related to both health and immunity – the two things that are the critical determinants for developing a good diet.

The Amalgamation of AI and What We Eat

In the present world, a popular food company was able to integrate AI with the food that is consumed by their customers. They introduced what is known as LIFEdata solutions[21] that are meant to engage with customers throughout the day to develop healthy eating habits that are customized for the specific user.

The platform works by understanding the user's lifestyle habits, external environment, motivational factors, and behavioral changes that go hand-in-hand with dietary habits. While it is not perfect, the platform currently has a mobile app that contains an entire database of nutritional data, varying recipes, and an integrated AI to provide smart suggestions.

The recommendations made to each user are based upon several self-report data inputs, including common surveys and detailed medical histories. By combining all of this data with eating habits and physiological reactions, personalized recommendations are made regarding dietary habits for each individual user.

Important features of this app include a simple method of selection between the correct food consumption to teach smart eating habits to children and entire families – based on their current medical and food consumption data. By following the smart suggestions provided by the AI, people can easily prevent chronic illnesses and choose to consume food that is especially healthy for their bodies.

Apart from that, the app also includes a voice assistant that can help people find recipes according to what they have available in their kitchens, as well as a step-by-step guide for recipe preparation.

The Mechanism of AI-Guided Diet Plans

Similar to the practical example of an AI-based solution quoted above, the mechanism of an AI-guided diet plan would also rely on machine learning and data analytics. With a deep understanding of the users' metabolic and digestive systems, the AI-based diet plan would be able to provide suggestions for ideal meals that would help your body rejuvenate.

This personalized diet plan is likely to contain the ability to save millions of lives per year. With diets that are specific to our bodily functions, preventing chronic illnesses such as diabetes, cancer, or heart disease would become much simpler.

Additionally, since many people resort to strict diets to lose weight, an AI-based solution will be much more effective in that aspect as well. By making use of big data and biotechnology, the AI-based diet plan would have a 72% probability of helping you lose weight.[22]

However, there is a critical downside to the use of AI-based diet plans that must be considered. Thousands of nutritionists across the globe may find themselves jobless if an AI-based diet plan system proves itself to be more efficient than these health practitioners. The likelihood of efficiency is extremely high in AI-based diet plans, especially since these machine learning systems will be able to process millions of bits of data within seconds[22] – something that the human mind cannot independently achieve.

Nevertheless, there is still an opportunity for existing nutritionists to expand their skillset and familiarize themselves with the applications of AI in the nutritional world. This would allow them to help people understand how the AI-based diet plans work and enabling users to make the most efficient use of such applications.

AI and Nutrition: The Future

While there are some developments in the field of AI for the food industry, they are definitely far from perfect. There are many more research areas that are yet to be covered before any significant developments can be made for customized diets using modern biotechnology as well as the different branches of AI.

However, there is no denying the usefulness of integrating AI with nutrition. In fact, an individualized and tailored diet will be able to promote a healthy lifestyle and allow our virtual assistants to take on a more significant role in our lives.

While a majority of AI-related dietary plans are still in their initial development stages, it is safe to say that technological advancement is fast enough for us to be soon testing personalized diet plans for ourselves.

We cannot know for sure what the future will bring for the food industry, especially with biotechnology and AI on the line now. However, we are certainly on the path towards creating increased access to legitimate information regarding dietary habits and implementing significant lifestyle changes. Hopefully, with AI-based diets, we would all be able to live healthier, happier, and longer lives.

References/Further Reading

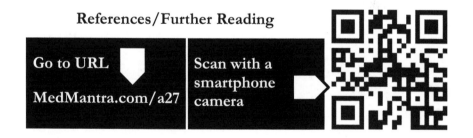

Go to URL

MedMantra.com/a27

Scan with a smartphone camera

CHAPTER TWENTY-EIGHT

RADIOLOGY

One of the important specialties of healthcare, radiology, is no stranger to involvement in medical advancements and AI integration. For many years now, computers have been an essential part of radiology. Therefore, it is no surprise that AI is now analyzing x-rays, CT scans, MRIs, and the like for abnormal readings, just like a radiologist would.

Yet, this also raises several questions about the future of radiology and just how important AI is to the progression of healthcare. In what ways can AI boost diagnostic efficacy in the radiology field? Will AI automate the tasks of radiologists? Will it be accurate and precise? One thing is certain: AI epitomizes potential for vastly improving medical examinations and diagnoses.

The Present State of Machine Learning in Clinical Imaging

Even with many start-ups or established research centers developing comprehensive AI-based tools for radio-imaging, it may be beneficial to understand how many of these applications are finally applied in the field and whether they really deliver the solutions they promised, outside of a trial set up.

A recent meta-analysis conducted by Rezazade M. and colleagues for the European Radiology Journal in 2020 evaluated all AI applications presented at the RSNA (Radiological Society of North America), ECR (European Congress of Radiology), and SIIM (Society for Imaging Informatics in Medicine) from 2017 to 2019, as well as trial studies and market research reports. They analyzed data from various sources to determine functionalities, focal modalities, targeted steps in the workflows, anatomical regions, and developmental and regulatory approval phases.

While North America and Europe took up most of the market share, at 41% and 22%, respectively, Asian companies also showed predominance, at 19%. Most of the applications are approved by the FDA or CE, while some countries, like Canada and Korea, have their own regulations for medical device approval. Fifty-four percent are built to retrofit with existing

PACS/RIS systems, while 25% are stand-alone. Seventy-four percent of the AI-based software analyzed was applied to CT, MRI, and X-ray images, while only 17% were meant to be applied in USG or mammography images. Breast screening data and diseases like the Big 3—lung cancer, COPD, and cardiovascular diseases—as well as brain imaging, are usually the focus of large-scale studies, and there has been tremendous growth in applications for the diagnosis of these conditions.

Eighty-seven percent of the AI-based algorithms are built to target reasoning and perception during the radiology workflow, that is, on improving the efficiency and speed of reporting images or scans.

Therefore, there is room to develop systems that help with areas like administration, the acquisition of machines, the processing of good-quality images, and transcription and reporting. Algorithms can be used to develop clinical decision-making support tools to determine which radiological investigations or radiation contrast dosages may be applied to individuals with common presenting features of conditions. Others may be used to monitor the downtime of machines, as well as maintenance or repair time, and to schedule tasks to balance the workload of the radiologists. Automated and AI-enhanced image processing enables clear, bright, and good-resolution images to be taken without skilled labor and without repetition, reducing the radiation exposure for patients and saving time for medical staff, with overall improved efficiency in operations. These innovations would truly make the applications of AI and machine learning systems in the field of radiology more comprehensive.[1]

Current Applications of AI-Based Radiology Systems

In 2015, a start-up based in San Francisco, *Enlitic*, flew software engineers to 80 clinical imaging centers throughout Central Asia, South East Asia, and Australia. These software engineers brought with them deep learning (AI) algorithm that had been designed to integrate with PACS, otherwise known as picture archiving and communication systems. Enlitic aims to use the algorithm to identify early stages of disease during clinical imaging sessions, including nuclear medicine, ultrasound, X-ray, computed tomography (CT), and magnetic resonance imaging (MRI). In 2016, Enlitic conducted a study that proved its AI software can improve the detection accuracy of radiologists in search of extremity fractures. According to its findings, the use of the Enlitic machine learning software alone aided in a 20% improvement in efficiency.[2]

Enlitic isn't the only up-and-coming software company with a hand in healthcare. Another San Francisco-based company, named *Arterys*, is making waves with its machine learning software. In November 2016, the FDA granted 501(k) clearance for Arterys 4D Flow software. 4D Flow is presently being used in cardiac MRI studies to improve the overall visualization and quantification of blood flow.[3]

In January 2017, another program, **Cardio DL**, was given the same clearance level. Similar to 4D Flow, Cardio DL is a cloud-based image processing technology that uses machine learning for the identification and segmentation of cardiac ventricles.[4]

To construct 4D Flow, Arterys formed a partnership with *Vios Works by GE Healthcare*. Arterys blended its cloud processing with the GE software for MRI machines. Though the product has not yet been released, already more than 40 hospitals are using the 4D Flow system for their research and have successfully used it in more than 10,000 cases.[5]

A Silicon Valley company called **RADLogics** is noted for creating **Alpha Point** software, a program that utilizes machine learning in preliminary findings, such as how a doctor would use medical records information and analyze the images from a radiology report. Already, the software has been given FDA clearance for chest CT scans and has been validated for chest X-rays. RADLogics is currently pursuing clearance for MRI scans as well.

During the 2020 Covid-19 pandemic, RADLogics deployed its AI-powered imaging software to analyze CT scans and X-rays from hospitals and clinics in the United States, Russia, Europe, China, and India, which greatly helped with patient triaging and rapid management. The application allowed for quantitative analysis of images, which could integrate seamlessly with existing software, making it scalable and offering global reach. Its accuracy has been validated in multiple clinical studies and, due to the rich influx of patient-related data, the machine learning algorithm has continued to improve and evolve.[6]

The co-founder of RADLogics, Moshe Becker, has stated that the software is meant to remove time-consuming measurements and other grunt work from the radiologist's workload. In fact, the software is more or less a virtual assistant. "Radiologists are valuable as diagnosticians. But, just as humans aren't that great in pixel counting or being a visual search engine, we're helping them go through the work more accurately, more consistently, and saving time." In fact, helping radiologists has become the company's primary goal.[7]

Meanwhile, other companies that aren't inherently medical have also begun dabbling in the healthcare setting. For example, **IBM has been working with its Watson system** to create **Watson Health**, which helps physicians with their diagnoses. From America to China to Europe to India and beyond, groups are endeavoring to revolutionize medical imaging with artificial intelligence.[8]

CAR AI Working Group

One of the latest and most extensive research groups is the *Canadian Association of Radiologists (CAR)* and the *AI Working Group*, founded in May 2017. Members of the working group include those in both pediatric and adult radiology as well as specialties in informatics, biophysics, and other research areas. The idea was to "discuss and deliberate on practice, policy, and patient care issues related to the introduction and implementation of AI in imaging." The primary goal was that radiologists could work together with AI developers to influence the way that such technology impacts their roles in the healthcare field. Other objectives include:

- Considering the potential impact of AI on radiology in Canada.

- Developing CAR policy regarding the usage and deployment of AI systems.

- Promoting and facilitating research in areas such as improving computer-aided design (CAD) systems, radiomics, computer-assisted reporting, natural language processing, and more.

- Offering guidance and support to help members incorporate AI systems into their practices in a way that will benefit patients and employees, such as optimizing workflow.

- Studying how AI learns through extensive research in elements like deep/machine learning and AI neural pathways, which are developed by relaying slightly different bits of information to the algorithms, creating a machine version of neuroplasticity.

- Looking into the social and ethical issues that the medical field may have to confront with the growing usage of deep/machine learning in healthcare.

While researching AI in multiple pathways, as well as how the machine learning software can evolve under certain conditions, the AI Working Group posed a powerful question: What is the impact of AI on radiology? Presently, AI is heavily impacting PACS, especially for tasks that are "prone to human error," such as detecting lung nodules (lung cancer) on X-rays or bone metastases on computed tomography (CT) scans. The working group concluded that while AI can improve the performance of clinicians, it cannot replace medical professionals. Another observation was that the pairing between clinician or physician and AI was better than either entity working alone.[9]

With this line of thinking, perhaps other countries should be establishing working groups for official radiology associations and allowing them to have a say in how AI is being integrated into the field. When miraculous medical advances are being made that benefit both physician and patient, and when radiologists are coming to realize that AI is not jeopardizing their position, better care can be delivered to patients worldwide.

How AI Will Change Radiology

One of the biggest challenges in the healthcare field presently is the amount of data being heaped on top of an already overwhelming workload for physicians and clinicians, including radiologists. Although electronic medical records (EMRs) have saved hospitals and doctors' offices from being flooded with papers and files, there are still exams, procedure reports, lab readings, EKG scans, pathology reports, and so much more. Through all of this raw data, medical professionals are expected to find the answer to a patient's discomfort.

That is where AI will change the entire healthcare industry, radiology included. Though AI cannot replace a human in many facets of healthcare, it can boost innate human comprehension to accelerate the discovery of the root cause of a patient's illness or pain. For example, a patient might be having chest pain. AI can look at computed tomography (CT) scan and single out the most relevant cause—or provide a narrowed-down number of possibilities. Thus, AI systems will improve medical imaging by doing the following:

- Scouring relevant data from prior medical exams with a focus on cardiac history.

- Looking into pharmacy information for drugs related to heart failure, coronary disease, COPD, and anticoagulants.

- Looking at previous chest CT scans to aid in analysis, including previous patient records, procedures, lab results, and pathology reports from similar cases.

In the end, the AI system might correctly weigh various causes that the doctors had been considering and put them on the right path. Without the aid of the AI system going through all this data within seconds, the patient's condition and health would worsen during the wait. In short, where humans are slow in scanning data and finding the answer, a computer can swiftly find the patterns and most probable causes.

A study was published in the **Public Library of Science** that reported on the development of a "collective intelligence" of radiologists that reduced the number of false positives and false negatives when reading mammograms. The Swarm AI was able to overcome "one of the fundamental limitations to decision accuracy that individual radiologists face," the researchers concluded. In other words, this "swarm intelligence" allowed groups of experts to come together and improve their decision-making skills. Everyone in the medical field knows that completing something a few seconds sooner can be lifesaving.[10]

Of course, AI will change the effectiveness of medical diagnosis in other ways, too. As seen with Arterys and Enlitic technologies, AI has already become an asset in radiology because it can accurately classify normal and abnormal MRI scans and x-rays with the same accuracy as a human. It doesn't matter if the clinical imaging is focused on intervertebral discs, torn ligaments, or cancer nodules—AI is capable of detecting these issues and reporting them to the radiologist. Not only does this improve the quality of the report, but it also improves the overall quality of care.

Why Radiologists Need AI

Going back to Enlitic for a moment—during the research, the engineers at Enlitic found that radiologists were hesitant to adopt the AI system. For example, during a lung cancer screening product trial, the radiologists would often overlook the analysis of the AI and instead use textbooks in search of rare cases. The Enlitic engineers noted how much time searching textbooks for information could take. When the AI system was used, however, the machine learning software would look for a history of lung nodules that were characteristically similar to what had been found on the image and make an appropriate detection that much faster.

There are more advantages to merging AI with medical imaging, though. Some of those benefits have been covered. Others are less apparent.

Let's take a moment to consider the experiences of **Mark Michalski, MD**, executive director of the *Brigham & Women's Hospital Center (BWH) for Clinical Data Science and the Massachusetts General Hospital (MGH)*. Michalski believes that AI can become the companion that radiologists have always needed—and sooner rather than later.[11]

In 2016, MGH paired up with **Nvidia,** an internationally renowned technology company, to employ a server made especially for AI applications called **DGX-1.** The MGH data scientists and Nvidia engineers were able to implement deep learning algorithms that took in 10 billion images from MGH records for training. Though much of the AI system is still in its infancy, the main algorithm that is being readily utilized is one to help radiologists assess bone age. How was it done? After exposing the deep learning algorithm to a plethora of (already interpreted) images related to bone age, it was able to learn how to conduct a satisfactory assessment. Now, radiologists enthusiastically use the AI system to aid them in their readings.[12]

Beyond having the benefit of an assistant that can carry out accurate assessments and enhance images, there is also the buzzword "automation" to think about. Many might recoil at the sight and sound of the word, but, in reality, automation goes hand in hand with AI. *Joerg Aumuller* from the *Artificial Intelligence and Decision Support Solutions department* at **Siemens Healthineers** stated, "The average radiologist is forced to interpret images quickly, potentially reducing diagnostic accuracy. When radiologists are rushed, their error rate rises... AI combines human and machine to be more powerful than the human alone".[13]

While the above statement is a nod toward the aspirations of swarm AI and software like RADLogics, one cannot overlook the main advantage: smoother workflow. For instance, AI could review chest X-rays and abnormalities in organs, and highlight these abnormal regions ahead of time, which would give the radiologist more time to study the images in full. An excellent example of this is the algorithm developed by **Predible Health (Bengaluru, India)** that can detect liver tumors. Without the AI, the time associated with segmenting out liver vessels, parenchyma, and tumors would be 45-60 minutes. Use of the AI dropped that time down to 5-10 minutes, leading to a faster diagnosis. The company worked with hospitals in India to access a rich mine of patient data in order to train the AI algorithm to develop two real-time applications. The first one is Predible Liver, which helps with the accurate planning that surgeons carry out before liver transplants or neoplasm resections. The second one, Predible Lung, accelerated lung nodule interpretation in CT scan images. Research is ongoing to introduce a platform for rapid stroke detection.[14]

AI vs. Radiologists

Naturally, these recent advancements in AI throughout several industries have raised the question of whether or not AI will one day completely automate the healthcare industry. In other words, will radiology become a job of a forgotten age? While it might seem that AI could overwhelm the healthcare field, it will not erase radiologists. Rather, it will enhance the efficacy of X-ray and MRI images, allowing radiologists to make more precise readings and analyses. However, before getting into why radiologists should be welcoming AI advancements rather than fearing them, we will review a few reasons why AI will change radiology for the better:

1. Humans Will Always Be Responsible

Despite automation's evolution throughout the years, it is mankind's desire for safety and communication. In other words, when legal responsibility is attached to the care of a patient, there is no fathomable circumstance in which the AI unit itself will be held accountable for a mistake. Someone must be there to take responsibility and offer recompense in some way. This means that it will always fall upon a human to check the analysis an AI system has made and finalize the decision. Although AI will aid the radiologist in developing clearer, more precise imaging, the AI system itself will be incapable of answering medical diagnostic questions 100% of the time.

2. Radiologists Look at More Than Images

Because radiology is more than looking at a single picture, there are dozens of tasks that an AI system cannot do. Many of these duties are designed for a human only. For example, a radiologist has face-to-face time with patients (such as discussing medical history details and providing directions during the examination period), must calibrate the machine and properly set the measurements, and must know how to choose the correct image type every time. Radiologists must also be able to identify certain types of readings (such as nodule detection or a hemorrhage), consult other physicians about diagnosis and treatment options, provide patient care (such as local ablative therapy), perform interventional radiology procedures, and tailor settings to a patient's condition. These are all things that only a flesh-and-blood person can do because they require emotional intelligence—which AI doesn't have—and hands-on action.

3. Machine Learning Takes Time

As mentioned previously in the section explaining the objective of the CAR AI Working Group, AI is not automatically all-knowing when it comes to the task it has been given. There are deep learning algorithms that form the brain, and it must learn through a flow of data. Someone will have to be there to figuratively hold the AI's hand and show it the way. Because no database of X-ray images is available to dump into the AI's brain, every new system will be starting from zero. The often-overlooked benefit of this, however, is that more radiologists will have to be hired to deal with the images and data being fed into the machine, especially when demand for AI-enhanced X-rays and MRIs increases exponentially in the next few years.AI might be able to schedule appointments and interpret images, but that won't cover even half of what a radiologist does daily.

Artificial Intelligence in Interventional Radiology

What Is Interventional Radiology?

Interventional radiology (IR) is a subspecialty of radiology responsible for performing many minimally invasive procedures.[15] These procedures are performed under medical imaging guidance, including x-ray fluoroscopy, ultrasound, magnetic resonance imaging, and computed tomography.

The primary goal of IR is to treat patients using the least invasive procedures available in the healthcare world. This minimizes the risk to patients and enhances the outcomes. IR procedures result in less pain, less risk, and less recovery time compared to standard surgical procedures.[15]

By integrating machine learning (ML) into diagnosis and treatment, AI can change the game for IR. It will empower healthcare professionals to efficiently offer the highest-quality care. Through AI, Big Data can be quickly analyzed to uncover new insights that aid radiologists.

Applications of AI in IR

1. Forecasting Outcomes

The biggest challenge IR faces is that professionals can't forecast the outcomes of treatment before performing it. They must devise an accurate method with a high success rate to reduce unnecessary interventions and procedures. This also reduces healthcare costs and risks to the patient.

Treatment efficacy must be measured before the patient agrees to the treatment. Such a challenge can be overcome with the help of AI, mainly deep learning (DL). The baseline diagnostic images of a patient's clinical data, and the outcomes of the planned intervention, can be used to teach the AI to work on a model that can learn the relationship between these variables and the procedure results.[16]

The results of the model would enable the prediction of the procedure outcome in new patients. Keep in mind that the characteristics of the intervention must be specified to obtain accurate results. DL-based AI can help interventional radiologists during the decision-making process.

2. Improving the Diagnosis

Another important application of AI in IR is to improve clinical imaging diagnoses. This involves DL-based classification of images, which helps radiologists. CNNs, also known as convolutional neural networks, are used to classify the hepatic masses on MR imaging, CT, and even ultrasound scans.[17,18]

Besides that, the higher the use of CNNs in the field, the more that healthcare specialists will learn about them and utilize them to enhance the patient care quality in IR. Keep in mind that CNNs function primarily as a black box. That is why an approach incorporating interpretability of the outcomes will help with clinical translation by allowing healthcare professionals to understand why decisions were made and predict why a decision may fail.

Creating such a model is tantamount in the field of IR. That is because it will enhance workflow and help IR professionals identify novel imaging

biomarkers for an accurate and effective diagnosis. Improved
significantly transform IR for patients and healthcare profes

3. Enhancing IR Procedures

There is always room for improvement, especially in the field of healthcare. Even in IR, radiologists must overcome challenges like high costs, slow decision-making, and more. These procedures increase patients' wait time and treatment costs.

Once AI is introduced in IR on a large scale, these procedures will improve significantly. The primary aim of AI in the healthcare industry is to reduce costs. The aim can also be achieved in IR, such as by automating many imaging and decision-making processes to significantly cut down costs.

Besides that, AI can enhance different aspects of IR. For example, remote catheter navigation assistance systems have been developed to improve the experience of interventional radiologists. The CorPath GRX Vascular Robotic System by Corindus (a Siemens Healthineers company) provides precise (sub-millimeter precision) device positioning from a distance during interventional procedures.[19-21]

It offers robotic-assisted control of guide catheters, guidewires, and rapid exchange catheters and provides radiation protection to the IR physician, as well as potentially reduces radiation exposure to staff and patients. In the same way, many new technologies can be developed to enhance various IR procedures.

ML models can run and offer results in milliseconds. These can allow for computations that improve the timing of decision-making processes in the field of IR. In the long run, both the patients and the radiologists will benefit from improved turn-around time and procedures in the field of IR.

4. Enhancing Patient Selection

Finally, AI in IR is also capable of enhancing patient selection. That is because ML can help professionals predict therapeutic outcomes.[22] This means more patients going through procedures in IR will receive the quality care they need.

⎣he best part about using an ML model is that fewer patients will be exposed to IR treatments that will not benefit them in any way.[16] Of course, that is just one way AI can improve IR when it comes to patient selection. The model can be expanded to many other cohorts to strengthen the entire process from diagnosis to treatment.

For example, before any therapy starts, AI mechanisms can identify nonresponders. When this happens, patients will be saved from unnecessary treatment and therapies. However, for the outcomes to be accurate, the AI must be fed with appropriate data.

Once the data is appropriate, the AI will make more accurate predictions and offer therapeutic recommendations that patients require. The data must also be validated and updated from time to time. Retraining the model is essential to get the most use out of it, as this affects the patients' experience when it comes to treatment.

Final Words – AI in IR

AI has many other potential applications in IR. Often, diagnostic radiologists are not available; this is an area that can drastically improve in the coming years. Besides that, AI has the power to provide higher quality care and a more accurate diagnosis.

Of course, AI techniques are at the stage where they are still evolving. The ethical problems involved in designing AI must be discussed and agreed upon by everyone involved in the process. In addition, more research is needed to create some of the best AI algorithms that the medical industry has ever seen.

Once all the proper steps have been followed, AI can drastically improve patient care and radiologist performance outcomes. The field of IR can significantly change once AI is in motion.

Conclusion

All in all, it is safe to say that the future of medicine and research lies in the virtual hands of deep/machine learning, also known as artificial intelligence. The revolution is happening now, all around us. Algorithms are interwoven into our daily lives, from Facebook's automatic face-tagging feature to the Amazon Alexa perched on the bookshelf. However, the biggest problem that AI faces is the hesitation of implementation that many medical professionals, including radiologists, have. Because many see AI as automation—and, thus, an adversary in the workforce—getting radiologists to adopt the technology that can help them is the current challenge.

What should be stressed is not the automation or how advanced the technology has already become, but how AI is more of an assistant that spots irregularities and reduces human error while simultaneously combining individual intelligence to accelerate diagnosis. AI will support radiologists in becoming a more evolved form of a medical professional than before, as they will have the time to completely examine the details of an image, communicate the results of the combined AI and radiologist findings, and play a more active role in the diagnosis of illness and disorders, as well as in the treatment of patients.

Perhaps, in the future, radiology and other medical fields will need to be renamed, but the human factor of healthcare will never change. The future of radiology lies within artificial intelligence, so let's allow AI to flourish and bring about a better future for everyone.

References/Further Reading

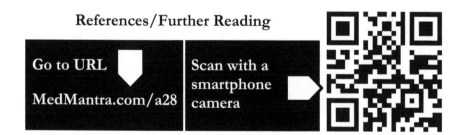

Go to URL
MedMantra.com/a28

Scan with a smartphone camera

CHAPTER TWENTY-NINE

PATHOLOGY

To take medical diagnosis and research to the next level, the latest advancements in technology, such as artificial intelligence (AI) and machine learning (ML), have to be considered.

The focus of the AI industry has unsurprisingly been on the applications of clinical diagnostics in fields like pathology. The idea is simple - to handover repetitive and time-consuming tasks to a machine so that the human experts can focus on more challenging and complex cases.

Data shows that low-income and middle-income countries (LMICs), which have a disproportionately large share of the global burden of diseases, have an inversely low number of trained professionals who can contribute to laboratory medicine services.[1]

Pathologists are a relatively small population of medical professionals in the healthcare industry. They could largely benefit from the support that AI technology could provide in order to tackle the growing threat of stronger, more resilient diseases, pathogens, and non-infectious disorders. While other healthcare sectors have adopted AI to take on tasks like regulating workflow or scanning data, its implementation in pathology has been fairly recent. However, the benefits that this budding partnership has already provided are undeniable and have brought about rapid improvements in the field.

The Growth of Digital Pathology

Climate change, industrialization, and other factors have long influenced the diseases and pathogens that affect humankind. Due to rising cancer rates as well as incidences of non-communicable diseases leading to chronic health conditions, there is an urgency to adopt digital pathology in clinical fields, with the hope to improve existing diagnostic measures and reduce costs associated with conventional methods.

In 2019, the digital pathology market was determined to be USD 767.6 million worldwide. It is predicted to grow at an 11.8% compound annual growth rate (CAGR) from 2020 to 2027 due to efforts made to improve the efficiency of workflows leading to rapid diagnostic tools. The Asia Pacific region will show a faster rate of expansion, expected to be at 12.9%, because of the rising popularity of digital imaging in growing economies.[2]

Whole slide imaging (WSI) captures images of tissue microscopy and uploads them into databases with specialized scanners. These databases are studied and analyzed to come to a diagnosis. WSI allows pathologists to visualize the data on a computer screen or a virtual microscope that allows for improvements in education, training, diagnostics, consultations, meetings, archiving, and more. According to the traditional surgical pathology lab workflow, after manual sectioning, several slides from the tissue specimen are sliced, and additional special stains or immunohistochemistry tests are applied. With WSI, pathologists make a series of whole slide images to use along with textbooks, medical records, and other previously collected molecular or lab data. However, due to the sheer data size of slides (2-3GB per image), they must be processed using an updated digital workflow. The data sets formed are enormous, and here lies the natural progression towards AI to help with analysis.

The adoption of AI in digital pathology requires the slides to be imported into a software program, which uses machine learning to spot subtle patterns and provide detailed information to the pathologist. Not only can specimens be analyzed by AI from different angles, but the workflow is also streamlined, and thus the efficiency and efficacy in reporting and diagnosis are increased.

Current advancements include whole slide imaging and robotic light microscopy, backed by ambient computing through fiber-optic communications, which work together to improve the applications of digitalization in pathology. Predictive and hybrid models used along with micro-arrays lead to efficient computer-aided diagnosis, along with estimations of disease progression and risk assessments, resulting in improved research and treatment initiatives.

Why does Pathology Need AI and ML?

Presently, cancer affects 1 in every three persons globally, which means that by 2030, more than half of the entire planet's population will have some form of cancer. However, pathologists cannot keep up with the demand for body tissue samples that require study. China, for instance, has about 20,000 pathologists in the entire country, but given the size of the total population, over 100,000 pathologists would be required to handle the workload.

More importantly, pathologists are constrained to what the human eye can detect in tissue samples put underneath the lens of a microscope to recognize patterns and correlate them with clinical findings. Even with digital whole slide imaging and other ways to collect visual data, there is a limit to the kind of information pathologists can obtain, on their own, in a time-bound manner. On the other hand, AI will be able to look at the details from a multitude of different perspectives, accessing new information from a wide range of disparate healthcare and research databases – inside and outside individual facilities. As such, there will be analysis made on larger data sets, revealing previously unobtained useful conclusions that can help solve cases faster, enabling the pathologist to move on to another case, thereby improving turnaround time.

This amalgamation of advanced imaging, automation, and powerful analytics like natural language processing (NLP), machine learning, and artificial intelligence (AI) in the field is bringing together the tools needed for accelerated diagnosis and earlier treatment options for patients.

In 2018, the UK established *The Path LAKE Consortium* as one of its 5 AI centers of excellence funded by UK Research and Innovation (UKRI). It brought together university and NHS partners committed to the creation of completely digital cellular pathology laboratories, along with an ethically approved data lake of anonymous scanned slide images, used to train and develop AI algorithms.[3]

Another large-scale digital slide library is *The Cancer Genome Atlas,* which allows researchers to access a large database of annotated pathology images linked with clinical and genomic history, which acts as training material for AI-based software in pathology diagnosis.[4]

The Future of Artificial Intelligence in Pathology

Though pathology departments have already integrated faster and more powerful technologies into their laboratories, the most exciting time for artificial intelligence and pathology is on the horizon. Many of the advancements go beyond the usefulness of WSI by incorporating the latest algorithms from deep learning to enhance the diagnostic capabilities of AI systems. These Deep learning systems create the possibility of machine-aided pathology or Computer-Aided Diagnosis (CAD).

This means that AI will be able to aid the pathologist in the following sections of work:

1. Formulating a hypothesis

Currently, pathologists arrive at a hypothesis by going through a systematic process based on what they know. They ask themselves what is relevant, and depending on their experience; they may overlook other possibilities. With AI support, thousands of pieces of data (from electronic patient records, ECGs, EEGs, MRIs, CT scans, etc.) will be scanned for the most suitable scenario. Since the AI will be able to classify common and uncommon patterns in certain images, it will become better and better at identifying diseases and other anomalies.

2. Detecting and classifying known features.

The large datasets that are formed with the cumulation from different sources can be overwhelming and difficult to analyze. Organization and classification of known features aids in better diagnosis. *The Joint Pathology Centre (JPC),* which is the pathology reference center for the United States federal government as well as a part of the US Defense Health Agency, selected **Huron's artificial intelligence-enabled** Lagotto™ image search engine to index and search JPC's growing digital image archive, unlocking the wealth of knowledge housed in the repository to enhance research and enable easier data sharing with researchers, diagnosticians, and educators. By connecting these rich datasets like pathology reports, treatment plans, patient outcomes, and even data from genomics, Lagotto sets the foundation for new applications, such as predictive algorithms for personalized treatment plans or improved drug discovery.[5]

3. Identifying unknowns.

A pathologist assisted by AI will be able to realize the presence of newer patterns or unexpected relationships that might not have existed before. This has the potential to help us arrive at new conclusions every time an AI algorithm searches through databases, biobanks, or electronic medical records.

A study by Hegde and colleagues in 2019 described Google's AI methodologies that helped to improve search results for similar features in digital images, irrespective of whether they had been annotated by trained pathologists or scientists. The experts who reviewed the digital slides marked them with their interpretations before feeding them into the database so that the AI algorithm can analyze and learn to differentiate cellular and tissue-based morphology from them. The algorithm named SMILY (Similar image search for histopathology) used datasets of unlabeled images to find morphologically similar images to recognize newer patterns to make more accurate predictions.[6]

4. Reducing errors

Since diagnosis in pathology often follows a path of repeated rejection of hypotheses until a final interpretation is derived, AI algorithms are able to rapidly and accurately sort through the various differential diagnoses and narrow down the most appropriate causative or prognostic factors for a particular disease. Robust algorithms may even be able to perform *"transfer learning,"* whereby the rationale used to diagnose a disease manifestation on one organ or tissue sample can be transferred or applied to another type of tissue sample. With the help of AI, applications not only can the WSI be analyzed automatically, but it can also be shared with or verified by experts globally, which ultimately reduces chances of errors and improves the accuracy of reports.

5. *Academic or professional training*

Lagotto™ is a patented, content-based image retrieval software that enables instant search for similar digital slides within an institution or a global data set and accesses the knowledge in corresponding diagnostic reports, patient outcomes, and metadata. With this software, users can find similar cases and read multiple pathology reports from subspecialty experts in real-time, providing a **"virtual peer review"** for pathologists, researchers, and educators.[7]

6. *Saving Time*

Pathologists who use AI systems report time-saving benefits during diagnosis, ensuring that they can spend more of their workdays on challenging cases and allow AI to take care of the labor-intensive, routine ones. In 2018, Google developed an AI algorithm *called Lymph Node Assistant (LYNA)* in order to report metastatic breast cancer on slides. In a study conducted by Steiner and colleagues, board-certified pathologists conducted a diagnostic simulation where the lymph nodes were reviewed for micrometastases of breast carcinoma cells in two phases, once with LYNA's help and once without. This laborious task was made easier with LYNA than without, as it cut the average slide review time in half. This also proves the potential of assistive technologies in reducing the burden of repetitive tasks for identification. The time and energy saved can be utilized by pathologists to focus on challenging diagnosis or clinical tasks.

The study also showed that pathologists using LYNA were more diagnostically accurate than either those who were unassisted or just the LYNA program when used alone, suggesting the ideal outcome was when the best of both the human mind and AI were used together.[8]

Evidence of Successful Applications of AI in Pathology

Applications in Microscopy

Despite the growth in AI research, the utilization of these tools in real practice is challenging due to prohibitors like the high cost of implementing the digitalization of sections using slides and scanners. To circumvent this, it was proposed to integrate AI directly into the microscope, i.e., the Augmented Reality Microscope (ARM), which overlays AI-based data points onto the microscopic view of the sample, relayed through the optical pathway in real-time, enabling seamless application of the algorithms into the microscopic workflow. The ARM can also be retrofitted into existing light microscopes using ready-made components, instead of investments in whole slide imaging technology. Currently, the program has been tried for breast and prostate cancers, but the potential applications are limitless. The ARM can provide visual feedback, like text, arrows, heat maps, or contours to help the pathologist narrow down on tumor-affected areas, helping to detect, quantify, and classify cancers rapidly and effectively.[9]

This helps to bring AI directly to the end-user, meeting them where they are most comfortable ... at their microscopes. The pathologist has ready access to deep learning as it moves away from the computer lab and into the medical lab.

Applications in Onco-Pathology

In the past few years, precision oncology has advanced significantly and moved towards predictive assays that can enable the stratification and selection of patients for treatment appropriately. The complex processes that lead to cancer formation and progression due to divergence of transcriptional or signaling networks that in turn disrupt the function of biomarkers based on gene expression or protein formation generate unique morphological features in stained tissue specimens. The large amount of permutational data generated from this has led to an interest in AI systems to help with diagnosis by teaching neural networks to identify tumor versus normal areas in tissue samples through digital whole slide imaging so that it can consciously refine its analysis on new data supplied.[10]

Deep Learning and machine learning applications are trained to look for particular morphological features through the analysis of digital pictures obtained by whole slide imaging (WSI) and scanning. Today, with the availability of powerful processors, cloud-based computing, and strong IT infrastructures, a workflow based on *pixel-pipelines* can be developed to create prognostic or diagnostic algorithms based on machine learning.[11]

A study conducted by Nagpal and colleagues in 2019 used a Deep Learning (DL) AI system to assign Gleason scores automatically after processing whole slide images of tissue resected from radical prostatectomy. When compared to the scoring done by general pathologists, with both sets of results checked by an expert genito-urinary pathologist, it was observed that the DL approach had an accuracy of 0.7 in predicting the Gleason score, whereas the pathologists had a mean accuracy of 0.6. This method of using the AI algorithm improved diagnostic accuracy, especially where specialist expertise is unavailable.[12]

While modern approaches to the treatment of breast cancer require classification of patients and disease profiles in order to provide tailored therapy and predict survival, this stratification is based on the interpretation of tissue slides, mitotic counting in cells, and histological grading with biomarker status, which has been delegated to AI-based software applied on WSI, to relieve the pathologists from time-consuming and labor-intensive tasks, which may have varied results due to their inherent subjectivity.[13]

Research conducted by Shamai and colleagues in 2019 used AI algorithms and a deep learning system to assess hormonal or biomarker status from tissue microarrays in patients with breast cancer, which was predicted with 92% accuracy. This suggests that deep learning models can assist pathologists with the molecular profiling of oncology cases.[14]

Applications in Inflammatory Pathology

Neoplastic pathology has always taken center stage in most deep learning studies while overlooking its potential in inflammatory conditions. A study conducted in 2019 by Martin and colleagues investigated the use of DL algorithms developed by *Indica Labs*[15] for non-neoplastic gastric biopsies when compared to the gold standard diagnoses by independent pathologists. The resulting sensitivity/specificity parings of manual screening accuracy versus deep learning showed that the algorithm could identify H. pylori at 95.7% and 100%, which suggests that a convolutional neural network (CNN) has the potential to be a good screening and diagnostic tool for H. pylori gastritis. *Indica Labs* provided the evaluation of the WSI, quantitatively, using HALO AI for analysis of the digital images and *HALO Link* for data management and seamless collaboration.[16]

Applications in COVID-19

Due to the global pandemic in 2020, the discovery of the novel coronavirus meant that healthcare systems around the world had to find easy ways to assimilate knowledge about how the virus affects different organs and body functions in a timely manner, to help with treatment efforts as well as research towards an effective vaccine. An initiative launched in May 2020, spearheaded by the US Federal Government with the support of Indica Labs, for computational pathology software and OCTO for IT systems support[17], aimed to build an adequate dataset of information about COVID-19. Blood and tissue samples were taken from patients who were either diagnosed with or succumbed due to the virus. Whole slide images were prepared from various organs, including renal, hepatic, and cardio-pulmonary tissue samples.

The digital images were annotated by expert pathologists. The metadata was compiled in a cloud-based repository, which can be utilized as an educational resource and for research and clinical trials aimed at discovering preventive or therapeutic alternatives for COVID-19. The repository is now hosted by the National Institutes of Health in the United States. The electronic database is augmented software from *Indica Labs' HALO Link™*, enabling collaboration and secure methods to analyze and share images.

Conclusion

In order to benefit from the many advantages that AI brings to the table, a general change in mindset is essential as pathologists and other medical professionals need to understand that it is their partnership and experience that is vital to the integration of better technology.

In addition, outdated IT infrastructures, storage space limitations for software and hardware, network latency, and lack of interoperability due to outdated EHR interfaces are real and significant barriers to large-scale implementation. Regulations and evidence-based validation of the tools that are developed are also required to promote buy-in from the medical community.

It is also evident that in spite of a few hurdles, AI is already making headway in its applications to improve digital and surgical pathology workflows and result outcomes, contributing largely to rapid, automated diagnosis and access to timely therapeutic interventions. It has the potential to disrupt conventional molecular and genomic-based testing, which are the standards for predicting re-occurrence and outcomes of treatment.

From the patients' point of view, AI tools can enhance the patient experience through applications and mobile devices, giving them access to their electronic health records, radiology, and pathology reports, and images, in a background of known genomics (precise, accessible genetic testing) and other population-based health data.

References/Further Reading

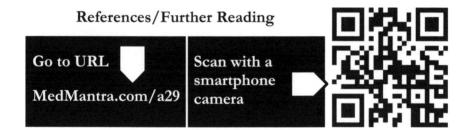

Go to URL
MedMantra.com/a29

Scan with a smartphone camera

CHAPTER THIRTY

SURGERY

In the coming decades, surgery done by humans will likely change dramatically, and the catalyst for the change will be the application of artificial intelligence in surgery, leading to faster and better patient care. Far from replacing surgical skills, AI-powered technology aims to ease the surgeon's burden and expand the possibilities of treatment.

The field of surgery in medicine itself has many specializations. Robotic surgery was introduced years ago to reduce the physical burden of practicing surgeons intra-operatively. AI, however, takes it a step further. The merging of AI applications with surgical robotics aims to reduce the cognitive burden as well by simplifying diagnosis and workflows with accurate and precise intra-operative maneuvers and the timely prediction of post-operative complications or morbidities.

Robotics in Surgery: The Foundation Laid

A surgeon's skill lies in finger dexterity and precise incisions. Their experience, obtained over years of training, is invaluable in the operating room. However, long and complicated surgical procedures are often physically demanding.

Surgical robots were invented and applied in the operating room, as they could execute multiple, repetitive surgical procedures precisely, under different levels of supervision, and could do so without fatigue. They also provided surgeons with a *"robotic wrist,"* which improved maneuvering and visualization within the surgical field. Ergonomics were also improved as kinematics were introduced, with large-scale human movements being scaled-down and converted into limited, complex, technical movements in the robotic hands. Robots could also avoid the very human tendency for unintended movements, hand tremors, or accidents that can have catastrophic results in surgery.

The very first robotic surgery, in 1985, was a simple neurosurgical procedure. A *stereotactic* brain biopsy was performed by a modified industrial robot called the **PUMA 560**. In 1994, **The Cyberknife** was invented, which used real-time image guidance, and a robotic arm to aim focused radiation beams for cancer treatment in patients who had inoperable or surgically complex tumors, using "stereotactic radiosurgery (SRS) as well as stereotactic body radiation therapy" (SBRT).

Since then, the area of surgical robotics has evolved rapidly to include **endoscopic** (the Zeus system in 1989 and the Da Vinci system in 2000), **bio-inspired** (the I-SNAKE and the CardioArm), and **micro-bot** models (capsule endoscopes like the PillCam). The development of **haptic feedback** technology, in which the robotic user interface could respond to touch, also introduced novel practical applications.[1]

However, the addition of AI to robotic surgery added a level of expertise that truly elevated the field and opened up a host of possibilities. The addition of different fields of AI like *Machine Learning (ML), Natural Language Processing (NLP), Artificial Neural Networks (ANN), and computer vision* has shown remarkable developments.

Applications of AI in Surgical Workflows and Robotics: The Future Built

While accuracy in robotics will greatly improve intra-operative surgical outcomes, the adoption of AI in pre-surgical and post-operative processes should also be considered in order to truly benefit patients going through surgery-based treatment modalities.

Machine learning (ML) applied to electronic health records (EHRs) has resulted in the design of a temporal prediction model that gives a data-based evaluation of patients for possible surgical site infections, based on an analysis of procedures, laboratory and radiological investigations, and patient symptoms, which gave remarkably accurate results as compared to traditional methods of diagnosis.[2]

Similarly, a Natural Language Processing (NLP) algorithm, the bag-of-words model, was applied to free text extracted from EHRs to diagnose the risk of anastomosis leakage after colorectal surgery, with 100% sensitivity and 72% specificity. This was done using surgeon notes about the operation, as well as predictive phrases that described patient symptoms or post-operative complaints.[3] Using Artificial Neural Networks (ANN) and Deep Learning, researchers were able to develop a clinical decision support system for surgeons evaluating a patient pre-operatively for an aortic vessel dilatation procedure, with 95.4% accuracy. Because the operation is very risky, the prediction of which patients are likely to develop complications or not survive the surgery is useful for reducing operational costs as well as post-procedure expenses due to expected morbidity. It gives patients the option for alternative treatments, knowing their predicted risk for surgical modalities, and helps to reduce undesirable post-procedure results.[4]

Computer vision algorithms can undertake an image-based analysis of patients' records that have surgical or diagnostic videos. Data absorbed from watching surgeons perform procedures, along with patient data from EHRs, can help to train machine learning systems to generate actionable information and even in identifying and predicting adverse events that may occur during or after surgical interventions in real time.

Fully Autonomous Systems: The Future Imagined

The first robot-assisted, trans-Atlantic telesurgery was conducted in 2001. It was termed "Operation Lindbergh" and involved gall bladder removal by a minimally invasive endoscopic procedure done while the patient was in an operating room at Strasbourg, France, while the surgeon operated a robotic console in New York, USA.[5]

To date, robotic surgery under teleguidance is an evolving prototype. Most systems under conceptualization do not leave decision-making to a robot, as they are performed with the surgeon's console within the operating room complex. Teleguided surgery is a more conventional option. A surgeon in the operating suite is at the local console, while an expert from another center not only visualizes but can even take over controls for certain crucial surgical steps. The implications of this technology in today's world are multi-fold. The doctor:patient ratio is drastically declining, leaving a dearth of specialty and super-specialty healthcare providers like surgeons. Therefore, it offers the ability for a clinically capable machine or robot to independently operate on patients in areas where human intervention is difficult, like those affected by natural disasters, endemic infections, or war zones, thereby maintaining both physician and patient safety, with good treatment outcomes.

In 2016, researchers initiated the **STAR trials (Smart Tissue Autonomous Robot)**, which used autonomous intestinal anastomosis procedures, employing only AI algorithms, with little or no human intervention at the controls. These trials gave AI its advent in surgical fields and provide a sneak peek at the future of truly intelligent machine applications in a skill-based, traditionally manual field in healthcare.[6,7]

Intraoperative applications of AI are, therefore, focused on guidance to facilitate improved visualization and localization during surgery. These are:

1. *Perception-based tools*: applications or software that trace the interactions between surgical tools and the environment, 3D reconstructions to show dynamic organ functions instead of static image displays, or instrument tracking and navigation.

2. *Localization and mapping of anatomical sites*: using **SLAM (Simultaneous Localization and Mapping) tools**[8], visual odometry and camera Localization, endoscopic navigation, and augmented reality.

3. *System modeling and control tools*: using kinematics, machine learning from demonstrations through reinforcement learning.

4. *Human-robot interaction tools:* using touchless manipulation or even intention understanding and prediction in the future.

In 2019, the **MicroSure** Robot, developed in the Netherlands for robotic microsurgery, used AI to suture small blood vessels in a patient with lymphoedema in order to reduce swelling.[9]

Early trials have been able to demonstrate that AI-assisted or controlled robotic surgery intraoperatively, or pre-operative and post-operative AI interventions, research-based guidance, or tools can help to reduce variations in clinical practice and procedures and thereby improve clinical outcomes. **Synaptive Medical recently tested its Modus V tool**, which is a fully automated, robotic digital microscope that can be used in operating rooms to visualize anatomical fields during the procedure.[10]

Proximie is a London-based web platform that allows doctors, especially surgeons, to communicate and collaborate through audio-video and augmented reality technology. Its AI-backed computer vision software enables surgeons to call upon data and images pertaining to the procedure and visualize it with unnatural clarity. "Proximie is now used by a third of all NHS hospitals, and the goal is to reach 40% penetration by the end of 2020" – Quote by Forbes magazine.[11]

Conclusion

Technology-based surgical practice can provide surgeons with the ability to improve care delivery. AI has the potential to collect and configure a vast database of surgical experience, similar to genomic databases and biobanks, to make clinical decision-making and complicated surgical techniques easier. Leveraging Big Data to create a "collective surgical consciousness" can lead to technology augmented and AI-controlled, real-time decision-making support, even leading to GPS-like guidance during an operation. Advanced AR and VR (Augmented Reality and Virtual Reality) systems can also step-up surgical training and teaching. If the technology is developed and implemented properly, AI can completely revolutionize the methods by which surgery is taught and applied, with the hope of a future primed to deliver optimum patient care.

References/Further Reading

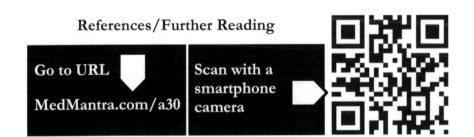

Go to URL
MedMantra.com/a30

Scan with a smartphone camera

CHAPTER THIRTY-ONE

ANESTHESIOLOGY

The field of anesthesiology is unique in medicine, as physicians involved in its practice must be equally involved with both their patients and other healthcare professionals, doctors, and nurses. Anesthesiologists must be familiar with drug metabolism, interactions, and timing while making critical decisions based on constantly changing patient variables and data inputs stemming from patient vitals and drug monitoring.

The introduction of Artificial Intelligence (AI) in healthcare aimed to make processes safer and more efficient for both physicians and patients. Anesthesia is no exception. Artificial Intelligence (AI) and Machine Learning (ML) can provide large quantities of highly accurate data, which can be processed efficiently, catering to patient-specific requirements.

AI has the potential to revolutionize the following areas in anesthesiology practice:

1. Depth of anesthesia monitoring

Distinguishing between awake and anesthetized states is one of the important problems in surgery. Vital sign parameters based on electroencephalogram (EEG) such as the Bispectral (BIS) - (Medtronic, USA) index have been used, as the EEG reflects brain activity to reveal information about different states of anesthesia that affect the brain, making it ideal for monitoring and predicting different depths of anesthesia (DoA).

Using recorded patient information as a data set for ML algorithms like LLE (Locally Linear Embedding) or ANN (Artificial Neural Networks), EEG signals can be classified into conscious and unconscious states for patients. Hence, researchers were able to develop a method for an EEG monitoring system that could assist anesthesiologists in accurately estimating the DoA during a surgery or procedure. Research conducted by Gu Y et al.[1] used ANN to analyze multiple EEG-based parameters like permutation entropy, Beta Ratio, and Synch Fast Flow to accurately distinguish between different patient states during propofol anesthesia. Similarly, Shalbaf et al. used data derived from EEG features to classify awake *versus* anesthetized patients during sevoflurane anesthesia with 92.91% accuracy.[2]

2. Control of anesthesia delivery

As the applications of BIS data derived from EEGs included being a key metric to measure the depth of anesthesia, researchers began to employ AI-based tools to achieve anesthetic control using BIS as a target measure. They also applied machine learning to regulate the delivery of anesthesia medications or mechanical ventilation. AI-dependent control systems that could automatically deliver drugs acting as neuromuscular blockades using rule-based hierarchy monitoring along with architecture framed with fuzzy logic control were used by Shieh et al., resulting in stable controller activity.[3]

Automated delivery of anesthesia by machine-based monitoring and weaning of mechanical ventilation has also been made possible through feedforward, feedback, or closed-loop systems.[4] Based on the patient's vital signs, the AI-based devices can automatically adjust DoA, which eliminates the need for the anesthesiologist to physically attend to the patient throughout a long surgical procedure. He may even be able to attend to multiple patients in adjacent OT rooms simultaneously, saving on manpower resources.

3. Event and risk prediction

The American Society of Anesthesiologists (ASA) has established a classification for the assessment of preoperative surgical patients for risk during surgery. Variations in interpretation have made uniform application of the ASA difficult, as often many variable patient factors must be considered, like the type of surgery, obesity, previous medical conditions, old age, etc. This leaves room for a considerable number of human errors. Hence, AI and deep learning algorithms were developed to guide physicians and surgeons through accurate allotment and interpretation of risk while using this grading system.

a. Collection of patient data

Anesthesia Touch™ is an AIMS (anesthesia information management and medication management system) for Android and iOS software that can enable automated and continuous charting of physiological data. Its user-friendly interface makes it comprehensive anesthesia documentation as well as a recorded patient electronic health record (EHR). Because AI-based monitoring devices can capture patient data automatically, the anesthesiologists need not write physical notes while attending to the patients.

Pharmacy Touch™ is a supplementary module that can automate documentation, thereby reducing drug errors, to support critical decisions in emergency situations at bedside care. This is integrated with **Synopsis Healthcare**, which specializes in the electronic preoperative assessment as well as anesthetic charting automation for the National Health Service (NHS) in the UK. **Synopsis iQ**[5] revolutionized the digital medication and monitoring role, making it clear and efficient. The platform reduces avoidable harmful events by improving consistency with interpretation. As a by-product, organizations can also reduce surgery or procedure cancellations with the efficient improvement of staff allocation and with increased patient turnover, decreasing unnecessary testing before procedures, and reducing malpractice risks.

b. Estimation of risk of difficult intubation

The preoperative identification of patients who exhibit signs of difficult intubation, through the use of automated, computerized assessments based on facial recognition software and trained AI algorithms, would reduce the incidence of adverse respiratory events due to anesthesia effects. A study conducted by Abdelaziz et al. used an ML algorithm called **Alex Difficult Laryngoscopy Software (ADLS)** along with the **Microsoft Visual Studio 2008** and **WEKA** (Waikato Environment for Knowledge Analysis) to identify intubations that were going to be difficult, with 76% accuracy.[6]

4. Ultrasound guidance

Artificial intelligence techniques have been used to assist the anesthetist in ultrasound-based procedures, most commonly undertaken to deliver medication. Hetherington et al. conducted a study based on a deep convolutional neural network (DCNN) to correctly identify vertebral levels to deliver epidural drugs. The algorithm discriminated between USG images of the lumbar vertebral spaces and bones with 80% accuracy. An augmented reality projection was displayed to show the anesthetist the vertebral level at the proposed puncture site.[7]

5. Pain management

Patient response to pain as well as to medication given to relieve pain can be estimated by AI-based neural networks to narrow down the specific drug and dosage required to lower pain scores, while titrating the amounts to prevent adverse reactions. This largely reduced trial and error methodologies, through predictive evidence-based algorithms, especially useful with post-operative pain, as well as patient-controlled chronic pain management.

Jose M et al. conducted a study using an analgesia monitor, the Analgesia Nociception Index (ANI) signal, to analyze the relationship between the ANI and drug titration made by the anesthesiologist, using machine learning techniques. The results, when cross-validated, can be used as an effective predictor for accurate dosages of pain management drugs.[8]

Procedure training by virtual reality

Simulation-based virtual reality training is rapidly finding its way into mainstream medical undergraduate as well as postgraduate courses. Traditional methods of training require immense time and resources from experienced and trained observers, which offers limited opportunities for learners to practice and hone skills for procedures. Virtual reality can provide repeated opportunities for the rehearsal of complex invasive procedures through simulation. The hardware required for VR training has also reduced in size, with the *Oculus* providing a cost-friendly and space-saving investment. Applied software like the *Anesthesia SimSTAT* is a screen-based training program developed by the American Society of Anesthesiologists and *CAE Healthcare*, which exposes learners to modeled pharmacology and live waveforms to help with anesthetic procedures for trauma, appendectomy, robotic surgery, and labor. The software is hosted on the Microsoft Azure platform, which also released its HoloLens 2, a wearable holographic computer, which allows for instinctual interactions with holograms, using AI algorithms to trace hand motions and eye gaze. This can train intensivists in case setups on emergency scenarios like cardiac arrest, strokes, and bloodstream infections.[9]

AI will reduce errors and increase efficiency and perfection.

The goal of any AI-backed system is to efficiently decrease the cognitive load on physicians while taking over manual, time-consuming, and repetitive tasks so that the anesthesiologists can focus their attention on patients as well as on truly complicated cases that require skill-based interventions. At the end of the day, it is the patients who will benefit from more reliable and vigilant care delivery.

With the help of AI-based decision support systems in anesthesia, human errors and variances in interpretations will decrease, and efficiency will increase. AI-based anesthesia information management systems (AIMS) have smart monitoring systems that will ensure continuous monitoring and alarms during and after surgery to limit the effect of human errors or post-surgical complications.

AI will not replace professionals but will assist them.

While anesthesiology will reap benefits by using AI-based devices, machine learning is not a substitute for knowledge and judgment and cannot replace trained 'anesthesiologists. Manual skills and work-based experience are essential for carrying out emergency life-saving decisions. Most of the studies conducted in this arena deal with the augmentation of the anesthesiologist's workflow, decision-making, and clinical care, without the replacement of the physician's role, which combines both clinical knowledge and physical dexterity to undertake even routine activities like tracheal intubation, venous cannulation, and neural blockade, among others.

"Anesthesiologists enjoy a good mix of cognitive and dexterity-based labor, and given that AI will primarily result in the automation of cognitive work, it may be that our hands prevent full automation of the specialty," said Alexander and Josh, Baylor University Medical Centre.[10]

Over the last decade, machine learning and deep learning systems applied in anesthesiology are advancing in scope and number, with many exciting potential opportunities to bring the field into the future.

References/Further Reading

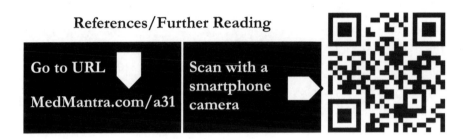

CHAPTER THIRTY-TWO

PAIN MEDICINE

Many of us don't do well with pain, especially after a medical procedure. We try to find as many ways as possible to manage pain, including abusing prescription medicines. That is because severe pain that is not relieved leads to mental stress, depression, and anxiety.

At this point, artificial intelligence (AI) is being used in all aspects of healthcare. It is also being utilized for pain management so that patients can deal better with their pain.[1] Here is everything you need to know about it.

The History of Pain Management

Pain management has been one of the most critical aspects of healthcare for a long time. Usually, the pain medicine is known as anesthesia and can be divided into four main categories:

- Anesthesia

- Intensive care medicine

- Critical emergency medicine

- Pain medicine

The primary aim of these four categories of pain management is to reduce sensitivity so that surgery can be performed without pain.[1] Before the development of modern medicine, various items were used as anesthetic agents, including:

- Belladonna

- Alcohol

- Narcotics such as opium

- Chloroform

- Nitrous oxide

- And many more

The problem with these early anesthetics was that they had several side effects.[2] These led to many complications and made the recovery procedure worse for patients. Of course, modern medicine has curbed many of these problems, but AI intervention is still required for better pain management.[3]

Use of Artificial Intelligence in Pain Medicine

Thanks to technology and AI, many companies are producing better solutions for pain management. Here are the many strides AI has made in terms of pain medicine and management:

1. PainChek

Did you know that around 50 million people worldwide have dementia? In the UK, 850,000 people and 70% of residents in care homes are affected by it. The main problem is that out of these people, at least 50% experience consistent pain.[4]

Dementia pain is one of the biggest challenges, as managing it can become complicated. That is because most of the time, the pain is undetected. When this happens, the pain is left untreated, which leads to psychological and behavioral issues that reduce patients' quality of life.

PainChek was created to help people with dementia manage their pain. It uses automated facial analysis technology and automation to help healthcare professionals identify pain in patients, especially when it is not easy to detect. PainChek can understand pain severity, monitor treatment impact, and optimize patient care quality.

The tool uses facial analysis technology and analyzes micro-expressions that indicate the presence of pain in a person. It detects a face, maps all the facial features, and applies different algorithms to detect pain. After all this analysis, it provides a pain score and intensity level.

Healthcare professionals can use this tool on iOS and Android devices even when they don't have an internet connection. After that, the data can be synchronized once the internet connection is available. That is why it is the perfect tool for detecting pain in patients across many clinical settings.

2. NeuroMetrix

NeuroMetrix has created a better version of its previous AI device (Quell) to provide treatment to users. Quell 2.0 is smaller than the previous one, but it is more powerful.[5] You can wear it on the leg regardless of where you are experiencing pain in your body. That is because Quell 2.0 is designed to send neural pulses to the brain that trigger a natural pain relief response in the central nervous system. You can easily get this device over the counter, after which you can track pain in your body.

Quell 2.0 was created to provide a better solution to patients dealing with pain. It employs the data of more than 70,000 users to determine the sensation threshold and administer the right dose of electrical stimulation. NeuroMetrix has applied Big Data to ensure that the administered dose is perfectly balanced.

People with chronic pain will benefit from this device the most, as, to experience pain relief, they will not have to depend on medications. The device will assess their pain intensity and then administer the perfect dose to help them in no time.

3. Kaia Health

Kaia Health is a startup that seeks to create an app for chronic pain management. The primary aim of this new approach is to offer painkiller alternatives. Kaia Health will do this by using technology to provide mind-body therapy for MSK (musculoskeletal) disorders.

The mobile technology will offer psychological techniques, guided physical exercises, and medical/health education. Mind-body therapy is currently incredibly expensive, and people who need it don't have access to it because of the costs.[6]

Kaia Health aims to change this, as the company wants people with MSK disorders to access this pain management therapy.

The startup has created many tools to help people obtain access to various pain management techniques. That is because the company doesn't want people to be dependent on opioid-based painkillers, which have significant side effects. We have yet to see how the new AI technology will help people with MSK disorders.

4. The DNA Company

The DNA Company is Toronto-based and bought My Pain Sensei (MPS), a pain management app, for thirty million dollars. The new AI technology combines genomic insights, Big Data, and conversational AI tracking tools.[7]

The platform can access more than sixty million electronic medical records. These records will help healthcare professionals understand:

- Symptoms

- Diagnosis

- Chronic pain treatment efficacy

- Chronic conditions

- And much more

The company aims to use this platform to develop various health apps that will allow people to take charge of their health management.[7] A range of apps will be designed to help people manage pain quickly. The company is also set to create many other healthcare tools, which we will find out about soon.

The Opioid Crisis and the Problem With Prescription Painkillers

It is necessary to understand pain management and medicine because of the people who abuse opioid painkillers daily. According to the United States Department of Health and Human Services, more than 115 million people abused prescription pain management medicines, which resulted in more than forty-two thousand deaths.[8] Ever since then, the number of people abusing these medicines has continued to increase.

That is why AI intervention is needed to provide people with access to other means of pain management. In the late 20th century, the medical community believed that these prescription medicines were not addictive and were an excellent solution for chronic pain management. Of course, the medical community couldn't have been more wrong, as the use of opioids has led to an increase in addiction and substance abuse.

The use of AI and Big Data is set to offer insights into addictive behaviors, relapses, early detection of substance abuse, and much more. The tools will offer support for rehab, recovery, and alternative sources of pain management.[8]

The problem with prescription abuse is that sometimes doctors can overprescribe medicines. They don't do this intentionally. That is because pain is a subjective experience. There are no set means or indicators to measure pain other than what the patient is reporting. Besides that, everyone has different pain thresholds. To provide prescriptions, doctors rely on the patient's pain perception and their own medical expertise.

Another common problem is that people with chronic pain develop a tolerance to the medications and require higher doses for pain management. All these problems lead patients to become addicted to painkillers. The most significant dilemmas that healthcare professionals face are the needs of the patient and the risk of addiction.

How AI Can Help With Prescription Abuse

The problem of prescription abuse can be overcome with the help of AI to manage pain more effectively. Patient data can be used along with machine learning to create better pain management solutions. AI aims to create a personalized pain management solution for the patient using Reinforcement Learning (RL).

RL is a form of ML that uses the patient's feedback to create better solutions. Such technology can help with pain management by adapting to the patients' changing needs. The feedback from the patients will include their pain intensity.

The pain intensity feedback, combined with population health data sets, will allow better pain treatment and management options to be created to meet the patients' needs in the best way possible. The problem of pain being subjective will be overcome with the help of such AI tools.

Another important thing to keep in mind is that the rate of opiate prescriptions varies from one state to another. Prescribers in some states write more than three times as many prescriptions per person than others. Because of this, patients who abuse these painkillers learn how to play the system to obtain more medications.

That is where the use of ML comes in. It can be used to track anomalies associated with a patient's prescriptions. For example, it can track when prescriptions are filled, the location, and known interactions with other medications being taken. The ML can track all these things and alert the patient's healthcare provider.

AI can offer support and constant intervention to users who abuse these prescription medications. For example, mobile devices or wearables can help individuals track their behavior and alert their healthcare professionals if something goes off track. In addition, such devices can offer alerts and reminders to patients so they can effectively manage their care.

The greater the number of patients who interact with and use these devices, the more data healthcare professionals will have to analyze and create better pain management solutions. Machine learning will become better, and people will not have to depend on painkillers to manage their pain all the time. Of course, cooperation from the patient is necessary for AI to work effectively and avert the opioid crisis.

AI and Chronic Pain Management

Besides prescription abuse, another significant problem is chronic pain, from which millions of people suffer. AI is highly capable of helping sufferers of chronic pain find treatment that will positively impact their long-term health. It can use patient data to provide affordability and remedy chronic pain with alternative methods.

AI can help chronic pain patients find medical assistance and doctors who have been proven to help people feel better without prescription medicine. Besides that, it can track pain intensity and duration to help patients take better care of their pain. Of course, much data and training will be required to create an AI tool that will effectively help each patient.

If such a technology is created accurately, it will have the power to help more than fifty million Americans suffering from chronic pain. It will also help millions of people worldwide. Pain management and medicine are some of the most important challenges of our times that can be overcome with the help of AI.

Conclusion

This was a complete guide to artificial intelligence in pain medicine and management. While we have a long way to go to overcome the opioid crisis and help people manage pain without abusing painkillers, AI has made strides in terms of pain medicine. Many tools and apps have been developed to help people worldwide manage their pain more effectively, so they don't become dependent on painkillers.

If the makers of such AI continue at this rate, soon an array of technology will be available to help people better manage back pain, chronic pain, post-operative pain, and other kinds of pain.[9]

Many people forget that pain is a symptom and not a disease. That is why you don't need to be dependent on medications to overcome it.

All you have to do is take the right steps to manage pain in the best way possible. Only time will tell if AI helps healthcare professionals and patients deal with pain.

References/Further Reading

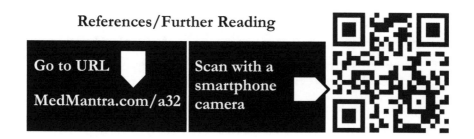

Go to URL
MedMantra.com/a32

Scan with a smartphone camera

CHAPTER THIRTY-THREE

PSYCHIATRY

Psychiatry is often thought to be reliant on human interaction. The psychiatrist sits with the patient or group of patients and listens to them speak about their troubles. From there, they address the situation with a diagnosis of a mental disorder or a similar mental health issue. Then, in a typical interaction, treatment with prescription drugs begins. Everything is done with a human psychiatrist at the helm—or is it? Similar to other medical fields, psychiatry is being quietly infiltrated by machines. The innovative technologies being born from advancements in artificial intelligence (AI) and machine learning are changing the delivery of psychotherapy that can be lifesaving for some patients.[1]

Mental Health Around the World

Approximately 792 million people have mental health problems globally, which translates to more than one in ten people. The National Institute of Mental Health (NIMH) has stated that 20% of adults in the United States, or 51.5 million people, suffer from at least one type of mental illness of various degrees of severity.[2] In Europe, around 83 million people have poor mental health, which is concerning because this includes people in some of the happiest countries in the world. Asia, too, has seen a sharp increase in people with mental illnesses. Aside from countries like Japan and South Korea having some of the highest rates of suicide in the world, Hong Kong has a population in which one in six people are afflicted by mental health woes. Unfortunately, due to the pandemic in 2020, this number is expected to grow in number and severity.

"There are huge unmet needs in psychiatry, with an acute shortage of psychiatrists and therapists in virtually every county in the U.S. and the shortage is even more dramatic in poorer countries," says Murali Doraiswamy, MD, professor of psychiatry and behavioral sciences and director of the neurocognitive disorders program at Duke University.

At the same time, there is a dearth of mental health professionals in the medical industry worldwide, and this shortage may lead to many people being unable to access psychiatric help when they need it.[3] Is this an area in which artificial intelligence (AI) can help? While many healthcare professionals, including psychiatrists, have different views when asked this question, recent developments suggest that AI may change the practice of psychiatric treatment modules for both physicians and patients.

Artificial Intelligence in Psychiatry at Present

The adoption of AI in psychiatry may be trickier than in other fields, like pathology or radiology, that deal with the recognition and correlation of images, patterns, or biomarkers to arrive at a diagnosis or formulate a treatment plan. Psychiatric symptoms cannot be tied down definitively to genetic codes, neuroimaging results, or brain activity patterns. The time and situational variances in brain functioning make it extremely difficult for technology to capture data.

The New Science of Human Behavior

In the realm of psychiatry, AI currently stands as a tool for assessment, with the initiation of a new branch called *"computational psychiatry."*

This field uses machine learning to increase data analysis and pull out the unknown factors beyond textbook mental disorders and illnesses or even much more unusual and extreme cases. In other words, AI makes it possible to mine psychiatric data and fabricate computer-aided experiments in which various personality traits and mental disorders are examined. There is also the potential to evaluate responses to medication in patients diagnosed with mental illnesses.

Use of AI in Mental Health Tools and Applications

1. mindLAMP

At the Beth Israel Deaconess Medical School, USA, the Division of Digital Psychiatry has developed an open-source project called *mindLAMP* ("Learn, Assess, Manage, and Prevent"), which uses a new technique called *digital phenotyping* through smartphone applications and sensors. The application gives clinicians and patients access to constantly updated real-time information regarding the patient's lived experience of mental illness, their true baseline, daily fluctuations, and reactions to life experiences, as well as responses to medications or treatment modules. The team has successfully secured their trial data and is using the app at their clinics. They have also managed to conduct surveys and cognitive tests through the software. With the application of machine learning algorithms to this data, researchers are looking to predict a patient's risk of serious mental illness or declining mental health status, and risk of relapse, so that adequate and timely interventions may be taken. The customizable application is currently available on both the Apple and Google app stores.[4]

2. Bi Affect

At the University of Illinois College of Medicine, the Departments of Psychiatry and Bioengineering created an application called Bi Affect, which has ingeniously analyzed an everyday feature in smartphones: the keyboard function. Studies have shown that patients suffering from bipolar disorder exhibit varying typing patterns depending on their change in moods. That is, during a manic episode, they tend to type faster, just like they would speak faster in person. Meanwhile, during a depressive episode, they tend to type shorter messages.[5]

Using this as a starting point, the team developed a deep learning algorithm (The *Deep Mood architecture*) which is applied to the keyboard metadata collected from the patient's smartphone. This captures and analyzes variations in typing speed, mistakes, pauses, backspace key use, etc., without collecting the matter that is being typed, in order to protect patient privacy. The analysis helped them to understand the correlation between mood swings and neurocognitive functioning.[6]

3. Cyberball Gaming Module

Cyberball is a computer game that measures social rejection. A subject controls one of the three players on the screen and believes that other people are controlling the remaining two, which are actually an AI-based algorithm. The researchers can then change the percentage of time the ball is passed to the human-controlled player to evoke feelings of rejection.

This type of algorithmic-based research has demonstrated how feelings of ostracism, social exclusion, or rejection may be different when comparing people with or without borderline personality disorders.[7]

4. Instagram Learning

They say a picture is worth a thousand words. Harvard University and the University of Vermont researchers believe this to be true, and so they took to Instagram with machine learning to seek out a means of improving depression screening. The AI diagnosed depression accurately in the trial participants, using photo metadata, color analysis, and algorithm-based face detection, and managed to outperform health practitioners' unassisted diagnostic success rate.[8]

5. Chat Bots

a. Tess by X2AI

Created by X2AI, Tess is AI software that asks all the questions people need to hear via text messages. The software can even administer psychotherapy to those afflicted with depression and emotional instability. According to X2AI's CEO and co-founder, Michiel Rauws, Tess is a psychological artificial intelligence that uses natural language processing to understand what the user is actually talking about, to pick up on human expressions like, "I don't want to wake up anymore in the morning." Then it delivers coping strategies or immediate aids for the situation.[9]

b. Woebot

Woebot is a digital cognitive behavioral therapist, accessible through smartphone mobile apps. The inbuilt AI algorithm is capable of having conversations with users to track their moods through videos and word games. After analysis, it devises recommended treatments based on scores and conversations. For instance, Woebot will ask, "How are you feeling?" and then proceed to emulate a face-to-face discussion with an actual human psychiatrist.[10]

6. IBM Research Through Watson

You might have recently read about ongoing studies that are looking into how people with various mental illnesses and problems verbalize themselves differently from others. The chances are that some of the latest research was assisted by AI. IBM has been collecting transcripts and audio clips from psychiatric interviews and paired this data with its algorithms, like Watson, to find patterns in speech. The hope is that having AI learn about these patterns can help with predicting and monitoring schizophrenia, mania, depression, and psychosis. Presently, IBM's AI needs to hear only about 300 words from a client before it detects the probability of psychosis, thus aiding in faster diagnosis and treatment.

Predictive Power

Researchers at Stanford's Center for Precision Mental Health and Wellness used an AI-based algorithm to interpret the brainwave patterns of people diagnosed with depression, before and after they were given medications for their symptoms, in order to predict which symptoms would change with the treatment given. In a mammoth task, individual patient symptoms were combined with individual electroencephalography (EEG) results at different points during the treatment. It was concluded that the algorithm could successfully identify patients with a higher risk of poor prognoses, such as suicidal tendencies, which may have otherwise been missed due to the subjective nature of traditional examinations. The validation of these processes, as well as large-scale implementation in resource-poor countries, may delay the adoption of the technology.[11]

Benefits of AI in Psychiatry

Using artificial intelligence as part of a psychiatric evaluation has a host of benefits. Looking briefly at other medical fields where AI is being integrated, there have been reports of streamlined workflow, earlier detection and treatment of diseases like cancer, and enhanced detection of abnormalities in radiology data (MRIs, CT scans, etc.). The advantages of AI to psychiatry would be as follows:

1. Easy accessibility

One of the biggest hindrances in the medical field for both healthcare professionals and patients is the lack of accessibility. According to studies, 56.4% of adults and over 60% of adolescents suffering from mental illness do not receive treatment. There is a global drought of psychiatric support systems.[12]

AI, however, could be a starting point for bringing psychiatric care to those who need it the most. Chatbots like *Tess* and *Woebot* can provide rudimentary consultations, while *online platforms like Ginger.io*[13,14], a partnership of machine learning and a clinical network, can provide suggestions or real-time support to users as well as an array of treatments through video-based therapy and psychiatry sessions.

2. Faster detection

Traditional psychiatric care was dependent on the patient's personal observations (or lack thereof) to make inferences on the issue, as well as professional observations and reporting. However, with AI created by IBM's Computational Psychiatry and Neuroimaging group, and research by universities and other technological startups, AI is now able to use methods like natural language processing (NLP) to use a patient's speech to predict mental illness or the onset of psychosis.[15]

3. Using AI for research-based tools to identify vulnerable populations

A team of MIT and Harvard University researchers used natural language processing algorithms to identify similarities in social media posts and thereby identify groups of people who expressed anxiety or isolation, referred to substance abuse, etc., during the last year. The number of people had significantly increased as compared to similar studies conducted in 2018 and 2019. This kind of analysis could aid in the identification of population groups that are most vulnerable to adverse mental health effects rooted in major events like the Covid-19 pandemic, political effects, or natural disasters.

If the algorithms were applied in real time to social media posts, they could be used to immediately offer online resources, like guiding people to online support groups, highlighting information on how to find mental health treatment, or even facilitating contact with a suicide hotline.[16]

Conclusion

AI and psychiatry can form a formidable partnership in the fight against mental illness and personality disorders. With digitization and automation of selected tasks, such as asking questionnaires, detecting various speech patterns, and thought processes, AI can aid those who need it most and also help psychiatrists detect problems faster than ever before. A multidisciplinary approach toward establishing a rigorous framework to evaluate new studies that deal with the applications of AI algorithms should be established for rapid and transparent validation. Though AI still has its limitations, the potential for the technology to improve the diagnosis and the delivery of mental health care is undeniable.

References/Further Reading

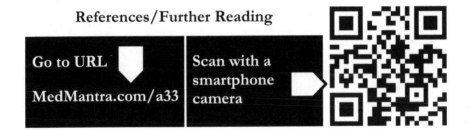

Go to URL
MedMantra.com/a33

Scan with a smartphone camera

CHAPTER THIRTY-FOUR

CARDIOLOGY

Cardiology and technology have always been intertwined. Without electrocardiograms, echocardiograms, cardiac catheterization, and similar modalities, cardiology would not exist as it does today. However, to meet the growing population of people with cardiac problems and ailments, cardiologists are finding that they need the help of computers so that they can become more efficient and effective in their line of work. When artificial intelligence arrived as a possible solution, it seemed like science fiction, restricted to far-fetched research projects. However, the rapid pace at which AI methods have progressed has resulted in the widespread adoption of these technologies, with many gaining market clearances from the FDA (U.S. Food and Drug Administration). With the incorporation of machine learning, deep learning, and other AI systems into healthcare, one may already be using and experiencing an AI system or algorithm for themselves, without even realizing it.

But just how far have AI and machine learning come in terms of cardiology? Moreover, what future developments can we hope to see within our lifetimes? In the field of cardiology, the future is now!

The State of Artificial Intelligence in Cardiology

Even though technology and medicine are gradually becoming dependent on one another, the idea of AI as an engineering tool for creating innovations in cardiovascular medicine has yet to truly catch on. However, progress is being made in these major areas:

1. Prediction of risk and outcomes

2. Imaging and diagnostics

3. Clinical decision support (CDS) after thorough validation

Here is a look at the latest innovations that came about due to the integration of AI with cardiology.

1. Prediction of Risks and Outcomes

Machine learning through AI is a robust and innovative tool that can help with cardiovascular risk stratification by incorporating nontraditional or unknown risk factors, thereby helping with preventive measures rather than curative.

a. Microsoft's Healthcare Next Initiative

Around March 2017, Microsoft launched the **Microsoft Intelligent Network for Eyecare (MINE)** in places like Australia, Brazil, India, and the US. MINE was renamed the AI Network for Healthcare because, soon after its launch, Microsoft partnered with Apollo Hospitals, one of the largest healthcare providers in India. The project became a part of **Microsoft's Healthcare Next Initiative**. The goal was to use AI to develop treatment guidelines and proven clinical algorithms in cardiology. The **National Clinical Coordination Committee (NCCC)** was also set up soon after, with the aim of constructing an India-specific heart risk score, in order to predict cardiovascular ailments for the Indian demographic, as opposed to using tools based on data derived from Western studies.

The corporate VP of Microsoft AI and Research, Peter Lee, stated, "By working side by side with the healthcare industry's most pioneering players, we are bringing Microsoft's capabilities in ground-breaking research and product development to help healthcare providers, biotech companies, and organizations around the world use artificial intelligence and the cloud to innovate".[1]

On analyzing a large database of patients with heart disease, the team was able to narrow down 21 risk factors that can predict the occurrence of cardiovascular events, which could change the way preventive health checks are done, as well as provide insight to physicians with early diagnosis and effective treatment plans.

Further, the team is working on an **AI-powered Cardio API platform** that could potentially predict a patient's heart risk score just by providing a detailed history, without investigations if not required, thereby streamlining operations. With an IT giant like Microsoft getting into biomedical technologies, one can anticipate many remarkable inventions.[2]

b. *Google's Verily Software*

Google's health-tech subsidiary *Verily* determined that it's AI algorithms could assess a person's risk of developing heart disease by reviewing scans from the back of a patient's eye, i.e., through a retinal scan. The algorithms could determine the patient's age, smoking habits, and blood pressure from the images, thereby predicting the individual's risk of cardiovascular disease, with almost 70% accuracy.[3]

c. *Wearable Sensors*

The application of remote patient monitoring in the evaluation of an individual's health has empowered patients to take control of their well-being. Smart bands or watches have been upgraded with ECG monitors that can pick up wave abnormalities and transmit the data in real time to treating physicians. Patient-generated data, when analyzed, can help create a database for future risk predictions incorporating a more diverse population group. A study conducted by *Tison and colleagues* attempted to passively detect atrial fibrillation using ECG reports generated from commercially available smartwatches, coupled with a deep neural network.[4]

At the *University of Nottingham in the UK*, researchers had AI teach itself, through machine learning, to find patterns in data and predict which patients would have a heart attack within ten years. The AI system scanned more than 300,000 patient records to make these predictions. At the end of the study, the researchers found that the AI algorithms predicted heart attacks with greater accuracy than the assessments created by the American College of Cardiology / American Heart Association.[5]

2. Imaging and Diagnostics

a. *Arterys MICA in Cardiac MRI*

One name that both radiologists and cardiologists are most likely familiar with by now is *Arterys Medical Imaging Cloud AI (Arterys MICA)*, which is an online medical imaging analytics program powered by AI. The system combines both cloud supercomputing and accelerated workflow to deliver results. The Cardio-based AI system has functions like 2D and 4D Flow blood imaging and 3D Cine for ventricular volumes. The algorithm is applied rapidly to perfusion datasets and signal intensity graphs from *cardiac MRI software* to deliver accurate, semi-quantitative segmental analysis that enables faster patient examinations by up to 30%, saving at least 25 minutes per LV/RV (left ventricle/right ventricle) function segmentation.

Presently, Arterys is partnered with Siemens Healthineers and GE ViosWorks. Interestingly, Siemens Healthineers is working alongside GE and IBM Watson to enhance medical imaging.[6]

b. *Caption Health in Echocardiography*

Caption Health (originally Bay Labs Inc.) is a US-based AI company devoted to using deep learning to help healthcare professionals in developing countries. The company brought deep learning to Kenya to help doctors identify rheumatic heart disease (RHD) and congenital heart disease. It previously tested its algorithms at the Minneapolis Heart Institute and Allina Health, Northwestern Medicine, Duke University School of Medicine, and cardiologists at Stanford University, to help cardiologists accurately interpret 2D echo studies.[7] The algorithm can automatically calculate ejection fractions while scanning from three cardiac views at the point of care, providing a quick visual assessment.[8]

c. *Convolutional Neural Networks*

In 2020, *Kusunose and colleagues*[9] used convolutional neural networks (CNN) to identify regional wall motion abnormalities in the cardiac musculature, from echo-cardiographic images, which demonstrated that the deep learning algorithm was able to diagnose the abnormalities as accurately as cardiologists or sonographers during the trial. This created the possibility of using CNN for automated diagnosis in echocardiography

Rima Arnaout[10], a cardiologist and assistant professor at UC San Francisco, created a deep learning CNN that applied an algorithm to categorize cardiac ultrasounds and detect congenital heart disease from fetal ultrasounds according to the type of view, with 92% accuracy as compared to 79% attained by human experts.

d. Analytics 4 Life

The Toronto-based company Analytics 4 Life has created the Corvista system, which is a new cardiac diagnostic platform. It is a point-of-care system that collects signals transmitted by the heart through leads while the patient is at rest. It is usually a three-minute recording that collects 10 million data points. This data is uploaded to the system's secure cloud database to create a three-dimensional image of the heart. AI-based machine learning algorithms are performed on the patient's data and help to determine the presence of cardiovascular disease through Phase Space Tomography. The test results are sent to clinicians immediately after the procedure for rapid intervention in cases of coronary artery disease, pulmonary hypertension, or heart failure. The device is being used in Canadian hospitals as a non-invasive diagnostic application.[11]

3. Clinical Decision Support

Point-of-care clinical decision-making tools are required as patient management becomes increasingly complex with the introduction of a variety of investigation and treatment options. Evidence-based guidelines are required to bring about good results, especially with the incredible range of electronic data available. Analysis of this data to arrive at actionable conclusions and recommendations has been a challenge for cardiologists thus far.

With the use of structured data sets like laboratory investigation reports, patient demographic information, and electrocardiography and physiology reports, machine learning algorithms have been able to accelerate diagnosis and predict risks and disease outcomes. With the addition of clinical narratives, through patient electronic health records (EHR), the data sets become augmented and complete, leading to better analysis. Extrapolating this information from EHRs was a challenge that was adequately resolved through the application of *natural language processing (NLP) algorithms* that add input to clinical decision support systems, making them more robust and accurate.

Weissler E and colleagues[12] applied trained NLP algorithms to patients' electronic health data in order to accurately diagnose peripheral artery disease, thereby leading to better interventions for patient care, while automatically estimating the prognosis. The Mayo Clinic has used data-empowered NLP software like *MEd Tagger*, which is an Open Health Natural Language Processing Consortium, for information extraction.[13]

Conclusion: The Future Is in the Research

Artificial intelligence and machine learning have led to a plethora of technological advancements in the field of cardiology. The studies that have recently been published bolster the already proven usefulness of AI systems. Yet, the future lies within the research.

Presently, many AI systems are based on imaging, reducing workload, and increasing both the productivity and the efficiency of medical field professionals. The enhancement of cardiac and other medical images provides doctors and surgeons with a sharper eye. AI is helping professionals make clearer, more informed decisions, leading to better patient outcomes with reduced mortality and morbidity rates. The challenge will be the adoption and implementation of this software in widespread clinical environments, when medical professionals realize that the real power of AI is to improve clinical efficacy by enhancing the clinician-patient interface, instead of replacing it. AI will become an indispensable partner in healthcare, especially when we get to the heart of the matter.

References/Further Reading

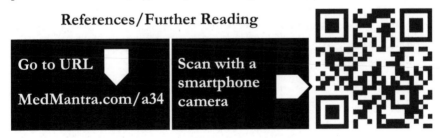

Go to URL
MedMantra.com/a34

Scan with a smartphone camera

CHAPTER THIRTY-FIVE

PHARMACY

In 2022, the pharmaceutical industry is thriving in ways it always has. Scientific discoveries influence the creation or reconstruction of certain medications, and new methods to quell epidemics, diseases, and other ailments affecting society are born. Yet, as new technologies beyond pharmacology are being introduced, the idea of what the "pharmacy" is and how it can evolve to better serve the future comes into question. How will advancements like artificial intelligence (AI) and machine learning (ML) alter the course of pharmacology and pharmaceutical company practices? As it turns out, AI is already having an impact on many realms of the healthcare system; pharmacy included.[1]

In fact, AI was woven into pharmacy more in 2020 than ever before. According to one of the recent trending topics, artificial intelligence has gained the attention of pharmaceutical giants like Johnson & Johnson, Merck, and GlaxoSmithKline. Each company has invested heavily in machine learning, hoping that AI will build "prediction models for potentially promising compounds." Right now, it takes up to 15 years for a new drug to be produced, starting from the moment of discovery to the proper execution—and that means over US$1 billion spent on the manufacturing and testing of a single drug type.

The hope is that AI will be able to manufacture new, more effective drugs with more celerity and for less production costs.

Current State of Artificial Intelligence in Pharmacy

But while investments from big enterprises is one step towards an AI-enriched future, what is happening between artificial intelligence and the pharmaceutical field presently?

The usefulness of AI is not solely limited to approximations and finding patterns. Presently, there are programs being developed that allow AI to detect specific symptoms or anomalies, add to the diagnostic process, develop treatment protocols, aid in medicine manufacturing, as well as monitoring and caring for patients. The main purpose of all these programs and deep learning algorithms is to lessen the burden on the human professionals and streamline the workload.

We see AI being incorporated into every facet of healthcare, ranging from

- Computers – faster data collection, better data processing

- Data recording in healthcare devices

- Creation of gene databases and pharmacogenomics

- Faster adoption of electronic health records and databases

- Systems with natural language processing capabilities to automate certain processes in the healthcare field.

What that means for pharmacies is that AI has already begun supporting researchers with making decisions about existing medications and drugs and various treatments. AI is also to be used to predict where epidemics may occur by having it learn the history of outbreaks through records and other media sources. However, it is safe to say that artificial intelligence and deep machine learning can be taken even further.

Future Hopes for AI and Pharmacy

Though much of the technology that will become more ubiquitous in the future is already under progressive development, the anticipation is that the integration of AI into the pharmacy and other fields in healthcare will expand rapidly by 2030.

AI and ML

Algorithms that can "learn" will play an integral role in the future, especially during drug development. Researchers will have access to a wealth of collected scientific data to work with, thanks to the efforts of AI gathering information from all over the world. Thus, research can be conducted quicker, aiding in the formation of new knowledge.

Benevolent Bio and its customized AI is the perfect example of this. Jackie Hunter of Benevolent Bio states, "The AI we've developed—embodied in the company's Judgement Correlation System (JACS)--is able to review billions of sentences and paragraphs from millions of scientific research papers and abstracts."

In other words, this system called JACS finds links in data and names it "known facts" about a specific condition or disease. Then these known facts are compiled, and further patterns or connections are made. The end result is that the JACS generates hundreds of hypotheses based on the criteria inputted by the scientists. Once the hypotheses are created, researchers discuss the most plausible and start testing the top 5 in the lab.

Streamlined workflow and a greater perspective of how and why ailments begin are a few of the major benefits of AI, and it's only to become more helpful in the future.

Personalized Pharmacy

In current times, a visit to the pharmacy means dealing with long lines, exorbitant prices, and no time to consult with the professionals behind the counter. One hope for AI in the future is to set up booths that allow for the patient to receive proactive care. For example, a system being utilized now is "Intouch Health," a telehealth network in remote locations of the US. Anyone using the system can access consultations for various conditions.

Additionally, AI and ML will increase the availability of personalized therapies. With the dissemination of cloud-based technologies and digitized healthcare systems, pharmacies will be able to receive information from primary healthcare providers and hospitals on-demand. This can even lead to advancements like the already FDA-approved epilepsy drug called Spritam that's made using 3D printers. The drug is layered, making it faster to dissolve than regular epilepsy drugs. Now imagine if pharmacies all had 3D printers to distribute necessary medication to those in need with the push of a button.

AI programs will be integrated into the electronic medical records, which will raise an immediate alarm if a physician tries to prescribe a medicine which the patient is allergic to or is incompatible with a medicine which the patient is already taking. AI programs will rapidly calculate the minimum possible but most effective dose of medicines after considering all patient-specific factors like body weight, biochemical results, other health conditions, etc.

That's the future of preventative healthcare. That's the future of pharmacy.

Conclusion

When it comes to a blending of artificial intelligence and pharmacy, there already are connections that have been made, even within the pharmacy management system, such as drug utilization data and clinical decision opinion screenings. AI is in the workflow, too. Thus, we are beginning to see a world where AI is shifting the focus away from the more mechanical side of pharmacy, such as the data collection and manufacturing of new drugs, and to the more human elements, like collaborating with other countries, optimizing health and wellness, and preventing catastrophic epidemics from spreading in the future. AI is already a major component of pharmacy, so it now comes down to accepting the advantages and implementing new methods of use.

References/Further Reading

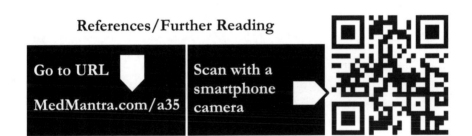

Go to URL
MedMantra.com/a35

Scan with a smartphone camera

CHAPTER THIRTY-SIX

DERMATOLOGY

Even though artificial intelligence applications are in the early stages of development in the healthcare sector, their current abilities are broad, and they are already improving the general state of healthcare.[1]

Furthermore, some centers in the United States have locally developed systems that give pop-up notifications to alert doctors when a specific drug or medication may not work with a patient based on some concrete reasons like genetic traits.[1]

These apps can also give physicians practical reasons; their major areas of specialization are skin image analysis and personalized skincare treatment.

Regarding Skin Image Analysis, AI-based dermatology companies are creating applications and devices using computer learning and machine learning to analyze photos to predict and prevent skin diseases from occurring.

Content-Based Image Retriever

Apart from predictive analytics and data management, artificial intelligence is used in the area of dermatology via the use of CBIR- content-based image retriever. The CBIR functions are culled from the skin image analysis.

DermEngine's Visual Search and Skin Vision are perfect examples of such dermatology apps. This intelligent dermatology software focuses on identifying skin cancer images and gives the medical professional visually similar pictures with the top diagnosis and the risk of malignancy of these past cases.

DermEngine's Visual Search

It uses deep learning and image processing technologies to aid medical experts in their clinical decisions, and it is also beneficial in training or to new physicians who want to specialize in skin cancer.

SkinVision

SkinVision is built solely to use machine vision to check for skin lesions for risk of cancer through photosynthesis.

It was founded in 2011 in the Netherlands; this app is sophisticatedly trained on a database of over one million images of skin lesions; the algorithm learns to recognize particular features like shape, color, and which one may indicate a higher risk of melanoma.

Skin10

Skin10 is yet another app developed to help dermatologists diagnose skin conditions; its algorithm is built on an extensive database of skin conditions, although the sources of database images are unclear.

How does it work?

All that the patients have to do is to download the Skin10 app and sign up for Skin10's network.

Secondly, users take pictures of the region of their body where they wish to analyze. However, the system can also process the entire body parts, and such scans can be integrated by using an overlay feature in the app camera. Skin10 can detect skin conditions like solar lentigo, lipoma, and malignant melanoma.

For the good of humanity

Artificial intelligence is making work easier for dermatologists; apart from skin image analysis, AI is also proving to be valuable in the area of personalized skincare treatments. Companies are building recommendation engines to personalize skincare treatment recommendations to user skin type.[1]

On a broad scale, access to high-quality data and incompatibilities between different electronic medical record databases are current challenges. However, AI-based Dermatology Company is an example of the perfect start-up company- cited by Eric Schmidt (Chairman of Alphabet Inc., the parent company of Google). Using crowd-sourced input from dermatologists, he imagined machine learning and deployed it via smartphone technology, which can create a highly accurate artificial intelligence diagnosis tool.[1]

Furthermore, an obvious concern is a possibility that AI may infringe on physicians' practice. The boundary between making clinical decisions and making recommendations remains to be drawn.

Nevertheless, at this development stage of AI in dermatology, we still cannot rely solely on a computer to tell us what to do; a medical judgment that involves a conversation with a patient is best left to the treating physician.[1]

References/Further Reading

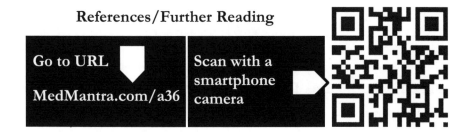

Go to URL

MedMantra.com/a36

Scan with a smartphone camera

CHAPTER THIRTY-SEVEN
DENTISTRY

Over the course of history, we have come to understand that communities always adopt the right and essential technology. One thing we are sure about is that artificial intelligence is positively changing the healthcare industry, including dentistry—and doing so faster than anyone could imagine.

This aspect of healthcare is not afraid or skeptical about implementing some of these new technologies. From management software to 3D printing to digital radiographs, dentists are the early adopters of these revolutionary inventions. Moreover, the next evolution of dental technology and its rapid adoption will be made possible through artificial intelligence-based products.

The Rise of AI-Based Technology in Dentistry

With the help of AI-based applications, it is now possible to detect the efficacy of various treatment methods considering anatomical conditions and distinct symptoms, using artificial intelligence and large datasets of diagnostic results, treatments, and outcomes. It is essential given the assortment of new dental techniques, materials, and technologies, which are introduced annually.

Applications of Artificial Intelligence in Different Fields of Dentistry

The last decade was considered the decade of vital achievements in the field of artificial intelligence. There are various practical applications of AI-based systems in dentistry:

1. **Artificial intelligence in patient management**

   An AI-based virtual dental assistant can perform different patient management tasks in a dental practice with more accuracy and less error. In departments such as oral pathology, oral medicine, and radiology, it can be used to manage patient appointments as well as to assist in diagnosis or to plan subsequent treatments.[1] It also works by notifying the dentist about the patient's complete dental and medical history, including details about alcohol consumption, smoking and tobacco use, oral hygiene habits, and food and other dietary habits.[2] Thus, a virtual database for each patient is developed to aid the dentist in prompt diagnosis and subsequent treatment of complex dental diseases.[1,2]

2. Artificial intelligence in the diagnosis and treatment of different dental problems

AI-based trained neural networks can be used to diagnose complex dental diseases having multifactorial etiology. This is a precious gift that artificial intelligence has given to clinical dental practice, as a correct diagnosis is a strong foundation for proper treatment. An example of this is the recurrent aphthous ulcer, which is a condition without a specific cause or with multifactorial etiology; trained neural networks can diagnose it based on the recurrence of the lesion and the exclusion of other factors.[3] AI can also precisely prognosticate a predisposition to oral cancer genes and tooth surface loss for a large population by using genetic algorithms of the oral lesions as well as the genetic algorithms of unerupted canines or premolars.[4]

3. Artificial intelligence in prosthetic dentistry

To render perfect prostheses for patients, various influencing factors such as esthetics, anthropological calculations, facial measurements, and patient preferences have been integrated by an AI-based system (RaPiD) for successful use in prosthetic dentistry. These AI-based systems integrate computer-aided manufacturing (CAM), knowledge-based systems, and computer-aided design (CAD) as a unifying medium for successful dental restoration with great accuracy.[5] CAD/CAM techniques are used in the manufacturing of inlays, onlays, crowns, and bridges.[6] AI plays a main role in the identification of the type of bone as well as the cortical thickness in order to make precise surgical guides for the placement of implants. It has replaced the time-consuming conventional methods of routine casting, thereby reducing the required time as well as errors.

4. Artificial intelligence in oral and maxillofacial surgery

AI software programs can help in the planning of oral and maxillofacial surgeries by providing the smallest details regarding vital structures around the craniofacial region in order to preserve them during the surgical procedures.[7] The extraordinary application of artificial intelligence in this field is the introduction of robotic surgery (in which human intelligence and human body motion are simulated). Removal of tumors and foreign bodies, oral implant surgery, biopsy, and temporomandibular joint surgeries are some common successful applications of AI-guided oral and maxillofacial surgeries.[8]

5. Artificial intelligence in orthodontics

AI-driven customized orthodontic diagnostics and treatments have revolutionized the field of orthodontic dentistry. AI algorithms and statistical analysis can be used in multiple orthodontics processes, from precise diagnosis to treatment planning and even to follow-up prognostic monitoring. AI-based intraoral 3D scanners and cameras can analyze different radiographs and photographs of relevant craniofacial and dental regions and aid in diagnosis as well as treatment planning.[9] From these photographs and radiographs, a data-driven algorithm can be developed. Final treatment outcomes, tooth movement, and pressure points for those specific teeth can be predicted by applying these algorithms and statistical analysis. Thus, AI-driven customized orthodontic treatment not only provides accurate treatment but also minimizes the chances of errors while reducing the treatment time.[10]

6. Artificial intelligence in radiology

AI-integrated imaging scans such as MRI and cone-beam CT may assess minor changes from normal that remain hidden to the human eye, e.g., artificial neural networks (ANNs) can localize minor apical foramen by magnifying the radiographs and aiding in the diagnosis of proximal caries.

In the last 5-10 years, image recognition in the radiology practice by using AI-based systems has shifted from science fiction to reality. AI provides an additional advantage in craniofacial imaging due to the distinctive ability of deep learning to identify minor deviations. AI algorithms can detect maxillary sinusitis on panoramic radiographs, and Sjogren syndrome on CT scans at early stages in order to prevent severe complications in the future.[11]

7. Artificial intelligence in periodontics

By using various radiographs and photographs, deep learning analysis tools can help in the diagnosis and treatment planning of complex periodontal diseases. AI can be used in the early detection of periodontal variations, bone loss, and variations in bone density, which helps in early intervention in dental implant systems.[12]

Convolutional neural networks can successfully detect periodontitis of premolars and molars. AI can also analyze the immune response profile of the patients and effectively categorize these patients into aggressive and chronic periodontitis. Thus, AI can guide dental professionals in optimum treatment protocols.[13]

8. Use of genetic algorithms to optimize dental implant systems

AI-based genetic algorithms work based on the "survival of the fittest" principle. Genetic algorithms can be used to optimize dental implant systems and determine the lifespan of restorative materials so that they can be chosen wisely. These algorithms can be applied to improve tooth color matching in prosthodontics. Statistical analysis based on genetic algorithms can predict dental caries at the initial stages to avoid future dental decay.[14] AI-driven genetic algorithms based on CAM/CAD can be used in the reconstruction of missing parts of the tooth and to maintain the overall smoothness of the reconstructed tooth surface.

9. Clinical decision support system in dentistry

A clinical decision support system (CDSS) based on inbuilt clinical knowledge supports dental professionals in making clinical decisions about the diagnosis, treatment, prognosis, and prevention of various dental problems. For example, when a patient with a toothache visits a dentist, the CDSS immediately analyzes all the relevant data through a short questionnaire filled out by the patient and automatically suggests a treatment plan.[15]

10. Artificial intelligence in endodontic dentistry

ANNs can be used to detect vertical root fractures as well as to localize minor apical foramen (*small* accessory canals at the tip or *apex* of some teeth roots) in the field of endodontic dentistry. ANNs can enhance the success of root canal treatment by increasing the accuracy of working length determination by up to 96%, which is greater than the accuracy attained by a professional endodontist.[16]

11. Artificial intelligence in forensic odontology

ANNs can be used to determine gender or age by using different dental parameters with minimal errors.[16] Automated techniques based on ANNs can be used effectively in forensic odontology to identify victims of child abuse, sexual assault, crimes, mass calamities, and other legal issues.

12. Artificial intelligence in pediatric dentistry

AI-driven CAD restorative design and manufacturing can be used in pediatric restorative dentistry to achieve great results in terms of time required and esthetics. The sizes of interrupted premolars and canines can be predicted during the mixed dentition period by using artificial neural networks.[17]

13. Prediction of dental problems by using ANN predictive models

ANN predictive models based on the association between tooth pain and daily brushing frequency, brush time, toothbrush replacement patterns, and other factors such as diet and exercise can effectively predict toothaches. ANN models can also be used to predict the expected timelines for dental extraction in orthodontic dentistry. Data mining analysis can determine the lifespan of restorative materials to choose them intelligently for suitable cases.

14. Artificial intelligence in community dentistry

AI-driven models can be used in community dentistry, including diagnostic recommendations for various dental problems, standard dental therapy protocols, personalized medicine, and even the prediction of epidemiological disease spread from a global perspective.

AI-based oral health mobile apps can track and educate a person about monitoring his/her dental health through an AI-based scanner in the app and regularly remind users about oral hygiene.[17]

15. Artificial intelligence in craniofacial cancer prediction

Using CT scan images, convolutional neural networks (CNNs) can predict areas in the head and neck with a high risk of cancer. Genetic programming (GP) can be used in the oral cancer prognosis by statistical analysis of different genetic factors.[18] Artificial neural networks (ANNs) can be used in the identification and grading of high-risk craniofacial cancer patients to plan a treatment regime accordingly.

Meet Some of the New Technologies

Orthy

Orthy was founded in 2016 by Patrick Y Lee. This AI-based tech claims to have the right elements to be the future of cosmetic dentistry with regard to invisible aligners. Without any doubt, Orthy has improved dental treatment by making aligner treatments more convenient and affordable. The app is built to predict the future smile of the patient after treatment. Users tap to request their snapshot for a 30-minute appointment with a dentist in the area. Then they get scanned and get X-rays done. If the patient is a good fit, in 24 hours, he or she can see the results in terms of his or her future smile.

Dentistry.AI

This is yet another benefit of artificial intelligence in dentistry. The digital health app is a cloud-based AI technology that physicians can use to detect dental caries on x-rays (bitewings).

The United States FDA has approved the caries detection software (by Dentistry.AI) for clinical use but as an investigational device. Moreover, Dentistry.AI and other top dentists are enhancing the AI-based caries detection software.[19]

Artificial intelligence allows Dentistry.AI to rapidly discover caries on dental x-rays. Furthermore, the AI-based technology seamlessly integrates with different X-ray sensors and detects caries within seconds.

Evidentiae

Evidentiae is creative and innovative cloud-based dental software with a streamlined virtual workflow. Its algorithm is created to pull information from dental and medical histories and charted exam results to generate a comprehensive overview of patients' dental health. It builds an in-depth diagnostics opinion for functional decision-making, biochemical parameters, dentofacial alterations, and, of course, periodical concerns.

Furthermore, Evidentiae is created to give dentists the most comprehensive documentation currently available, with the ability to use the provided information in the event of a presentation.

Advantages of AI in Dentistry

a) AI algorithms can perform various dental tasks in less time as compared to conventional methods.

b) It helps in achieving a greater degree of accuracy and precision by reducing human errors.

c) AI can store and keep patient data regarding dental problems in a single place and enables the dentist to make a more accurate diagnosis.

d) Prediction of various dental problems can be made by using databases containing millions of symptoms and diagnoses of particular dental diseases.

Limitations of AI in Dentistry

a) Its setup requires immense expenses due to the use of new and complex machines.

b) Properly trained professionals are required.

c) Most of the time, the outcomes of AI do not apply to real-world dentistry.

In conclusion, the world will experience the birth of AI-based technologies in the healthcare industry, including dentistry. These technologies will eliminate virtually all the repetitive manual and digital tasks. AI models can be applied for quick diagnosis and treatment of complex dental problems. AI has a bright future in both maxillofacial radiology and general dentistry. Very soon, we will see AI being applied in most tasks in endodontics, orthodontics, and restorative dentistry.

References/Further Reading

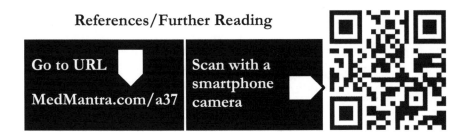

Go to URL
MedMantra.com/a37

Scan with a smartphone camera

CHAPTER THIRTY-EIGHT
ORTHOPEDICS

Machine learning intended to derive information about treatment patterns and diagnoses has already been utilized in more massive digital databases of Electronic Health Records (EHR) in the UK and has enhanced the data-based prediction of drug effects and interactions, the discovery of comorbidity clusters in autism spectrum disorders, and the identification of type 2 diabetes subgroups.

The United States is not left behind either, as the IBM Watson Health cognitive computing system (IBM Corp., Armonk, New York) used machine learning (ML) approaches to develop a decision support system for doctors treating cancer patients in order to improve diagnostic accuracy and reduce costs using large volumes of patient cases and more than one million scholarly articles.

Furthermore, within musculoskeletal medicine, active shape modeling and machine learning are influential in the comprehension of orthopedics, biomechanics, robotic surgery, bone tumor resection, and prediction of the progression of osteoarthritis based on anatomical shape assessment.

Over the years, we have come to realize that machine learning and deep learning are changing the present medical, and especially the musculoskeletal, landscape. Moreover, through the power of search engines, voice recognition, spam filters, and, of course, autonomous driving vehicles all rely on machine learning technologies and are presently part of our lives, no matter which industry sector we belong to. Furthermore, medicine seems particularly receptive to machine learning solutions, and it has been the center of interest in developing technological economies like those in Silicon Valley.

Artificial intelligence and orthopedics

According to the Bone & Joint Research, significant improvements have been seen in all phases of the medical imaging pathway, from analysis and interpretation to acquisition and reconstruction.

Segmentation

Segmentation, which is the division of digitized images into homogeneous partitions concerning specific borders of regions of interest, is frequently used in the evaluation of cartilage lesions.

Traditionally performed manually

Conventionally performed manually, it is a time-consuming and difficult task with limited standardization. Fully automated machine learning analysis segmentation of wrist cartilage, hip, and knee MRI images has transformed this process and promises to bring automated segmentation into the mainstream of research and clinical practice.

Complex user-dependent image analysis techniques

User-dependent image analysis techniques—for instance, ultrasound for developmental dysplasia of the hip—are specifically amenable to deep learning techniques. Unskilled users can image people in geographically distant or remote locations; these patients can be accurately diagnosed and then directed to professional care at an earlier stage in the natural history of the disease, possibly transforming outcomes.

Kenneth Urish has been developing an AI that can determine the progression of cartilage loss in osteoarthritis by evaluating MRI images.[1] There is evidence that AI can ease the grading process of lumbar disc pathology with 95.6% accuracy. The use of AI in estimating the age of human bones and finding joint and other bony pathologies has a great degree of precision when combined with the work of a trained radiologist.[2]

MyRecovery

One of the artificial intelligence applications created for orthopedics is *MyRecovery*. It was founded by Axel Sylvan and Tom Harte and is a brilliantly designed app for orthopedic patients. Furthermore, the London-based company's app contains information developed and approved by surgeons who seek to help orthopedic surgery patients feel more informed about their pre- or post-operation care and treatment plan.

The digital health app improves patients' experience by enhancing the flow of information from surgeons to patients. MyRecovery includes tips and advice for patients; it allows them to track their progress on the road to recovery. Moreover, all content is approved by the patient's surgeon, which makes the information specific to the patient instead of depending on a one-solution-fits-all model.

Prediction of the clinical outcome

Patient database, genomic mapping, and radiographic imaging can be utilized by AI to predict the risk and prognosis of the disease outcome. The machine learning abilities of AI can provide personalized patient care by foreseeing the possible complications in various orthopedic surgeries such as lumbar fusion surgery[3], knee valgus[4], etc. Similarly, according to Christopher P. Ames, from the University of California, San Francisco (UCSF), AI can predict the risk of postoperative complications, readmission, benefits, and particular surgical intervention by analyzing the patient's medical and demographic details.[5,6]

Use in the treatment of traumatic injuries

Badylak and colleagues are developing an AI application that can help reduce the duration of wound healing of musculoskeletal tissues by almost half.[5,6] The process involves the use of smart bandages that can analyze the rate of healing of wounds by measuring biomarkers and suggesting an appropriate intervention to hasten the process.

AI-assisted robotic use

The use of robots in orthopedic surgery began in 1992 with the application of ROBODOC in the treatment of total hip replacement.[7] Some recent advancements in the robotic field with the advent of the Mako system have enabled us to efficiently perform complex operations such as arthroplasty of the hip and knee.[8] Most spine surgeries done today implicate the use of Renaissance and Rosa robots, which have the finest precision—far better than that of human hands.[9] AI-based spine surgery has greatly helped surgeons to minimize the damage caused to neurovascular bundles during operative procedures such as placement of screws. In 2019, 5G-enabled remote surgery was performed for the first time by Prof. Wei Tian with a higher degree of safety and efficacy.[6] This clearly shows the universality, acceptance, and promises of the use of AI in orthopedics.

AI in computer-assisted navigation

Robotics have been extensively used in accurately positioning the screws and prosthesis or an implant during orthopedic surgery. An AI-operated device called *Optotrack 3020* can precisely locate the bones using infrared rays, which can prove helpful in any bone surgery or grafting. A similar AI, called *Robodoc*, developed by the Curexo technology, uses the intelligence of AI to drill a canal for prosthesis utilizing CT scan images.[10]

Total hip surgery has shown significantly better outcomes using computer-based technology compared to conservative approaches. The cup placement during the implantation of a prosthesis is reported to be more accurate with the use of AI. AI-based use of modern technology has dramatically improved the process of aligning the prosthesis in the course of total knee replacement. Evidence suggests that there is a 32 percent lower risk of the wrong implantation of screws with the use of AI compared to traditional surgical approaches.[11]

Similarly, AI has reduced the complications of ACL reconstruction.[12] It has also been used to surgically treat fractures and dysplasia of the shoulder joint by making use of the advanced navigation system.

AI-aided radiograph analysis

The AI radiographic analyzer was developed by researchers at the Royal Institute of Technology in Sweden. The use of machine learning has proven advantageous in analyzing radiographic images to diagnose subtle abnormalities, which can be highly useful in an emergency setup.[13]

Multiple pathological images were sent to the computer network. The machine-learning algorithm correctly analyzed thousands of such radiographs and, hence, was primed to diagnose the pathology. The accuracy of fracture diagnosis was 83%, while the accuracy by a human is around 82%. In another group of images, the computer network demonstrated 99% accuracy in determining the body part included in the radiograph. This is almost comparable to the accuracy of a top-rated human-level performance. The future of AI in the field of orthopedics is fascinating, with skyrocketing advancements made every day.

Conclusion

The use of AI has only begun to advance. Although it has revolutionized today's healthcare system, it is still not perfect. The promising boon of AI is accompanied by philosophical, financial, legal, and technical challenges. The use of AI comes with an achingly high financial burden to the patient and the country overall. Expensive healthcare again presents the question of affordability and accessibility. It requires a very high degree of skill to operate AI-powered devices. The cost and time of training are also tremendously increased. While empathy, communication, and emotions are the core human qualities in any field of medicine, the use of AI may hinder a strong doctor-patient relationship.

The recording of a patient database can create the risk of breaching patients' confidentiality. This, again, presents a distinct set of ethical issues to consider. Another philosophical dilemma regards the replacement of human jobs by AI because of the latter's higher efficiency in every human discipline. Also, in the event of medical mishaps arising from the use of the AI device, there are legal implications as to who—i.e., the doctor or the manufacturer—will be responsible for the negligence. These questions should be properly addressed before we move to the real AI age.

References/Further Reading

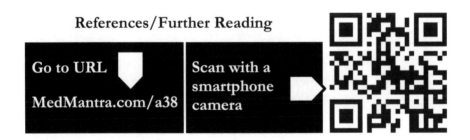

Go to URL
MedMantra.com/a38

Scan with a smartphone camera

CHAPTER THIRTY-NINE
OPHTHALMOLOGY

Ophthalmologists are using artificial intelligence, deep learning, and machine learning to verify read images, disease diagnoses, improve surgical results as well as for perfecting IOL calculations, as these modern techniques become more commonplace in the area.

According to Aaron Y. Lee, MD, of UW Medicine, "Most recent breakthroughs have been in the field of deep learning." He further stated that the breakthroughs in computer vision have allowed near-human performance on many tasks in the last 4 or 5 years.[1]

He pointed out that "the Food and Drug Administration (FDA) has recently approved the use of machine learning algorithm for the purpose of automated diabetic retinopathy grading." This is excellent news because it paves the way for AI-based tech to deliver care to a more substantial number of people. Lee believes that the algorithm will play an innovative role in the delivery of healthcare and the way optometrists practice ophthalmology.

Google's Algorithm

The tech-giant Google is not keeping still in the artificial intelligence for improving the practice of ophthalmology. Research teams at Google's AI laboratory successfully trained an algorithm to diagnose a commonly occurring eye disease, as well as an experienced ophthalmologist.[2]

According to Will Knight in "An AI Ophthalmologist Shows How Machine Learning May Transform Medicine," "Google researchers have developed a retinal scanning algorithm to discover out on its own with the much-needed help from humans. It is created to find a common form of blindness; Google's algorithm shows the possibilities for artificial intelligence to change medicine in the near future positively," he said.

Furthermore, Google's new algorithm can scan the retinal images and diagnose and grade diabetic retinopathy, which affects almost a third of diabetes patients, just as a professional ophthalmologist can do. Nonetheless, we can use the machine-learning technique created by Google to tag web images.

In Will Knight's article, he wrote, "Diabetic retinopathy is caused by damage to blood vessels in the eye and results in a steady degeneration of vision. However, if detected early, it can be treated, but the patients may experience no symptoms in the early stage, which makes the screening essential. Diabetic retinopathy is diagnosed in part by an expert who examines the images of the sufferer's retina, captured with a specialized device, for signs of fluid leakage and bleeding".

Artificial Intelligence-based model vs. Traditional model

Lee further stated that the most exciting areas of AI applications in ophthalmology are the areas of personalized medicine and future prognosis. Unlike the traditional statistical models used for risk prediction, AI deep learning models are more flexible and powerful. For instance, deep learning models may have the ability to read a Humphrey visual field and predict how fast they can go blind or understand an Optical Coherence Tomography and predict who will develop wet macular degeneration.

Furthermore, the birth of artificial intelligence has given rise to other possibilities to take place in the healthcare sector, especially in ophthalmology, such as simple deep learning with convolutional neural networks (CNN), automated detectors, disease feature-based versus image-based ("black box") learning, basic machine learning, and advanced machine learning.

References/Further Reading

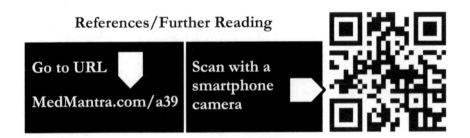

Go to URL

MedMantra.com/a39

Scan with a smartphone camera

CHAPTER FORTY

CRITICAL CARE MEDICINE

Critical care medicine, which deals with the study of diseases and conditions that are life-threatening and need urgent intervention, requires prompt decisions in practice.[1] AI can prove to be an essential element in aiding the overall process of critical care medicine in the healthcare system.

The Importance of AI in Critical Care Medicine

Currently, there is a huge dependency on human experience to make decisions in the ICU setting. This has led to the possibility of variations when it comes to decision-making. Every doctor or clinician has a different experience and applies systems based on their understanding of the situation.

AI picks up the algorithms and offers a great range of data, allowing for better implementation by the human workforce present in the healthcare system. Following are the uses of AI in critical care medicine.

a. Mortality prediction and scoring

Scoring systems have been implemented in ICU departments to effectively deal with complex cases. While the severity, outcome predictions, and other parameters are recorded, the current scoring and prediction system is found to be less effective in considering the demographical, geographical, and other differences present in the system.[2]

With the advent of AI, it will be easier to gather data much more effectively and come up with better predictions and severity scoring. Predictions and scoring can be made on an individual basis, and therefore can prove to be much more effective.

b. Sepsis prediction

It is common to overlook the possibility of sepsis, therefore leading to a late diagnosis or misdiagnosis. Currently, the methods used to predict sepsis do not produce effective results. However, implementing AI in this scenario can make things much easier. For instance, a range of predictive markers can be used to collect the data, ensuring earlier diagnosis and effective treatment for the patient as opposed to having to wait for the test results.[3]

c. Mechanical ventilation

AI is highly effective in ensuring the right amount of sedation medication and also makes a wise decision regarding the time for removal of ventilators. Because there is currently clear evidence of variations in the system, introducing AI into critical care medicine can surely overcome the limitations present. AI makes use of algorithms, so it has proven to be better than the clinical practices followed. Through AI, there is improved and accurate measurement and analysis over time of vital signs like oxygen saturation percentage, heart and respiratory rates, and body temperature.[4]

Overall, AI is set to make a difference in critical care medicine because it offers improved data handling to draw better conclusions more quickly. Because critical care medicine is highly dependent on data, it is essential to have accurate data in the system. Introducing AI into healthcare, especially critical care medicine, allows for better decision-making and dealing with complexities.

References/Further Reading

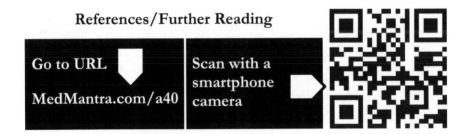

Go to URL
MedMantra.com/a40

Scan with a smartphone camera

CHAPTER FORTY-ONE

EMERGENCY MEDICINE

AI in emergency medicine can surely be a boon especially considering the time limitations that prevail while diagnosing and managing emergency cases.

Present Uses of AI in Emergency Medicine

Decision-making processes should be very quick and accurate in the emergency department (ED), where the clinician has little time to arrive at a diagnosis and start appropriate management. Diagnostic, decision-making and treatment processes in the ED are based upon the usage of large quantities of data, the recalling of which would be very difficult for any human being.[1] On the other hand, an AI-based system can fetch the relevant data from various sources, make accurate decisions, and suggest further plans of action in no time. This can phenomenally improve the effectiveness of the patient care process. AI can effectively triage patients in ED based on their level of emergency, with the most urgent cases given priority over less- or non-urgent ones. Also, a large number of patients can be simultaneously managed if AI is used wisely in the ED.[2]

To make the AI implementation effective, a system must be in place for constant surveillance of the public to acquire their health data. Using this data, AI can update their medical records in real time. This will help in giving them the correct treatment for their condition in a very short period in case of a medical emergency, as no time will be wasted in history taking, physical examination, and measuring vital parameters.

A range of speculations has been put forward as to what might be beneficial for emergency medicine in terms of the incorporation of AI. However, there are no clear indications of any implementation of these practices in the current systems. Therefore, more work must be done to figure out more effective ways to handle emergency medicine.

The Future Possibilities of AI in Emergency Medicine

There is a great emphasis on the development of AI in emergency medicine because of the current limitations that exist.

By incorporating AI into emergency medicine, the clinicians present on-site will have a much easier time addressing the issues at hand because there will be adequate data to work with. The real-time data will allow doctors to work more effectively and with accurate diagnoses and treatments for patients in the ED.

References/Further Reading

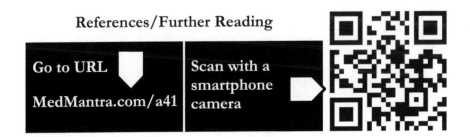

Go to URL

MedMantra.com/a41

Scan with a smartphone camera

CHAPTER FORTY-TWO
ENDOCRINOLOGY

Medical practice as we know it could experience a revolution sooner than expected. The rise of automation and the adoption of artificial intelligence systems across varied fields in healthcare have resulted in a plethora of studies, with a collaboration of scientists and engineers coming together to alleviate chronic conditions that truly hamper the quality of life and raise morbidity and mortality rates. Variations in hormone balance can disrupt body functioning AND are often responsible for life-long illnesses. Therefore, it is not surprising that AI efforts have targeted endocrinology and its associated disease spectrum.

1. Application in diabetes and its co-morbidities

In 2019 it was reported that around 463 million people (20-79 years old) were currently suffering from diabetes and that diabetes had caused 4.2 million deaths worldwide. It was also projected that by 2045 the number of patients would increase to 700 million.[1]

a. AI in the diagnosis of diabetic retinopathy

Diabetic retinopathy is a common complication of longstanding uncontrolled diabetes.

Corneal confocal microscopy is often used and is a non-invasive imaging method for the retina that can identify peripheral as well as central neural degeneration. To help with a rapid and accurate diagnosis, Williams and colleagues developed a deep learning algorithm with convolutional neural networks (CNN) to quantify nerve fiber properties that could diagnose diabetic changes in the retina by comparing observations with a validated and automated data analysis program. The software demonstrated accurate performance for the localization and quantification of nerve biomarkers in the cornea.[2]

b. AI in diabetic self-management

Awareness of predisposing factors like diet, exercise, and lifestyle has improved. The global community is moving toward better eating habits as they become more mindful about the prevention and control of diet-borne diseases like type 2 diabetes mellitus. Tracking food intake through phone applications is a popular but often time-consuming and inconvenient task. The "Snap n Eat" smartphone application uses an image-based food monitoring system that estimates caloric or nutritional content without user involvement. It could detect 15 categories of food items with 85% accuracy.[3]

Exercise goes hand in hand with dietary restrictions for people living with diabetes. Researchers have used symbolic reasoning along with machine learning to recognize and evaluate patients' lifestyle history using data captured through their smartphones, with an accuracy of 83.4%. This was an easy way to track activity rates without burdening the patients, thereby improving compliance with both diet and exercise regimens.[4]

c. AI-controlled glucometers

Artificial intelligence programs are being used at every stage of chronic disease management, such as the recording of patient physiology (like temperature, heart rate, number of steps, hours of sleep, hydration, and even geolocation), made possible through the integration of smartphone applications with wearables or remote patient monitoring devices. Machine learning principles have been used to build algorithms that help to predict risk for the development of diabetes. They also allow for continuous and easy monitoring of blood glucose levels, biomarkers, and data from insulin pumps to facilitate better glycemic control, which is the advent of data-driven clinical decision support and precision care.[5]

Leveraging the power of the Internet-of-Medical-Things (IoMT), the "Intelligent Glucose Meter" (i.e., iGLU) was based on machine learning models and infrared sensor-based spectroscopy. It was developed as a point-of-care testing device for accurate but non-invasive testing of blood glucose levels. IGLU has also been used and validated in hospital settings, with patient values backed up in a secure server that endocrinologists can access and monitor remotely.[6]

d. AI in the management of type 1 diabetes using an artificial pancreas

In 2019, a French medical device start-up called Diabeloop secured €31m in funding for its 'artificial pancreas' which uses AI to predict the need for intervention and automatically facilitate personalized treatment for patients suffering from type 1 diabetes using continuous blood glucose monitoring, reinforcement learning algorithm-based smart controllers, and closed-loop insulin control pumps to deliver insulin dosages based on regimens calibrated to suit the patient's immediate needs.[7,8]

2. Applications in thyroid disease

Integrated bioinformatics and genomics, backed by deep learning methods, helped researchers to analyze different gene expressions that resulted in anaplastic thyroid carcinomas.[9]

3. Applications in pituitary gland disease

Machine learning methods used to augment mass spectrometry (MS) imaging have shown potential in differentiating pituitary adenomas into hormone-secreting and non-secreting types, thereby identifying normal gland architecture at a molecular level in under half an hour. This would enable real-time tumor resection intra-operatively to improve outcomes.[10]

Conclusion

Given the large amount of patient data to be monitored over long periods, endocrine disorders and their chronic nature have proven to benefit greatly from AI-enriched technology, leading to precise investigations and diagnostics and a reduction in healthcare expenses as well as facilitating databases for research.[11] With the widespread implementation and through adequate awareness and funding, modern clinical endocrinology can evolve into a technologically smart and sound treatment pathway in the future.

References/Further Reading

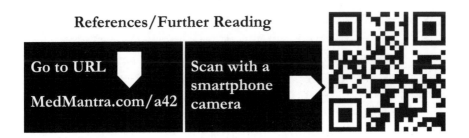

Go to URL

MedMantra.com/a42

Scan with a smartphone camera

CHAPTER FORTY-THREE

GASTROENTEROLOGY

Introduction

AI has been widely used to augment various diagnostic modalities in the field of gastroenterology. Besides gastrointestinal radiology, it is also applicable in procedures such as endoscopic analysis of lesions, like in the detection of cancer, gastritis, polyps, gastric ulcer, etc.[1] AI, under proper guidance and supervision of a human brain, can diagnose liver fibrosis, differentiate pancreatic cancer from pancreatitis, and establish prognostic factors and predict responses to treatments.

How Effective Is the Current Implementation?

The current implementations of AI in gastroenterology are highly effective in diagnosing a range of abnormalities. However, the implementations are limited to CNNs (convolutional neural networks) for the augmenting of endoscopic imaging.[2] While this alone is highly effective, it is not enough when it comes to the range of challenges or pathologies that exist in gastroenterology.

Other aspects, such as the use of AI-based medication management, will prove to be highly effective, but they are currently not used. Given that there are variations in the disease presentations and that two patients may not always have the same problems, at the current stage, it is difficult for human doctors to get into the details of each and every case.

What Are the Future Possibilities?

AI seems to be highly useful in gastroenterology. More importance should be given to the use of AI tools rather than traditional methods, wherever feasible. For instance, the use of AI should not be limited to the implementation of CNNs in endoscopies on certain occasions.[2] Instead, it should be used regularly in practice with all examinations. There should be a standardized AI-based procedure for all patients who have similar diseases so that the diagnosis and treatment become streamlined, thereby significantly reducing human error.

References/Further Reading

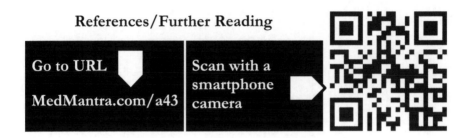

Go to URL
MedMantra.com/a43

Scan with a smartphone camera

CHAPTER FORTY-FOUR

HEMATOLOGY

The rapid growth of AI and machine learning in healthcare has created benefits for patients and physicians, as they have access to accurate and timely therapeutic interventions. Diagnostics play a large role in patient management, and the field of hematology is no exception. The analysis of whole blood through largely automated systems has completely revolutionized a branch that was initially extremely labor-intensive. Highly sensitive cell counters and coagulometers can give accurate readings, along with a differential interpretation and flags to draw the pathologist's attention to slides that require scanning. Whole-slide imaging has become predominant in histopathology, making digital and telepathology more mainstream in the last few years, where the identification of tissue patterns and cell differentiation stages are the mainstay of diagnosis. Similarly, blood cell imaging, through either blood smears, bone marrow smears, or flow cytometry for hematological conditions ranging from the humble malaria infection to neoplastic conditions like leukemias and lymphomas, are some of the major investigations conducted in the laboratory. These auto-analyzers generate large data sets that, when combined with pathologist interpretation and clinical findings, can be used to train artificial intelligence systems.

The application of AI-based software to hematological investigations has the potential to vastly improve both the accuracy of diagnosis and the turnaround time of specialist-dependent interpretation and reporting, which may be prone to discrepancies. AI algorithms trained in the identification of abnormal blood cell morphology can filter out normal or routine blood smear results from those with abnormal findings that warrant specialized testing like flow cytometry or karyotyping, necessary to identifying neoplastic states.

A machine learning algorithm trained in the interpretation of multicolor flow cytometry findings through a study conducted by Bor Sheng Ko and colleagues was clinically validated in its diagnosis of acute myeloid leukemia and myelodysplastic syndromes with an accuracy of 84.6% and 92.4%, respectively.[1]

Myelodysplastic syndromes (MDS) are notoriously difficult to interpret on slide imaging, which makes the correlation between the phenotype and the genotype of blood or marrow cell morphology challenging. Another study conducted by Nagata and colleagues provided inputs like cytomorphology and clinical features through patient records and molecular and genetic approaches with genome sequencing and used them to train a machine learning algorithm to identify distinct types of MDS profiles, thereby segregating patients based on their staging and prognosis. This provides a multi-dimensional approach to diagnosis from the first step itself.[2]

Cell Population Data (CPD) can provide blood cell parameters that, in turn, are utilized for differential diagnosis of hematological conditions. Machine learning (ML)-based applications have played a major role in modifying medical diagnostics based on hematology. Research conducted by Syed-Abdul and colleagues tested a new approach, using ML algorithms and CPD to screen for malignancies in blood. It was observed that the system achieved 82.8% accuracy and precision with 93.5% recall.[3]

Rajaraman S. applied pre-trained convolutional neural networks (CNN) to extract diagnoses of parasite infiltration, like malaria rings, schizonts, and gametocytes, in whole blood thin smear images. Widespread application of this software could greatly impact the health of countries with rural endemic areas prone to malaria infections where adequate skilled human staff are not available for accurate screening and diagnosis; this would eventually lead to faster and improved therapeutic interventions.[4]

The innovations tested and the promising results obtained indicate that the penetration of AI-backed interpretation into hematology practice is just the beginning, with much to look forward to in the near future.

References/Further Reading

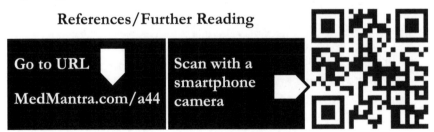

Go to URL
MedMantra.com/a44

Scan with a smartphone camera

CHAPTER FORTY-FIVE
INFECTIOUS DISEASES

Infectious diseases are disorders caused by organisms such as bacteria, viruses, fungi, and parasites. Their tendency to cause diseases in human beings depends upon different factors like the immunological status of the host, the virulence of the organism, and environmental factors.

Being the era of COVID-19, this year has made us all too familiar with the notion of infectious diseases. They are a threat to our survival, especially when they spiral out of control and turn into a pandemic. It is perhaps the most significant health crisis of the 21st century.

Of course, technology has come a long way, and with the help of artificial intelligence (AI), the healthcare industry is making strides.

What Do Infectious Disease Specialists Focus On?

Infectious disease specialists perform various functions like prevention, diagnosis through clinical features, microscopy or culture, and management of infections. They use laboratory data, data from cultures, and the microscopy of body samples to make their diagnoses. All the data is collected, integrated, and analyzed to devise a treatment plan.

Clinicians recommend different types of treatments for infectious diseases. These include:

- Antiviral therapy

- Antibiotic therapy

- Antifungal therapy

- Anti-parasitic therapy

The choice of the treatment plan depends on the infection you have and what your body can take. Many infections are present in a mild form and can be managed with a short course of antibiotic therapy. However, there are lethal infections as well, like malaria, pneumonia, HIV, diarrheal diseases, and tuberculosis, which may require more intensive work-up for management. Patients with infectious diseases can be treated anywhere from outpatient facilities to the ICU.

Current Role of Artificial Intelligence in Infectious Diseases

In the field of infectious diseases, AI can be used to identify different aspects of a disease, like ecological and epidemiological patterns, and the tendency and possibility of an outbreak to occur, and thus the measures to cope with outbreaks like an epidemic.[1]

For this, a huge amount of data regarding particular infectious diseases is analyzed by AI-based computerized systems. These predictions help ecologists, government officials, public health experts, and the general population to act beforehand in order to cope with upcoming epidemics and thereby minimize loss and disruptions. Also, talking about the present scenario, while everyone is focused on COVID-19, AI can keep an eye on other possible outbreaks around the world.

Practically, there have been only limited uses of AI in infectious diseases.[1] Many clinics and health organizations are using both machine learning (ML) and deep learning (DL) technology. However, they are not being used in an organized manner globally.

Of course, this doesn't mean that there is no potential. If health organizations start deploying AI for infectious diseases, much good can be done. Conditions can be diagnosed beforehand, and infections could be prevented from spreading.

Right now, the focus is more on data collection. Big datasets are being collected from health exchanges, electronic health records, and many other sources. In the traditional setup, data was derived by the public health sector from labs, which was costly and time-consuming.

There are many electronic health data sources, but there must be a proper strategy for data collection. Once this data is organized, reviewed, and analyzed, it can help create insights that can be used to learn more about infectious diseases.

AI makes intelligent inferences from the data and, thus, obtains conclusions directly linked to patient care.

The Future Role of AI in Infectious Diseases

Much remains to be done in this area, but here are the many ways that both ML and DL will be used for infectious diseases.

a. Early diagnosis

The key to the prevention of disease is the early identification of the underlying causative factor(s). For this, AI will be used in the future. It can be used for earlier diagnosis at present as well, but more organization of a tremendous amount of data must be done to diagnose more diseases early. In the future, AI has the potential to sound the alarm about the disease in its initial stage.[1]

One prime example of AI's use in the field of infectious diseases is BlueDot.[2] This is a health monitoring platform in Canada that sounded the alarm for COVID-19 before any other AI entity. The platform was created after the CEO of BlueDot wanted to track diseases after the SARS outbreak in 2003.

BlueDot launched six years ago, and it uses various algorithms to conduct surveillance of infectious diseases, predict the emergence and spread of the infectious disease, and provide warnings. BlueDot sent a message to its clients about a virus in China on December 3, 2019.[2]

This was even before the WHO let out an official warning on January 9, 2020. AI is being used for the surveillance of outbreaks at present but only in a handful of places. If such technology is employed on a larger scale, AI will easily give early warnings, and epidemics can be prevented, or their effects can be minimized.

b. Tracking the spread of diseases

Infectious diseases can lead to large outbreaks. COVID-19 is perhaps the biggest current example of infectious diseases that are spreading like wildfire. AI can help detect new diseases and then track where they are spreading.

For example, once COVID-19 started spreading, BlueDot analyzed the airline ticketing data and accurately predicted that the virus would travel from Wuhan to Bangkok, Seoul, Taipei, and Tokyo.

We can now see that contract tracing apps are being used to understand disease patterns.[3] AI algorithms determine the risk of infection and then alert smartphone users of this risk.

Someone near an individual who already has COVID-19 can be alerted about the disease. AI and big data have a great potential to track the spread of diseases before they are uncontrollable. Of course, in the end, it is up to us to try to contain the disease so it does not spread the way COVID-19 did.

c. **Allocation of resources**

If an infectious disease spreads, it is up to the government to control it in their country. That means the government must allocate resources efficiently. They need to make tough decisions so that the disease can be controlled in the best way possible.

AI can help make these decisions in a much better way by using the data available and also helping to make accurate predictions and guide resource allocation to solve the problem.[4]

For example, AI can accurately predict where the infectious disease will travel next. Officials can create checkpoints in those places and also ensure that hospitals in those areas have enough resources to deal with the crisis.

Also, researchers can combine AI with simulation models to assess how effective the policy response is. This will help in determining how effective a certain action is in controlling the infectious disease.

These algorithms can also help in determining the populations that will benefit from public health communications and measures to slow down the spread of an infectious disease or even prevent it.

Such an algorithm exists right now. The USC Viterbi School of Engineering has created an AI algorithm like this.[5] The school used real-time tuberculosis data to create the algorithm, which considers the transmission of the disease and the patterns of human behavior.

Many other public health officials have used similar algorithms to prevent infectious diseases such as Hepatitis C and HIV. So, there is a lot of potential in this area that can be utilized in the future.

d. Vaccine development

Developing a vaccine requires an immense amount of data and time. A lot of research into an infectious disease must take place before a promising vaccine can be developed. Even these vaccines need to go through a trial period, so their effectiveness can be tested before they are launched for the general public.[6]

AI algorithms help in analyzing virus genomes so that a vaccine can be quickly developed. Using AI, scientists can detect the mutations in bacteria or viruses as they emerge in a short time and can then take steps to deal with those mutated pathogens.

e. Prediction of future outbreaks

For the past four to five decades, 75% of documented infectious diseases have been zoonotic. This means they spread from animals to humans, just like in the case of COVID-19. Before the advancement of AI, researchers could identify the animal host at a very late stage.[7]

The disease would have already spread to thousands of humans before the animal host was identified. However, AI is used to identify both epidemiological and ecological patterns that lead to outbreaks, and the preventive and control measures can be started early.

These mathematical models are based on ML that analyzes significant amounts of data to understand and predict the next source of infection. Such predictions can help researchers and ecologists to monitor host species so that future outbreaks can be prevented.

Many such models are being invented. One example is the Cary Institute for Ecosystem Studies.[8] They have created a computer model that chooses different species of rodents that have a high potential of carrying an infectious disease.

The computer model scanned approximately 2300 species of rodents and found almost 60 potential hosts. Further research shows that two of these were confirmed to harbor pathogens. That is not all the institute did.

They also used ML and AI to predict the types of bats that can carry filoviruses such as Ebola. The model that predicts this uses 57 factors to make predictions, such as ecology data, life history, etc.

Challenges in Creating AI for Infectious Diseases

Many challenges accompany creating AI for the prevention of infectious diseases. The biggest challenge is the effectiveness of the data that creates these models.

AI is completely data-driven. If the data is incomplete or inaccurate, the insights from it will not be accurate. Such errors can lead to a lack of applicability, as well as to misclassification and false negatives.

A strict check and balance must be placed on the mode of data collection. The datasets are responsible for designing learning algorithms. If the data is inaccurate, the learning algorithms will be of no use. It becomes a waste of time, money, and resources.

An even bigger challenge that we face regarding data is data ownership and privacy. We are familiar with the fact that our data can be exploited for political and commercial gain. The case of Cambridge Analytica is the biggest example of this.[9]

Medical data is even more sensitive, and its exploitation can lead to grave consequences. People don't want to give up their privacy like this, and nor do they want their data to be exploited in any way. So, there must be some type of regulation that protects people's privacy.

Many experts have suggested that patients should have ownership and control of their data. Once they have this data, they can consent to the use of data regarding their health for the development of AI algorithms. Of course, this will not be easy, either.

There must be transparency, discussion, and regulation by public officials to safely develop the AI algorithm without misusing or abusing data. Every individual has the right to privacy, and this must be safeguarded by the healthcare system.

In short, containing and preventing infectious disease outbreaks using AI is not an easy task. Much needs to be improved upon in this field before data can be made available on such a large scale. Unless something can be done to effectively protect patients' privacy, the role of AI in infectious diseases will be limited.

Conclusion

That was a complete guide to the current and future role of AI in infectious diseases and its challenges. Remember that AI can sometimes overlook small things, such as data clusters. Therefore, we are far from having a perfect model that will provide us with everything we need.

The key is to experiment, see what works, and then use it for the people's good. Of course, this is ideal thinking, but there is much hope in the direction AI is headed. Right now, the focus should be on the collection of accurate data. Once it is collected, it can be put into different ML and DL models for accurate predictions and insights.

References/Further Reading

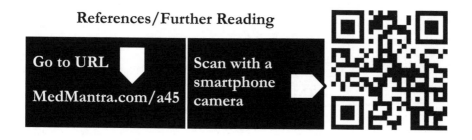

Go to URL
MedMantra.com/a45

Scan with a smartphone camera

CHAPTER FORTY-SIX

FAMILY MEDICINE/PRIMARY CARE

The use of artificial intelligence has proven to be a transformational force in the primary care industry. Many experts concluded that the use of artificial intelligence in primary care could transform the patient/physician relationship.

The Use of Artificial Intelligence in Primary Care

1. Digital health coaching

The use of artificial intelligence in primary care has revolutionized the way we take care of ourselves. Many companies are offering digital health coaching to customers. They are used for keeping a check on hypertension, obesity, diabetes, and many other chronic conditions.[1] These programs are integrated into the health systems. The use of these programs has resulted in a drastic reduction in the number of visits by patients to primary care providers.

2. Device integration

Many wearable devices are available to keep track of your health and check other vital signs. All you need to do is wear them, and they will take care of your health in ways that you never imagined. The most common example of this case is the Apple Watch. The health kit in Apple Watch integrates data from different devices.[1] This helps the care team to detect deviations from the routine, which may suggest the presence of illness.

3. Medical advice

The use of AI in the field of primary care is not restricted to health coaching and device integration. Many companies have even developed AI doctors. The job of these AI doctors is to provide health advice to patients.[2] This can help users obtain primary care for their common symptoms without making an appointment with the actual doctor. This will also free up time for patients who have more serious problems and need immediate attention.

4. **Clinical decision-making**

Artificial intelligence involves much more than checking your heartbeat or blood pressure. It also provides advisory services to primary care physicians. These advisory services help in making the best clinical decisions. Therefore, it is beneficial for both patients and doctors.[3]

5. **Diagnostics**

AI algorithms can diagnose some diseases that even the most experienced primary care physicians cannot. Whether it is detecting skin cancer, congenital diseases, lung cancer, and many other conditions, it can all be done with the use of AI applications that analyze skin/face photographs, chest X-rays, and other images.[4]

References/Further Reading

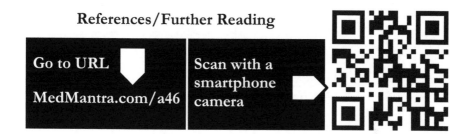

Go to URL
MedMantra.com/a46

Scan with a smartphone camera

CHAPTER FORTY-SEVEN
NEPHROLOGY

While the diagnosis and disease risk and prevalence of nephrology and urology conditions have been analyzed as Big Data groups to train Artificial Intelligence (AI) systems, the implementation of AI solutions in treatment was still at its nascent stages until multiple research initiatives spearheaded the effort to introduce deep learning systems with artificial neural networks (ANNs) to revolutionize treatment options, with a focus on automating dialysis, along with conditions that arise due to chronic kidney disease.

AI has been applied in various areas to help physicians navigate the management of these conditions. For example:

1. Sounding the Alarm – Alerting Systems for Kidney Injury

The incidence of Acute Kidney Injury (AKI) has been increasing at the rate of 11% per year, predominantly among indoor and ICU patients. This has been known to increase the average length of stay at hospitals, with associated increased mortality and morbidity rates and patients deteriorating to end-stage renal disease. Therefore, early diagnosis of AKI and the provision of timely management are important.[1]

Koyner and colleagues developed a Gradient Boosting Machine (GBM) algorithm that predicted kidney injury by correlating serum creatinine levels with data from patients' electronic health records, including demographics, locations, vitals, and radiological and laboratory values, as well as preliminary interventions. The algorithm managed to predict stage 2 acute kidney injury with 84% sensitivity and 85% specificity.[2] Another study by Zimmerman and colleagues demonstrated that ML models could accurately predict AKI onset following intensive care admission [3].

2. Finding the Root Cause – Diagnostic Assistance

Computer-aided diagnosis (CAD) was used in the diagnosis of hereditary Autosomal Dominant Polycystic Kidney Disease (ADPKD) by evaluating CT and MRI images for Total Kidney Volume (TKV) computation. Most recently, van Gastel MDA and colleagues developed an automated segmentation that uses a deep learning neural network to automatically calculate TKV, which correlated highly with manually traced TKV.[4]

In addition, Wei and colleagues developed an automated, algorithm-based quantification system for measuring interstitial fibrosis in kidney biopsies, while Kannan and colleagues developed a deep learning framework to identify glomeruli in biopsies, based on a CNN segmentation model.[5,6]

3. *Showing the Way – Guidance for Clinical Decision-Making*

a. Hemodialysis

Innovative dialysis devices are automated systems based on AI networks to enable real-time monitoring of equipment alarms, patient parameters, and electronic health record data. This data set is used to train the algorithm to produce instantaneous changes in the dialysis prescription. Most recently, wearable artificial kidneys (WAK) have been introduced; if backed by AI, they would be a game-changer for ·patients on chronic dialysis treatments. These systems work based on the predictions that AI-based software can make about the probable incidence of secondary anemia, body water composition, or hypotension during dialysis, thereby ensuring patient safety. The automatic, instantaneous biofeedback made possible with the AI systems will allow continuously changing dialysis orders, thereby benefitting patients through accurate and time-saving interventions.[7]

Barbieri and colleagues developed a multiple endpoint model that maintains the delicate balance between adequate fluid removal and the risk of intradialytic adverse events. This model predicted session-specific fluid volume removal, ECG, and blood pressure and heart rate readings along with patient characteristics, previous hemodynamic responses, or any adverse reactions prompting changes in dialysis prescription in the past.[8]

b. Anemia management

Computational intelligence software run on patient records and lab investigations has been used to predict the selection of doses of erythropoiesis-stimulating agents, which leads to better anemia management, hopefully decreasing the number of transfusions.[9]

c. Nutrition-based approaches

AI was used to automate the method and improve the accuracy of assessing the dry weight of patients on dialysis through the design of an ANN that utilized bio-impedancemetry and blood volume and that monitored blood pressure values as data inputs, to create a calculated output of dry weight. In many cases, the predictions made by the AI system outperformed that of expert nephrologists, showing promising results for the application.[10]

d. Peritoneal dialysis

AI algorithms and machine learning have also been applied to decisions about peritoneal dialysis (PD), including which PD techniques to use, the risk of infections, or the prediction of cardiovascular events, based on patient history and response trends.

e. Kidney transplant

Transplant databases are run more efficiently with management systems that use ML as pretransplant organ-matching tools. They also help to predict graft rejection and evaluate tacrolimus therapy modulation or the presentation of dietary issues.

4. *Evaluating the Effect – Analysing Prognosis*

As a sequela of long-term dialysis, patients may develop hypertension with decreased vein function and fistula collapse. Predictive AI models help to reduce repeated USG doppler testing for the viability of the fistula by evaluating data points that describe the health of the fistula and thereby predict its lifespan so that interventions can be carried out proactively.[11]

Conclusion

In the future, we can expect to see AI being used actively in surgical interventions like urolithiasis, where it is used to analyze urinary stone composition or the severity and prognosis of prostate enlargement.

Radiological applications of AI algorithms in the nuclear grading of renal carcinomas, cystoscopy-led diagnosis of bladder cancers, and the calculation of Gleason score are just a few ways that AI is projected to impact the fields of nephrology and urology.[12]

References/Further Reading

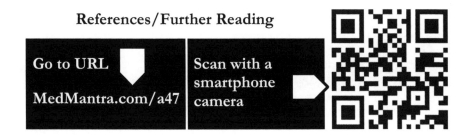

Go to URL

MedMantra.com/a47

Scan with a smartphone camera

CHAPTER FORTY-EIGHT

NEUROLOGY AND NEUROSURGERY

Neurology and neurosurgery are important fields in medicine and surgery, respectively, where the use of AI has proved to be invaluable.

Neurology

AI has been shown to be highly effective in dealing with large quantities of data which are usually present in fields like neurology. The use of the human brain in making calculations and deriving results with interpretations from the vast amount of data is not able to eliminate significant unavoidable biases and errors, as the amount of data that a human brain can retain is limited. Thus, obtained results are less trustworthy, which affects the overall health outcome in neurology.

On the other hand, AI/deep learning uses a streamlined system of algorithms and can store a tremendous amount of data, unlike a human brain. The simultaneous use of multiple datasets is easier with AI; thus, the conclusion derived is unbiased. Also, the time consumed by AI is quite a bit less than that consumed by a neurologist working on his own. The conclusions derived are directly linked to the patient's diagnosis and treatment.

For example, for the diagnosis of stroke, AI-based assessments of CT scans can be used, which helps in early and effective lesion detection[1] and quantification of increased bleeding.

Also, AI can detect the early warning signs of ischemia on CT scans and measure the extent of early ischemic changes so that emergency intervention can be planned. This has a positive effect on the outcome of the intervention.

Clinical Judgments and AI

Let's assume a scenario in which a patient walks into a clinic with some complaints and is observed by both a doctor and an AI-based system. With the use of vast experience, the doctor narrows down the list of causes of the problems that the patient might be facing.

The doctor takes a history of the patient, examines him/her, and performs some investigations to narrow down the possible causes in each step.

The AI-based system runs a series of steps like receiving the patient's history and performing an examination with a camera and provides an output with a narrow list of possible causes that the patient might be facing—just like the doctor but in a much shorter time.

On the one hand, the output presented by AI is much quicker than that presented by the doctor; on the other hand, the results presented by the doctor are more likely to be erroneous than those of the AI because humans cannot retain excessive information. Furthermore, it is difficult to analyze and interpret the vast amount of data presented to the human brain.

A neurologist, however, must be the core part of the process of patient care, as he needs to analyze the output from AI and make plans to proceed further. Hence, the focus should be on the combined effort of AI and the doctor so that healthcare practices can be more systematic, easy, and effective.

Neurosurgery

AI has been used in carrying out surgical procedures for neurological problems and has been found to be useful, just like in neurology. Using different techniques[2], AI has surpassed the traditional methods of decision-making in neurosurgery, in which predictions, diagnoses, and prognoses are made with the human brain working alone.

AI has been proven to be highly effective in diagnosing and managing various problems requiring neurosurgical intervention, like brain tumors, epilepsy, trauma, cerebral vasospasm, disc herniation, and more.

For example, a robot with the help of AI may be used to place screws in the spine during a neurosurgical procedure. The screw placement by the robot is quicker and potentially more accurate than that by a neurosurgeon[3].

Uses of AI in Neurology and Neurosurgery

AI has proven itself to be a wise, effective, and trustworthy companion for a neurologist or neurosurgeon. Following are the different subspecialties of neurology and/or neurosurgery in which artificial intelligence can be used as a gift from modern technology to mankind:

Neuro-oncology

Neuro-oncology deals with the study of different aspects, including the prevention, diagnosis, and management of tumors of the brain and spinal cord. AI can be used to make an early diagnosis of brain tumors by employing different methods of investigation like AI-based CT or MRI scans that have high sensitivity.[4] This is done by training the AI system so that the AI 'learns' and 'understands' the normal patterns and variations in the brain morphology. This has a positive effect upon the patient's health because when the tumor is diagnosed in its earlier stages, there is a higher chance of its complete cure. Also, the accuracy of the diagnosis prevents patients from receiving wrong or unnecessary treatment. AI has also been used to predict the survival timing of the patient and is found to be highly accurate in most cases.

Neurodegenerative diseases

Neurodegenerative diseases are incurable and debilitating conditions like Alzheimer's, Parkinson's, and multiple sclerosis in which neurons progressively die or degenerate, causing problems with movement, memory, etc.

AI can be a major help in understanding whether a person is developing any form of neurodegeneration at an earlier stage. With the use of various algorithms through which thousands of data samples are assessed, the mechanism allows for the identification of all the markers that are abnormal in neurodegenerative diseases.[5] So, AI helps in making a timely diagnosis of these diseases for early and outcome-based intervention and assists in predicting the course of these diseases.

Neurovascular diseases

AI offers a range of applications in the neurovascular subspecialty. Through AI-based CT scans, a hemorrhagic or an ischemic lesion can be detected; this technology can also predict the future possibilities of the patient having a stroke. This prediction can be very helpful for making necessary arrangements before the attack occurs.

Also, patients who have already received treatment for a stroke can be placed under post-treatment monitoring through AI mechanisms. According to

Leibovitz from Montefiore Medical Center and AiCure, patient monitoring can become easier for doctors, as algorithms can be installed on their phones to assess whether or not the patient is taking the required medication.[6] This also allows for understanding the patient's behavior and figuring out the extent to which the patient is following the treatment plan.

Traumatic brain injury

Researchers from Finland discovered that an algorithm developed in an AI system allows doctors to understand and predict the mortality rate in patients with traumatic brain injury. In this system, algorithms are set for measuring and recording cerebral perfusion pressure, mean arterial pressure, and intracranial pressure. The outcome data of these parameters are used to predict the probability of the patient's recovery. Moreover, these researchers placed a secondary algorithm where the motor functions of the brain, like eye movements, were assessed in a traumatic brain injury patient.[7]

It was found that about 80% of the predictions made with this system were correct. So, the AI predictions can be used in planning the future course of treatment that the patient will have and in formulating and following necessary precautions to prevent a worse outcome.

Spinal cord injury

Spinal cord injury happens in road traffic accidents, other accidents, homicidal assaults, etc. Injury to the spinal cord causes paralysis or loss of sensation or both in the part of the body below the level of the injury. Different research has shown that intra-cortical recorded signals sent with the aid of an AI-based system help in the activation of muscles that were paralyzed due to different causes. Therefore, AI mechanisms may be implemented to figure out the underlying pathology and to overcome paralysis due to spinal cord injuries.[8]

It was proved that a 24-year-old man who was paralyzed due to spinal cord injury was able to overcome his paralysis through the implementation of this mechanism. The algorithms were set so that signals were sent to his brain. This triggered his brain, just like a natural impulse does, and therefore he was able to use his muscles.

Future Possibilities of AI in Neurology/Neurosurgery

AI, as mentioned above, has proven itself to be an important part of modern medicine in neurology and neurosurgery. Its uses in neurology and neurosurgery range from making an excellent diagnosis of a stroke before many neurons die to diagnosing and resecting a brain tumor that would otherwise kill the patient.

Many of the algorithms that can be used for neurological diseases and conditions not mentioned above are in their developmental stages.

With the possibility of AI-based technology to assist in these aspects of neuroscience, there are sure to be a range of benefits that come with it. The most important benefit of AI-based systems, among others in the case of neurology and neurosurgery, is advanced imaging technologies like CT scanning and MRI, which are very useful in making early diagnoses of stroke (hemorrhagic or ischemic), tumors, and other neurological diseases, with a higher percentage of precision as mentioned above.

Hence, by having different qualities like effectiveness, accuracy, and efficiency in all forms, AI in neurology and neurosurgery is sure to be highly beneficial and rewarding in the future.

References/Further Reading

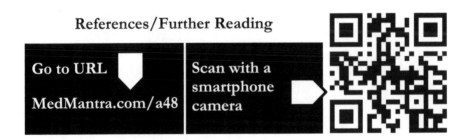

Go to URL
MedMantra.com/a48

Scan with a smartphone camera

CHAPTER FORTY-NINE
OBSTETRICS AND GYNECOLOGY

Reproductive medicine, much like other segments of the healthcare sector, is highly dependent on the clinicians' presence.[1] Most issues arise based on the variations found in the system that is run mainly using human efforts. AI can limit the number of problems and wrong treatments put forward in the system. There are other issues at hand that AI can help with as well.

There is an increased development and need for AI in the case of in vitro fertilization (IVF). With a success rate of 40%, the treatment gives hope to women seeking to get pregnant and start their families.[2]

To ensure the effectiveness of IVF, it is essential to ensure that the embryo is healthy and of high quality. However, there is a lack of methods showcasing successful embryo selection. With few to no details about the quality of embryos, sperm, and other reproductive factors used in the procedures, there is a major gap in the system. This gap can easily be filled with the implementation of AI-based mechanisms.

Because infertility is a major issue and people are always looking for ways to overcome it, AI has proven to be the ticket through which this issue can be managed more effectively. The main driver for this is the need to find solutions and prognoses for patients who suffer from infertility.

By making use of large and complex data sets available in the system, doctors can more easily perform their activities in the obstetrics/gynecology department than ever before. This can be done only by incorporating AI mechanisms and utilizing the massive data available at hand, and then making the right use of it.

The Current State of AI in Obstetrics/Gynecology

AI is essential to a series of departments in the healthcare sector, and reproductive medicine is no stranger to this. Current AI practices keep developing to ensure that the most effective and efficient version is made use of for the department.

Currently, a mix of three practices is heavily used in reproductive medicine. These include machine learning (ML), natural language processing (NLP), and robotic surgery. ML is essentially making use of all the data (imaging and other clinical data) about the patient to provide useful insights into his/her health.

NLP is much more detailed, as it makes use of unstructured data and converts it to structured data. This data will eventually be used by ML techniques to figure out health issues. Lastly, robotic surgery is the use of technological advancements such as remotely operated cameras and surgical instruments to perform surgery in patients.

Uses of AI in Obstetrics/Gynecology

There are different ways in which these AI-based mechanisms are used and implemented in real life. There are three common ways that AI is used in obstetrics/gynecology. These are Pap smears, ultrasounds, and electronic medical records (EMR).

Through the application of AI to these aspects of the department, it has become easier to understand whether or not something is wrong with the patient. AI offers pattern recognition. Through this, making a diagnosis and treating the patient becomes easier.

Pap smear

Pap smear (scraping from cervical mucosa) tests are widely conducted to screen women for cervical cancer. AI can automate the analysis of Pap smears and quickly produce more accurate results as compared to human technologists.[3] The use of microscopes, image processors, and data collection allows for a smooth process, avoiding human errors.

Ultrasound

Another major focus of AI in obstetrics/gynecology is ultrasound examinations. Ultrasound is the most commonly used screening imaging technique to detect pathologies associated with female pelvic organs. Also, ultrasound examinations are routinely performed on pregnant women to check the growth of their babies.

The incorporation of AI into this field will make life easier for radiologists and sonographers. There are certain things, such as measuring a fetus's head or femur length, that a doctor/sonographer must do on their own. However, with the implementation of AI-based mechanisms, it will be possible to completely/partially automate the task of taking and analyzing various fetal measurements.[4]

Also, with the advent of AI, doctors can more easily arrive at conclusions. Without AI, the sole responsibility for diagnosis and decision-making lies in the doctor's hands. AI-based mechanisms make it easier to reach conclusions, as doctors get help from the AI-based clinical decision support system.

Electronic medical records (EMR)

When AI is incorporated into EMR systems and used for all data needs, it becomes easier to assess which patient might be high-risk and which could go through normal birth. This happens automatically when clinicians input the relevant data into the EMR.

Once the relevant data is added to the EMR, the AI-integrated mechanism analyzes the data and automatically suggests what the issue at hand might be.[5] For instance, it can help indicate whether or not a mother might have to go through pre-term delivery. Through the wide collection of data within the records, it becomes easier for the algorithm to pick out details and present solutions that would help the doctor understand the best course of action.

Moreover, with the implementation of AI, clinicians can improve their effectiveness. Through AI algorithms, the system can monitor the risk factors that it picked up from earlier cases.

Future of AI in Obstetrics/Gynecology

In the future, there is a possibility of using an AI-enabled fetal monitoring system. This will take care of subjective variation in different clinicians, as a much more standardized and effective measure will be put in place. However, this doesn't mean that the role of clinicians will end. Instead, there will be more accurate and faster diagnosis and treatment when both AI and clinicians work together.

AI-based systems in place will remove the burden on the human workforce, thereby allowing for a much more proactive interaction between doctors and patients.[6] More than that, there is a great possibility that advanced monitoring will be much more effective, as it will ripple down to at-home monitoring as well. With such quality monitoring in place, there is a better possibility of accurate decision-making.

AI tools will allow clinicians to practice much more efficiently and precisely when it comes to the management of obstetrics/gynecology patients. AI tools will further ensure that monitoring is effective and non-invasive, along with ensuring that any obstetric/gynecological pathologies are dealt with efficiently.

References/Further Reading

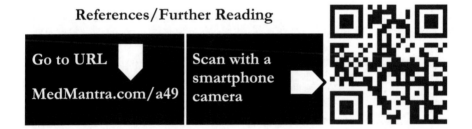

Go to URL

MedMantra.com/a49

Scan with a smartphone camera

CHAPTER FIFTY

ONCOLOGY

Introduction

The use of artificial intelligence in oncology has brought about many changes in the way cancer patients are treated.

Oncology is one of the major fields in which AI is expected to make significant changes. Finding the most suitable treatment for an individual cancer patient is a time-consuming job for an oncologist. However, ever since the introduction of AI in the field of oncology, doctors have received great help in quickly understanding and knowing which treatment method to prescribe for a particular cancer patient.[1]

AI is used in various stages of cancer treatment. It can help both the patients and the doctors in many ways. Some of the uses of AI in the field of oncology are mentioned below.

AI is used as a diagnostic tool

One of the major benefits of using AI in the field of oncology is that it can be used as a diagnostic tool, from the early-stage diagnosis to the prognosis of cancer. A major example of it can be seen in the context of breast cancer. The use of AI in mammographic breast screening has significantly reduced the false positive and false negative diagnosis, thereby avoiding further unnecessary tests and reducing overall program costs.[2]

AI reduces the rate of misdiagnosis

Much research has concluded that the use of AI in the field of oncology has drastically reduced the rate of misdiagnosis. AI helps in diagnosing the disease at an early stage, and treatment is started as soon as possible.[3] For this reason, Google has developed an augmented reality microscope. It uses software based on artificial intelligence to help doctors detect cancer. This can also help in reducing time-consuming activities such as the manual counting of cells.

AI is used in clinical decision support tools

With the development of technologies, numerous therapies are introduced to cure cancer. This is the reason why the complexity of cancer management has increased significantly. AI helps clinicians determine the optimum treatment strategy and the steps to be followed with the main goal of improving the quality of care.[4]

AI helps in the genomic characterization of tumors

Apart from its use in the diagnosis of cancer, artificial intelligence is also used in identifying specific gene mutations. This identification is carried out using pathology images instead of genomic sequencing. There are many examples of this in the field of oncology. The most common one is the research that was carried out by NCI-funded researchers from New York University. These researchers used deep learning to observe the pathology images of different lung tumors. The images were obtained from the Cancer Genome Atlas. According to the findings of the research, this method is able to differentiate between the most common subtypes of lung cancer simply by looking at the pathology images.[5]

AI is used for precision medicine

Artificial intelligence has huge potential for precision medicine in the field of oncology. Although it offers great advantages for both patients and doctors, the AI system has some shortcomings. We are still short of the range of drugs that can effectively treat all the patients suffering from various cancers. For this reason, many AI developers are trying to expedite drug development using AI applications. It is a huge opportunity that has attracted a large number of AI developers and pharmaceutical companies.[6] According to an estimate, an approximate number of a hundred start-ups are using artificial intelligence for drug discovery.

AI helps in reducing trial costs

With the use of artificial intelligence in oncology, researchers can now obtain insights from real-world data and apply this data to the designing of clinical trials. As a result, it can help in reducing the cost to a large extent.[7]

This is extremely important because the recruitment of patients alone can represent 30% of the total clinical trial cost.

Challenges Faced in Using Artificial Intelligence in the Field of Oncology

Though there are many benefits of using artificial intelligence in the field of oncology, some challenges and limitations are present as well. The oncologists and patients must keep in mind the limitations and challenges present in using artificial intelligence to cure cancer. If the oncologists and patients keep these limitations in mind, they will be able to get a better outcome.

Data scientists face a major challenge while using AI in oncology. They must deal with electronic medical records containing unstructured data from multiple sources. This data requires a lot of costly processing before it becomes suitable for use by AI algorithms.

The Future of Artificial Intelligence in Oncology

The future of artificial intelligence in oncology looks quite bright and promising. There is great potential in artificial intelligence in improving the quality of care of oncology patients, patient outcomes, and also the operational efficiencies of oncology practices. This will eventually lower the cost of cancer treatment as well.[8]

Conclusion

Artificial intelligence has many potential applications in the field of oncology. All these applications are being developed to support oncologists for the screening, diagnosis, and management of cancer. AI helps oncologists process and analyze big data and also helps them make clinical decisions. Although AI in the field of oncology is still improving, many platforms are already in use in some areas of oncology, such as the screening and diagnosis of cancer, setting trends for treatment, and evaluating large databases. So, it would not be wrong to say that the future of oncology with AI seems promising.

References/Further Reading

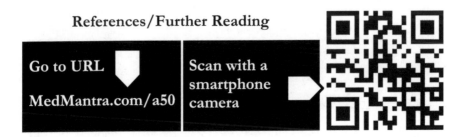

Go to URL
MedMantra.com/a50

Scan with a smartphone camera

CHAPTER FIFTY-ONE
PEDIATRICS

The use of artificial intelligence in pediatrics has an expansive history dating back to 1984.

1984 - 2008

The first-ever paper about artificial intelligence in pediatrics was published in 1984. The paper introduced a decision-making system known as SHELP in the field of pediatrics. This computer-assisted program helped to diagnose inborn errors. SHELP helped to diagnose metabolism-related inborn errors as well. Thus, it would not be wrong to say that the software played an important role in diagnosing and treating pediatric diseases.[1]

Up until 2008, the major research work that was done on artificial intelligence in the field of pediatrics included the use of applications that were controlled by knowledge-based systems, genetic algorithms, artificial neural networks, and, in some cases, decision trees.[1] These AI applications were useful for the extraction of information, decision-making, premature birth, cancer, neuroblastoma, and lesion treatment.

2009 - 2012

From 2009 to 2012, the implementation of artificial intelligence in the field of pediatrics became more advanced than ever. This also meant that things became more complex than ever. AI was used for logistic representation models, diagnosis of diseases, support vector machines for prediction, and discrimination and analysis. Additionally, AI helped in processing pediatric images and speech.[1] Some common pediatric diseases that were treated with the use of AI included infections, seizures, and prematurity.

2013 to onwards

Next came the period that started in 2013 and is prevailing today. During this time period, some incredible developments have been made using artificial intelligence in the field of pediatrics.[1] The most famous of these developments include the use of AI for diagnosing and treating asthma, pneumonia, epilepsy, and neurological conditions like autism.

The Uses of Artificial Intelligence in Pediatrics

The primary focus of implementing AI in pediatrics includes developmental disorders, oncology, brain mapping, gene profiling, and much more.[2]

Let's take a look at some of the AI applications in pediatrics.

Reduces the risk of false alarms

Did you know that about 75% of clinical alarms are false? As a result, the patients who are in dire need of care and attention suffer. False alarms are one of the major problems in hospitals. They lead to many problems such as alarm fatigue, a condition in which the alarm signals increase at a disturbingly fast rate. As a result, caretakers get exhausted and overwhelmed. This can lead to a delay in responses as well. As a result, the efficiency of caretakers declines. They may sometimes completely miss the alarm. This is where artificial intelligence helps pediatrics.

Before the implementation of AI techniques, the doctors completely depended upon other methods to reduce the risk of false alarms. It was not helping them much. As a result, their efficiency decreased as well. However, ever since AI was used, it has completely revolutionized the use of alarms. Machine-based algorithms were used and played an important role in classifying signals as genuine or fake. As a result, the efficiency increased as well.

Helps in clinical diagnosis

With the help of AI-based processes such as vector machines and neural networks, accurately diagnosing various pediatric conditions has become easier than ever. Researchers have also introduced machine-learning algorithms. These algorithms are used in the prediction of leukomalacia after cardiac surgery.[3] Apart from this, artificial intelligence has played an extremely important role in pediatric radiology. This includes the automated detection of diseases. AI algorithms can even identify abnormalities in images that a human eye cannot detect. This is why it would not be wrong to say that AI has revolutionized how diseases are diagnosed in the field of pediatrics.[3]

Helps in wearable technology

Wearable technologies are getting popular these days. Smartwatches equipped with various sensors collect useful health and medical data in real time. Apart from this, the technology is used to record a patient's visit to the physician and check the patient's heart rate, heart rhythm, respiration, etc.[4]

Additionally, wearable technologies help in many other ways, such as in sleep studies, controlling obesity, and helping children who have movement disorders.

Thus, the use of artificial intelligence in pediatrics through wearable technology has helped both the patients and the doctors.

Helps in robotic technology

The use of robotic technology can help children with autism learn several new things.[5] According to a survey, children enjoy completing tasks more with a robot than they do with an adult. The robots can help them learn different things in a fun-filled environment.

Apart from this, robotic technology can significantly help physicians. Physicians can use a robot-assisted arm to improve the muscular activities in a patient. These activities are important in cases in which the patient has suffered from a stroke.

The Future of Artificial Intelligence in Pediatrics

Much ongoing research is related to artificial intelligence in the field of pediatrics. Much more will come in the future, which will revolutionize the way things are done and improve patient care.[1] Although the implementation process may take years, it will certainly revolutionize the field of pediatrics and optimize the treatment of patients.

Conclusion

The use of artificial intelligence in the field of pediatrics has not only revolutionized treatment methods but also improved one's whole lifestyle as well. With the introduction of algorithm-based processes, every aspect of healthcare has improved. Apart from improving patients' lives, these methods are less prone to errors. This is why the use of AI is increasing rapidly and is sure to take over old methods.

References/Further Reading

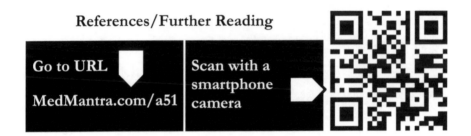

Go to URL

MedMantra.com/a51

Scan with a smartphone camera

CHAPTER FIFTY-TWO

PULMONOLOGY

Researchers have proved that a deep learning algorithm that was used in an AI-based system succeeded in classifying fibrotic lung disease, picking up malignant lung nodules, diagnosing chronic obstructive pulmonary disease (COPD) in smokers, and predicting acute respiratory disease events and mortality.[1]

Also, AI is utilized for MRI and CT scans of the chest and bronchoscopy that have been proved to diagnose lung diseases like cancer at an early stage. For example, in the screening for lung cancer, AI models showed the ability to identify pulmonary nodules.[2] They were also able to distinguish between malignant and benign nodules.

According to a 2018 review published in Nature Reviews Cancer, studies of NSCLC (non-small cell lung cancer) used radiomics to make predictions about distant metastasis in lung adenocarcinoma and tumor histological subtypes. It also predicted somatic mutations, disease recurrence, and gene-expression profiles.[3]

Chest radiographs (X-rays) constitute almost 26% of all diagnostic imaging studies.[4] In 2018, researchers developed and tested a DL-based algorithm to classify the results of chest radiographs. The data was acquired from different patients with pulmonary diseases such as pneumonia, active tuberculosis, pneumothorax, and malignant pulmonary neoplasms. In the last few years, many researchers and start-up companies from various parts of the globe have developed and tested different AI algorithms to classify images from studies like chest radiographs and chest CT scans.[4]

These are the uses of AI in pulmonology at present. The focus is on imaging right now, but there is potential for significant growth in other areas. However, a plethora of potential use cases can be implemented, and more AI models based on ML and DL can be developed to improve this area of healthcare. Let us explore the future potential of this.

Future Role of AI in Pulmonology

Here are the many ways in which AI can help in the field of pulmonology in the future.

Improved detection of lung cancer

Lung cancer is a common and highly fatal disorder for which people seek treatment in pulmonology. AI can enhance patients' and doctors' experiences, as it can carry out qualitative interpretation of lung cancer imaging.

The imaging by specialists can include extrapolation of tumor genotype, volumetric delineation of tumors, and prediction of clinical outcome, and the analysis of the impact of the disease and treatment plan on different organs inside the body near the lungs.[5]

All of this can be based on the DL model, as it offers the possibility of eliminating nodule segmentation. That will happen as whole-body imaging data will be developed and worked on so that all organs can be examined and analyzed.

Early diagnosis of respiratory diseases

Different fields of healthcare may use AI algorithms to achieve early diagnosis of different diseases. In the field of pulmonology, an earlier diagnosis of respiratory illnesses may be achieved through this technology.

Currently, a few technologies are in place that allow for self-monitoring of COPD through devices that one can utilize at home. These devices are also remotely accessed by clinicians so that they can interpret the data.[1]

Such technology can be taken further in the future, and newer imaging techniques can help pulmonologists with the data required to use these AI systems. Visual images are just as crucial as other data in making predictions and creating insights.

Interpretation of pulmonary function tests

Pulmonary function tests are not easy to conduct, as they gather a lot of information that pulmonologists need to interpret. Interpreting such information takes time, and often more tests must be undertaken before doctors can reach a proper diagnosis.

AI has a much superior performance compared to that of human beings in this field, so it can provide robust and fast analysis of these tests.[6] It can be used by specialists to improve their practice and as a decision support tool.

Two hospitals in Belgium are already using AI software that improves these tests' interpretation and helps with diagnosis. The technology allows them to diagnose early, fast, and with high accuracy.

However, remember that AI cannot completely replace pulmonologists. That is because doctors can see a broader perspective provided by the clinical data other than the pulmonary function tests. Therefore, AI can be more of a support tool rather than a tool that the doctors depend on entirely.

Challenges of Using AI in Pulmonology

The most challenging aspect of this AI software is the transferability of the models. This means that the algorithm may perform excellently in one hospital but not in another. To overcome this challenge, specialists will have to include a heterogeneous and representative set of images while these algorithms are being developed and trained by data scientists.

Another challenge is the complexity of lung and chest diseases in which the imaging patterns overlap, as many diseases have the same imaging pattern. So, it can be challenging to determine what condition an individual is going through.

Thus, in the future, pulmonology will not rely solely on AI systems.

Conclusion

Limited research studies are being done in the area of pulmonology. However, as ML and DL models are being utilized more, this field will also show excellent progress in the use of AI. Researchers are working on new technologies and trying them in hospitals to test their effectiveness. Thus, we can hope to see AI support technologies in this specialty soon.

References/Further Reading

Go to URL

MedMantra.com/a52

Scan with a smartphone camera

CHAPTER FIFTY-THREE

RHEUMATOLOGY

Rheumatology deals with long-standing illnesses and their complications, leading to variations in disease progression and treatment. The discovery of phenotypic factors that may affect the incidence of diseases like osteoarthritis, lupus, or Sjogren's syndrome is also accompanied by fluctuating and inconsistent results resulting from traditional medications. This has made the application of precision-based treatments and AI-backed personalized medicine more appealing to rheumatologists.[1]

Machine learning algorithms can collate data from laboratory investigations, patient case studies, research and trial results, and medical and radiological scan images, as well as genetic data to arrive at predictive conclusions that can guide clinicians toward optimal treatment strategies targeted at individual patients. The applications of artificial intelligence principles in rheumatology are comprehensive in scope, ranging from diagnosis to management.

1. Electronic diagnosis:

The use of chatbots has grown tremendously with websites or health applications that interact with patients and respond to the questions or imported data interactively. These de facto symptom checkers have evolved from simple systems to deep learning systems that depend on patient experience to collate and exploit data. The Symptomate Chatbot is one such application.[2]

2. Disease identification and staging:

Machine learning has been applied to electronic medical records, with medical coding and billing data, to successfully detect patients with rheumatoid arthritis with an AUC (area under the curve) score of 0.97, thereby showing its potential in many research activities that require expansive sample sizes, to evaluate symptoms and disease progression.[3] A large-scale study in the United Kingdom by Zhou and colleagues used random forest methods to mine data from primary electronic health records, keeping track of diagnostic codes used for RA or medication codes used in the prescription of DMARD (disease-modifying anti-rheumatic drugs). This data-driven exercise achieved an accuracy of 92% while identifying patients with RA in the testing set of more than 5,000 patients.[4]

3. Imaging modalities:

The interpretation of diagnostic imaging from simple X-rays to sonographies and MRI scans has used AI methods like segmentation and the extraction of specific diagnostic and prognostic features to classify diseases and stages. These take into consideration findings like bone erosions, cartilage loss, tenosynovitis, bone marrow edema, and vasculopathy obtained through various imaging modalities, comparing and collating data to produce a predictive and actionable report in rheumatoid diseases.[5]

A recent study by Anderson and colleagues evaluated the results obtained by applying convolutional neural networks (CNNs) to the scoring of arthritic features based on sonography images, with 86.4% to 86.9% accuracy. Similarly, Rohrbach and colleagues conducted bone erosion studies in RA patients using CNNs with X-ray images and found no significant differences between the conclusions derived from the AI system and human experts.[6]

4. Treatment pathways:

Large multi-centers have funded studies that investigated the applications of artificial intelligence in specific pathogenicity faced in primary Sjogren's syndrome as well as large cohorts of patients suffering from similar systemic autoimmune diseases (SADs).[7] Machine learning methods have been efficient in using patient data sets to understand the disease course, thereby allowing clinicians to draft treatment pathways to bring about remission while also knowing when to de-escalate medications or interventions.[8]

5. Genetic profiling:

In rheumatology, the genetic predisposition for inflammatory diseases is significant and is seen in the increased incidence of chronic inflammation. Efforts have been made to trace these expression patterns with the help of cytokine signatures like IFN (interferons) and other biomarkers. In 2019, a machine learning algorithm was applied to the genetic profiles of psoriasis patients, using 200 genetic markers. The AI software revealed new gene loci for the incidence of psoriasis, as well as predictive analysis for the incidence of cutaneous psoriasis with 90% precision and 100% specificity.[9]

Conclusion

The future of AI in rheumatology seems bright, with the application of AI-based tools poised to increase the speed and accuracy of image-based diagnosis, as well as medical records-based data to determine the efficacy of treatment modalities, remission rates, and disease progression. The aim toward precision-based personalized medicine is achievable with robust efforts to collate data sets, followed by user validation, to ensure acceptance and widespread applications by both clinicians and patients.

References/Further Reading

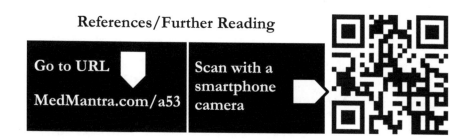

Go to URL

MedMantra.com/a53

Scan with a smartphone camera

CHAPTER FIFTY-FOUR

NURSING

The profession of nursing has started utilizing AI technology to generate a systematic clinical system comprising electronic medical records, integrated pieces of medical equipment, and a backing system.

Apart from collecting medical information, artificial intelligence is being used to interrogate the clinical data and answer the awaited questions. The technology is also capable of deducing the possible prognosis for patients' suffering based on the identification of specific trends in the patients' data. Nurses can elevate their working capacity by making use of AI, which enables them to rapidly process a significant amount of information and thereby make recommendations, prognosticate results, and help with decisions.

Comprehending a complex computer program can be a great struggle, especially when you are in the field of medicine. To make the process less intricate, nurses should keep one thing in mind: "Algorithms" are the core basis of AI. Algorithms are a set of well-constructed and chronological rules or commands that allow AI to self-learn. These algorithms, when used in a healthcare system, are referred to as "clinical intelligence." Clinical intelligence is the uniquely designed algorithms specific to diagnostic and treatment processes to deliver correct treatment to the correct person at the suitable recommended time interval.

Role of Artificial Intelligence in Nursing

Machine-driven cognitive skills benefit the critical thinking aptitudes of nurses in the following manner[1]:

Visual recognition

The visual recognition technology of AI evaluates images and videos for identification and diagnostic purposes. With the aid of this technology, nurses can analyze and detect wounds, monitor breathing rates, and detect unidentifiable pain as well as anxiety and depression.

Speech assistance

The voice assistance skill of AI is responsible for projecting the voiced commands to identify the relevant data when required. This AI skill is used in nursing for many reasons, like setting timers and reminders for the nursing tasks, restoring patients' information, and answering their queries about their scheduled appointments or any other probe related to their disease.

Neural networks

The neural network, also known as machine learning, works in two ways. First, it scrutinizes the information and other data by making use of multifaceted algorithms, followed by robotically improving it based on learned experience. Through this technology, nurses can identify a patient's program or arrange follow-up appointments. Also, they can estimate the cost of supplies and facilities used for treating a particular patient.

The role of nurses in a healthcare system is known to be amongst the most significant of all, and along with the utilization of artificial technology, healthcare organizations have become more systematized.[2] Command centers have been built in hospitals, based entirely on artificial intelligence to provide hospital staff (doctors or nurses) with beneficial data that would enable them to regulate and put forward new policies so that they can augment their supplies and resources to even the patient flow.

The command center lays out the following data:

- It detects and provides information about the hampering of the scheduled surgeries or appointments.

- It provides notifications about the reasons for patients' troubling conditions.

- The command center helps the nurses by providing complete details regarding the number of patients and in which units they have been called in sick.

What More Does Artificial Intelligence Have to Offer in the Future Regarding the Profession of Nursing?

The line of nursing will be impacted because efficient artificial intelligence technologies will analyze and interpret the tasks that nurses perform. These technologies will greatly influence the way nurses work by scheduling and monitoring most of their tasks. One may assume that due to highly proficient cognitive and programming skills, the role of nurses may slowly and gradually diminish. However, they are not eliminated in either way, as they will learn to integrate artificial intelligence into their practice of providing care and supervising patients; hence, the human factor is not reduced.[3]

Through a highly technologically driven system, nurses will increase their knowledge and capability only by learning new and productive methods of thinking and processing. These creative skills will ramp up the proficiency level of nurses, as they can operate as health coaches, information experts, and so on, as AI would save their time by managing many of their time-consuming tasks—for instance, bladder scanning or vein detection.[4]

The future of nursing in line with artificial intelligence is optimistic and promising. Artificial intelligence (AI) has greatly influenced healthcare systems by making them more structured and systematic and has helped clinicians and nurses make prompt decisions for patients. Hence, in this field, it will be a combined effort of machines and humans. Lastly, the clinician will always have the final say.

References/Further Reading

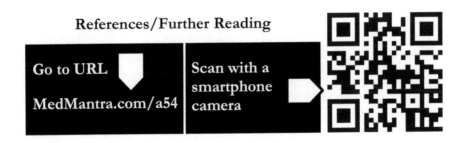

Go to URL

MedMantra.com/a54

Scan with a smartphone camera

CHAPTER FIFTY-FIVE

PHYSICAL THERAPY

Artificial Intelligence with Motion Sensors in Physical Therapy

Artificial intelligence is not all about smart robots like in the movies. It is about computer programs that can integrate with physical sensors to improve our lives. With modern-day technologies, physical workouts have improved, and people are noticing huge changes in the results. This is mainly because artificial intelligence offers the perfect solutions to healthcare and fitness problems by making us do the things that are best suited to us. This innovative method of engaging in physical exercise and staying fit has caught the attention of millions of people. It is better, safer, and more efficient than the traditional ways. The user will still need to complete the actual exercises, but this time they will be monitored by the ultimate professional with all the knowledge. AI used in physical therapy is often accompanied by motion sensors that help the program with decision-making.

How It Works

When it comes to physical therapy, artificial intelligence uses motion sensors and the data it receives through an innovative program that monitors sessions.[1] These motion sensors detect movements in muscles and can let us know if anything needs to change. In detecting the strain on muscles, they can image the position of the user to check if things are done in the right manner. Integrated software can collect the data received from the motion sensors and process it for the user to see. It will also tell the user about areas that require more work and how to go through with it. Having access to such technology, people around the world have started to adopt and include these intelligent setups as a part of their physical therapy. Modern-day programs can also communicate with the user during a physical training session. Through voice notes, the digital therapist can let the user know how to work out properly.

Benefits of AI in Physical Therapy

Here are some of the ways AI has changed the world of physical therapy.

Data collection

Most AI programs have enabled data collection that can allow the program to save relevant data regarding the physical therapy sessions. This data gives the software enough information about the user to make recommendations for improvement. The data that the program collects can also be seen by the user, which is a great way to keep track of the physical therapy sessions. Collected data can also help the AI to plan out sessions for the future and let users know what is best for them.[2] This helps in long-term improvements for the users.

Best results

It is well known that AI's smartness is beyond our imagination. Within seconds, AI programs can make decisions that are best suited for an individual. Physical therapy programs with AI have been proven to create the best results for millions of people. This is because AI can simulate all the workout scenarios and select the best plans for each user.[3] It also helps the user work on their mistakes and thereby improve their training regimen. For this reason, AI in physical therapy can offer the best results to users.

Constant monitoring

Another great thing about AI is that it can provide constant monitoring for users. This means that users will no longer need to get appointments or complete workout sessions on their own. With a digital trainer constantly watching their every move, users can achieve the perfect fitness level. Motion sensors that allow the AI to monitor physical therapy sessions work at all times, and users can get feedback after every set of exercises.[4] This enhances the results for users and keeps them fit and healthy.

Helps doctors and physical therapists

AI integrated physical therapy is not only beneficial for users but also provides insight for doctors and physical therapists. The intelligent programs can help the professional keep track of a patient's fitness level. It can also assist them in determining the best possible workout routines for their patients, ultimately improving the healthcare provided. Furthermore, physical therapists can monitor the patients remotely and make decisions with the data that AI has provided to them.[5]

Implications for the Future

Artificial intelligence has made its mark in the health and fitness fields and will continue to enhance physical therapy. The prospects of intelligent programs are bright, and we can expect more innovations as the years go by. With all the information AI can process in seconds, it is imagined that healthcare will only get better. As time passes, modern-day technologies like artificial intelligence will see their roles in physical therapy increase. This will ultimately improve the way of life for everyone. People who utilize AI's benefits to stay healthy and fit through physical training will continue to make it a part of their lives.

References/Further Reading

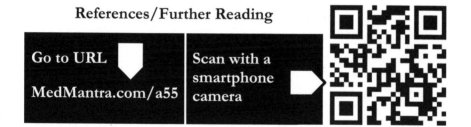

Go to URL

MedMantra.com/a55

Scan with a smartphone camera

CHAPTER FIFTY-SIX
VETERINARY MEDICINE

Veterinary medicine has always been a subbranch of medicine that does not receive as much attention as it needs. Artificial intelligence can change this and pave the way to an improved healthcare system for animals.[1]

Training and practice programs

First, artificial intelligence has impacted the training regimes of many professions. Simulations and augmented reality can help many veterinary doctors with training and practice. An improved training system for vets will result in a better healthcare system for animals. Even experts and already-trained medical personnel can benefit from simulations and practice in augmented reality before the real procedure. This can be done as all-out training before practicing medicine or simulations based on every complicated case a vet may encounter. In either case, artificial intelligence has brushed up the training programs and recruitment for vets.[1] We can expect this to continue, as it will result in more experienced and qualified individuals in the field.

Data collection and analysis

Data collection and analysis are crucial in the medical profession. They help professionals study various scenarios and come up with effective solutions. This is a common practice for doctors who work with human patients. However, veterinary doctors and surgeons are unable to take advantage of this technique, as not enough data is collected and analyzed. This prevents the vets from accessing or keeping a record of notes from their previous sessions. Most of the time, the little data collected manually is lost at some point. With the help of artificial intelligence, this can change, and animal doctors and surgeons can benefit from it.[2] Artificial intelligence can help with tracking the data and collecting it as well as saving all the notes. This can result in an improved standard of animal care and more knowledgeable healthcare systems.

- ### *Assist in diagnosis*

  Artificial intelligence paired with modern-day equipment and computers can help veterinary doctors with diagnostics as well. One of the most difficult things about being an animal doctor or surgeon is that the animal can't communicate to discuss symptoms, causes, and problems. This increases the dependency on the outer condition and medical scans. Artificial intelligence can assist the vets in determining the condition of an animal as well as the diagnosis of disease.[3] It can tell the vets about areas they need to work on as well as the root cause of the problem. Vets can make a better decision with this information, ultimately enhancing the medical help provided.

- ### *Suitable procedures and decision support*

  On top of diagnosis, artificial intelligence can help the vets through other parts of treatment, such as surgery procedures and decision-making. The ultimate decision will still be with the professional doctor, but AI can help with suggestions. This can be extremely beneficial for the animals, as artificial intelligence will go through all the resources such as data and notes before making a decision backed by data and statistics. This will not only help animal doctors come up with effective solutions but also provide them with relevant information that led to the suggested decision.

- ### *Reduces workload for professionals*

  The primary aim behind artificial intelligence is to assist humans in a better way than traditional methods. Most of the time, extensive work and lack of time to rest can result in stress and reduced productivity. To reduce the burden on healthcare workers, AI can be used to effectively assist them and reduce the workload. Bringing artificial intelligence to the field of animal medicine can allow doctors and healthcare workers to relax.[4] It will reduce the workload on professional vets by assisting them in various parts of the treatment, such as diagnosis and decision support. Artificial intelligence can work as an assistant for vets and take some of the burdens off them. This can improve the healthcare services that vets provide to animals.

Reviews Published on AI in Veterinary Medicine

Not many reviews have been published on artificial intelligence in veterinary medicine. This makes it difficult to understand the impact AI can have in this field. However, the few reviews that have been published convey the same message. They stress the importance of AI for animal healthcare systems and how it can be beneficial. Analysis of data collection and decision support can also be seen in these reviews. This provides a comprehensive idea of the significance of artificial intelligence in veterinary medicine and how it can improve in the years to come.

Future Prospects for AI in Veterinary Medicine

It is safe to say that the future of artificial intelligence in veterinary medicine is promising. The use of AI is on the rise and is improving many areas of the medical field. Many methods and uses of artificial intelligence in human medicine can be expected in animal healthcare as well. Improvement in diagnostics and data analysis, as well as artificial intelligence, can help vets with decision-making. The future also promises improved programs and software that will allow veterinary workers to enhance their treatments and offer better service to animals.

Artificial intelligence and the benefits it offers to veterinary medicine should not be overlooked. By assisting vets with data and diagnostics, artificial intelligence can save the lives of many animals. It can also help professionals with surgeries, increasing the success rates of animal operations. By reducing the burden on healthcare workers, artificial intelligence can also provide effective support for decision-making. All things considered, the positive reviews published on the impact of AI in veterinary medicine show us that it can pave the way for a brighter future.

Conclusion

Some diseases, like chronic kidney disease (CKD) in cats, are quite difficult to diagnose and are diagnosed only when the disease is at an advanced stage. AI, however, makes use of biomarkers of renal function, like symmetric dimethylarginine (SDMA), to find the disease earlier.

Also, AI is used to collect and analyze a huge array of data and obtain meaningful results in less time. Like human health, AI is crucial in animal health as well, as it makes use of advanced diagnostic and treatment techniques that are far more promising than traditional ones. The advancements made in this field might cover more diseases in the days to come.

References/Further Reading

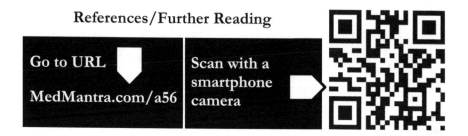

CHAPTER FIFTY-SEVEN
HEALTHCARE ADMINISTRATION

The role of artificial intelligence in healthcare administration has moved from luxury to a necessity. Many healthcare organizations have started using artificial intelligence for their administrative departments. From using AI to improve operational efficiencies to extracting important data from old files, AI helps a healthcare administrator with virtually everything.

Artificial Intelligence in Healthcare Administration

The use of artificial intelligence in healthcare refers to the use of algorithms to perform specific tasks. The tasks performed using the algorithm are carried out in an automated fashion. When the data is fed to the computers, the AI algorithm reviews the data, helps the admin staff interpret the data, and suggests solutions to certain administrative problems as well. This is why AI has endless applications in healthcare administration.

Research done by HIMSS (Healthcare Information and Management Systems Society) Media concluded that while 59% of hospitals utilize AI to overcome operational inefficiencies, 48% of them are using it to maximize administrative operations in the healthcare industry.[1] Other research shows that the use of AI in administrative tasks can result in $18 billion savings in the healthcare industry.[2] According to the American Hospital Association, the use of AI will completely change the way things are done at hospitals within the next five years.

The Importance of Artificial Intelligence in Healthcare Administration

The revenue margins for hospitals are expected to tighten more than ever in the future. For this reason, the use of AI in healthcare administration has become more important than before. The use of AI-enhanced robotics and AI-powered tools will make it easier for hospitals to reduce errors, improve efficiency, increase productivity, and reduce costs in healthcare practices.

Let us take a look at some of the ways AI has changed how things are run at a hospital.

Helps in prior authorization

During a survey, 85% of doctors reported that the administrative burden in the hospital had increased a lot during the last five years. It has become impossible to manage this administrative burden alone. This is how AI has helped them overcome this problem. As most of the admin staff in hospitals deal with hundreds of authorizations each day, AI helps the healthcare executives with the automation of the prior authorization.[2] As a result, it saves them a lot of time and personnel cost as well.

Helps in information management

The use of AI in healthcare is a great tool for managing information for both doctors and patients. Patients can get to the doctors faster when the information is managed using AI.[3] As a result, valuable time and money will be saved, and the strain on both the patient and the doctor will reduce as well.

Helps in claims and billing processing

It is very tiresome for the admin staff of a busy hospital to handle the claims processing themselves. Not only is it time-consuming, but it can also get expensive. According to an estimate, the billing and processing cost alone can make up 13% of a physician's earning, whereas it can consume 85% of a hospital's earnings, which is a huge amount. This is where AI can help the hospitals and admin staff.[4] It saves on a lot of costs and eases the duties of the admin staff as well.

Helps in clinical decision support

The use of artificial intelligence in healthcare administration can be extremely useful for both doctors and patients. The doctors can leverage the easy availability of patient data and AI-based clinical decision support systems to make better (more accurate and precise) decisions.[5] This saves a lot of time while arriving at the diagnosis, in turn giving patients a chance to recover quickly.

Increases productivity

The back office is not the only place in the hospital where administrative tasks take place. Administrative tasks include a lot of other tasks such as recording patient summaries, documenting chart notes, and writing prescriptions and test orders. All of these tasks can be managed by AI at present. In this way, it increases the productivity of the providers by eliminating most or all of the manual and repetitive tasks. The use of AI is estimated to save almost 5% of the time for nurses and almost 17% of the time for physicians.[6] They can use this saved time to do other productive tasks.

The Future Possibilities of AI in Healthcare Administration

Though AI offers a lot of benefits to offer healthcare administration, whether, in a hospital or a clinic, some administrations are still reluctant to use it because of the initial setup cost. Apart from this, they are concerned about privacy, data integrity, and the presence of many organizational silos. What they do not realize is that the use of AI can completely change the way things are done presently[7], leading to significant cost savings in the long run.

It is said that the future of artificial intelligence and the future of healthcare administration are deeply connected. The rise in the popularity of artificial intelligence will change the whole outlook of the healthcare industry. Up until now, we have only scratched the surface of what artificial intelligence can do for healthcare administration. When we explore it deeply, we will get to know how much the healthcare industry can save by implementing the system in their administration.

Conclusion

Overall, AI is all set to have a huge impact on healthcare administration in the next five years. All the staff and departments of the sector will be highly dependent on the use of artificial intelligence for the execution of their duties.

References/Further Reading

Go to URL	Scan with a
MedMantra.com/a57	smartphone camera

"If an AI possessed any one of these skills—social abilities, technological development, economic ability—at a superhuman level, it is quite likely that it would quickly come to dominate our world in one way or another. And as we've seen, if it ever developed these abilities to the human level, then it would likely soon develop them to a superhuman level. So, we can assume that if even one of these skills gets programmed into a computer, then our world will come to be dominated by AIs or AI-empowered humans."

- Stuart Armstrong

A REVIEW OF SOME ADVANCES IN TECHNOLOGY AND THE IMPLICATIONS FOR MEDICAL APPLICATIONS

CHAPTER FIFTY-EIGHT

A REVIEW OF SOME ADVANCES IN TECHNOLOGY AND THE IMPLICATIONS FOR MEDICAL APPLICATIONS

A. Introduction

Technology advances apace and seems to be accelerating. Hardly a day goes by without the publication of a notable paper announcing some important advance or new clue to our understanding of the natural world. Progress for progress' sake is fine, but the real benefits are reaped when these advances are applied to the real world.

This chapter looks at some recent developments in communications, computing, and AI, providing examples of their applications to medicine, whether in patient care, diagnostics, or research.

B. Telecommunications

5G Cellular Communications

A lot of nonsense is said about 5G networks. Even setting aside the ridiculous conspiracy theories, public (and, in some cases, expert) understanding of the benefits of 5G is not good. A lot of this can be blamed on the cellular operators not communicating their plans properly; however, the pundits must also take some share of the blame; essentially, they just make up stuff and set false expectations. Things that 5G will NOT do:

- Provide infinite data rates to all consumers all the time

- Replace all consumer broadband internet services (making fiber almost irrelevant)

- Have massively increased coverage compared to existing cellular services

- Be more reliable than existing cellular services

5G is an evolution of 4G. 4G brought true internet service speeds to the mobile device marketplace. 5G extends that. 5G provides three basic sets of services:

- **MBB (Massive Broadband)** – This is the higher data rates bit. Yes, 5G will provide individual users with potentially very high data rates, using spectrum more efficiently.

- **Differentiated Services** – The ability to support differentiated service types over the cellular network. Essentially, this means the cellular quality of service (QoS). Some traffic will take priority over other traffic on the network. Typically, these will be premium services.

- **eMTC (enhanced Machine Type Communication)** – A set of special protocols designed for Internet of Things (IoT) sensors. Typically, these will be lower speed, extended-range services.

Low Earth Orbit (LEO) Satellite Internet

SpaceX (Starlink), Amazon (Kuiper), and OneWeb are developing a constellation of LEO satellites to provide space-based internet.

SpaceX intends to provide satellite internet connectivity to underserved areas of the planet with very low latency and at speeds better than 4G. This technology will provide some of the advantages of the 5G network to improve medical and healthcare practice in previously underserved rural and remote areas where 5G is not feasible. It can also function as a backup internet connection.

It should be noted, however, that the first tranche of devices and terminals associated with these platforms is likely to be large and expensive (compared to traditional mobile handsets or routers).

Advances in communications systems promise to bring a great advantage to healthcare, such as remote monitoring of patients in real-time, decentralization of health services, provision of remote telemedicine services to remote locations or disaster/war zones, and effective implementation of medical robotics in our hospitals.

Tele-assisted surgical operations

Due to low latency networks and the provision of high-speed differentiated services, 5G technology allowed the first remote surgical operation in Spain to be successfully carried out at the Hospital Clínic de Barcelona.[1]

Robotic surgery

Beyond the necessary evolution in surgical robotics, to develop machinery that is increasingly effective and functional, it is necessary to have the support of telecommunications technologies that secure a stable connection to the internet, ensuring their functionality.

In this sense, 5G allows for a constant connection without interruptions, eliminating the risk that the robot could "disconnect" halfway during surgery. Robotic telesurgery has already been demonstrated.[2] For practical, scaled applications, the PRIMARY connectivity between surgeon and robot would likely be achieved by high-capacity fiber-optic networks with appropriate QoS; 5G would be a backup against fiber failure. This approach of backing up fixed networks with cellular is commonplace in enterprise networks.

Decentralization of medical care

High-speed optical and cellular networks, now driven faster by the COVID-19 pandemic, are delivering the rapid adoption of teleconsultation services. Although occasionally controversial, this is one of the regular uses of telemedicine today. By leveraging satellite broadband services, this approach to telemedicine can drive modern diagnosis and consultation in remote and previously inaccessible locations – or into disaster areas and war zones.

Additionally, specialized medical devices are being designed[3] to deliver both specialized care and online telemetry into these remote locations.

C. Centralization of medical data

Data storage and analysis are increasingly important for medical practice. Equally, medical records require both security and persistence in storage, best achieved in modern data centers. Medical records (in a formatted, normalized, and consistent form) also serve as a basis for, for example, certain artificial intelligence systems to make predictions about the development or evolution of a disease.

D. Virtual, Augmented, and Mixed Reality

This is a spectrum of experiences enabled by a set of similar technologies.

At one end of the spectrum, Virtual Reality (VR) environments present the user with a fully synthesized world and interactions. Augmented Reality

(AR), on the other hand, overlays the real world with virtual objects, labels, and textures. In the middle, we have mixed. In Mixed Reality (MR), the real and the virtual world are interconnected, allowing interaction with digital objects and preserving a sense of presence within the physical environment.

All of these have significant implications for both the practice and the teaching of medicine.

Whether in the discoveries, the improvement of medicines, or the evolution of learning techniques and the monitoring of patients with the prevention and treatment of diseases, the area has leveraged the benefits of AR/VR and MR.[4]

AR plays an important role in allowing doctors to seamlessly blend real-world sensory experience with digital data. Thus, they will no longer need to look away during treatment to obtain vital information, as the data will be superimposed on the patient, enabling anatomical structures to be identified and highlighted by AR in real-time, thereby assisting in diagnosis and procedures. The use of this technology in diagnostic, surgical, and treatment procedures can save lives.

Many medical students do not have a chance to participate in real operations and gain insight into a professional's line of work. However, with Virtual Reality, the trend is that this will change, as surgeries with a high level of detail can be transmitted globally.

Thus, future doctors would be able to observe all the details of the human body, the surgeon's actions, and, hundreds of kilometers away, learn how to perform surgery.

E. Artificial Intelligence

This is a huge field, one in which advances are being made all the time. Made more popular by the hype surrounding it, and with the development of cloud services enabling open-source communities to access huge computing resources at low cost, AI is positively sprinting forward. The demand for AI and data science graduates is outstripping supply – truly, this is a fertile field for invention, innovation, and development.

The definition of AI is a fuzzy one, as the field is so huge. At one level, AI has been defined as "Machines which have the ability to perform an, often narrowly defined task, which would normally require a human being." That narrowly defined comment is important – you are never going to hang out at the coffee machine with the AI that examines your smear tests. However, AI can be found that comes very close to besting a Turing test (though the same machine would not do well with smart tests).

Machines that statistically encode complex algorithms (such as chess-playing computers[5] and missile guidance systems) have been described as AI. However, most of the focus of AI research in the last few years has been on Machine Learning. That is the ability of machines to learn from data[6] and to make inferences about new data sets based on previous training on other data sets. Within this, again, there are sub-specialties, including Deep Learning and Reinforcement Machine Learning.

The development of AI/ML products is a deeply mathematical field, requiring a comprehensive understanding of advanced statistical analytical techniques. The number of tools for analyzing and visualizing data has exploded in the last few years, and practical applications are now entering the public domain with a performance that approaches if not exceeds, human capability.[7]

Artificial intelligence has already played an important role in diagnostic tests and diagnostic imaging, making the process faster and more accurate, as well as less invasive.

Cloud Artificial Intelligence

Artificial intelligence cloud computing is the amalgamation of AI and machine learning capabilities with cloud-based computing environments. The "pay-as-you-use" commercial model of cloud providers makes vast computing environments accessible to developers and end-users at low cost, thus lowering the barriers to innovation.

Digital helpers like Amazon Alexa, Siri, and Google Assistant join a seamless flow of cloud-based computing resources and AI technology to enable users to access a range of services by providing contextually-aware voice analysis services, e.g., to play a song instantly, make purchases, or adjust a smart thermostat.

Neural Networks and the Capsule Network

Neural Networks (NN) are among the foundational capabilities of AI/ML products. NN are software structures that replicate the operation of a biological neuron. Each neuron (software or fleshy) is conceptually simple – lots of input levels are consolidated (non-simplistically) to a single output value. These outputs are then connected to the inputs of other neurons. These large structures of neurons can be assembled into NN, which can then accomplish tasks (if appropriately trained).[8]

The Capsule Network, also known as CapsNet, is one of the innovative deep Neural Network designs that was suggested lately by Hinton et al. Hinton has been prolific in several fields, especially in natural language processing and image recognition.

CapsNet has not yet been added to studies related to drug discovery. In the first attempt, they used CapsNet to improve classification models of hERG (human Ether-a-go-go-Related Gene) blockers and non-blockers. Restricted Boltzmann machine-capsule network (RBM-CapsNet) and the Convolution-capsule network (Conv-CapsNet) are the dual capsule networks that were introduced. The convolution and restricted Boltzmann machine (RBM) were employed as characteristic extractors.

They are noticeable signs of progress in deep learning processes because a quick studying algorithm for deep confidence nets was introduced in 2006 by Hinton et al. They have widely been used in many fields, especially biometrics, speech recognition, machine translation, computer vision, audio identification, natural language dispensation, social network filtering, and other games in which they have produced a reasonable outcome that is, in a way, greater than human effort. Lately, deep learning was introduced into drug discovery, and it has shown its capability. Moreover, a few problems face the implementation of deep learning in drug research and discovery. An example is that deep learning requires a huge number of samples for its model training.

Improved Productivity

Artificial intelligence is used to streamline the workload and automate repetitive tasks within the IT infrastructure, which will effectively and efficiently increase productivity. This case study examines how AI has benefitted productivity in a radiology department.[9]

Harnessing Big Data

With artificial intelligence, deep learning algorithms digest vast amounts of data because the more the data they consume, the smarter they become at identifying patterns, automating complexity, and making predictions.

The use of artificial intelligence in the computing infrastructure means more processing power for Big Data analytics, which could streamline disease prediction and much more.[10]

Fuzzy Cognitive Maps

Fuzzy cognitive maps (FCM) are AI tools that represent knowledge graphically based on a causative perception of the state of a system. Unsurprisingly, FCM is a combination of Cognitive Mapping and Fuzzy Logic. Fuzzy Logic is a branch of mathematics that, instead of encoding data as 1 or 0, incorporates several states. There are obvious parallels between FCM and NN.[11]

A representative application of FCMs in medicine is MDSSs (medical decision-support systems) that help physicians to make a proper decision. This is very important. Through the merging of the properties of Neural Networks and Fuzzy Logic, FCMs are among the most efficient, recent, and powerful AI methods for illustrating complicated systems.

The foremost arrangement for every application in medicine can be presented by researching the attributes of FCMs' structures. To examine the ability of different FCM versions in organizing MDSSs, medical implementations are grouped into four main areas: prediction, decision-making, classification, and diagnoses. The differential diagnosis and difficulties affecting decision assistance that were addressed by fuzzy cognitive maps in recent years are now reviewed to bring in different types of FCMs and also determine their contribution so far.

As a result of the uniform requirements of fuzzy cognitive maps in combining human skill and knowledge and equally encountering computer-assisted methods, they are amongst the instruments for the design of MDSSs. Shortly, FCM within MDSS will have a vital purpose to play in medicine.

Generative Query Network

A generative query network (GCQ) can "imagine" hidden scenes with a new outlook and with remarkable accuracy. When the scene is depicted, and new views are formed, sharp images are taken without predetermining the laws of perspective, obstruction, or illumination. This is achieved by having two distinct networks: a representative network that makes observations and a generative network that turns observations into predictions.

GQN representation enables robust, and data-efficient reinforced learning. Combined with compact GQN representations, advanced, in-depth learning agents learn to perform tasks on data more efficiently than basic agents without a model.

The GQN representation can learn, enumerate, locate, and categorize unlabeled objects at the object level. Even if its representation can be very small, GQN's predictions for the query are very accurate and often indistinguishable from the truth. This means, for example, that the display network accurately discovers the correct configuration of the blocks that make up the following scenes.

A generative query network can represent, measure, and decrease uncertainties. It can explain the uncertainty inherent in its beliefs about the scene, even if its content is not fully visible, and it can combine several partial views of the scene into a coherent whole. It expresses its uncertainty through the variability of the model predictions, which gradually decreases as it progresses through the maze. This will facilitate Neural Network training and induce an impact on medical imaging.

The utility of GQN can best be explained by example, such as this paper[12] describing a GQN operation on medical imaging data.

Hypergraph Database

HyperGraphDB is an open-source, extensible, portable, distributed, embedded, and universal data storage mechanism. It is a graphical database created especially for projects in the fields of artificial intelligence and the semantic web.

HyperGraphDB is derived primarily from a carefully chosen name: a database for storing hypergraphs. Although part of the general graphical database family, HyperGraphDB cannot be easily classified as just another database because much of its design allows information to be managed in a layered structure with arbitrary complexity.

For example, an object-oriented and relational data management style can be imitated. As a graphical database, HyperGraphDB offers unlimited and much greater generality than any other graphical database we can find.

Bioinformatics projects[13] are a very complex category of software that not only benefits from data management such as HyperGraphDB but can also be seamlessly integrated into it. These projects often have to deal with very complex descriptive information based on structured taxonomies (or ontologies) and large experimental data sets. Furthermore, sophisticated algorithms work with experimental and ontological data to derive interaction networks at different levels of biological organization. HyperGraphDB is built to simplify these activities.

Low-Shot Learning

Machine learning has grown significantly in recent years. Factors contributing to the amazing growth include the increasing complexity of learning algorithms and models, the increasing computing power of machines, and the availability of Big Data. As its name suggests, low-shot learning relates to the practical method of providing ideal learning with a very small quantity of training data, as opposed to the usual practice of consuming a big amount of training data.

This technique is more commonly used in the field of image processing, in which the use of an object categorization model without multiple training patterns always leads to adequate results.

In certain cases, one-shot learning will be useful in biomedical systems, as regular convolutional Neural Networks (CNNs) are based on Big Data and labeled data sets, which may not be scalable for certain diseases.

Neuromorphic Computing

Neuromorphic computing is a form of computing in which the components of a computer are designed to model the human nervous system. The name refers to the arrangement of computer hardware and software components.

Neuromorphic computing has two general aims (sometimes called neuromorphic engineering). The primary intent is to build a tool that can learn, store information, and even draw logical conclusions, just like the human brain. The second aim is to increase current information about the operation of the human brain.

Traditional Neural Networks and machine learning computations are well-matched to existing algorithms. They usually concentrate on speedy computing or reduced power usage, most of the time completing one at the cost of the other.

Neuromorphic systems permit speedy computation and less power usage. They are also massively parallel, which means you can perform multiple tasks at once. They are event-driven, which means they react to happenings based on changing ecological circumstances and require only the power of the computer components used. They also have high compliance and elasticity, which means they are very flexible; can generalize; and are fault-tolerant, which means they can often continue to operate and deliver results even after a component failure.

Additionally, neuromorphic systems present a current chip design that connects memory and processing to individual neurons, rather than allocating a different area to each.

Swarm Intelligence

Swarm intelligence (SI) concerns the aggregate learning encoded within decentralized and self-organizing systems.

SI systems generally comprise simple agents that interrelate locally with each other and with their environment. SI is stimulated by biological systems. Agents follow very simple rules. There is no centralized management formation that would ascertain the behavior of an individual agent. Still, local and sometimes arbitrary agent interactions lead to the arrival of certain intelligence undisclosed to each agent. Some natural examples of SI are ant colonies, bird populations, grazing animals, bacterial growth, and fish school. For a strikingly beautiful example of SI, please look into Starling Murmuration[14] – an annual swarming of starling birds in the autumn.

In addition to implementation for traditional optimization problems, SI is used in many areas, e.g., in library material collection, communication, medical document classification, dynamic control, and systems design.

SI can be useful to a wide-ranging field in basic research, medicine, engineering, commerce, and the social sciences.

The main purpose of this exceptional intelligence is to supply the combined intelligence of the swarm with a high-quality philosophy that addresses the main challenges and that answers many queries associated with medicine and healthcare. The application of swarm intelligence reflects emerging trends in advanced algorithms.

Transfer Learning

Simplistically, Transfer Learning (TL) uses the knowledge gained for one task to solve another. In AI, TL refers to taking a trained model that is already in use and repurposing it for a different task. For example, if you are using a simple classifier to predict whether an image includes a backpack, you can use the knowledge gained during the training to identify other objects, such as sunglasses. The task is similar: Identify objects of type X in images of format Y. The task now becomes: Identify objects of type Xn in images of format Y. With TL, we essentially try to examine what we have learned in one task to improve the generalization of the other – moving the weights that a network has learned in "Task A" to a new "Task B."

Transfer learning is used primarily for computer vision and natural language processing tasks such as sentiment analysis due to the high computational load.

Transfer learning has aided in grouping retinal images for macular degeneration and diabetic retinopathy.[15]

F. Blockchain and Cybersecurity

As in AI, there has been incredible hype regarding blockchain over the last few years.

The goal of blockchain is to offer a model that adds confidence to unreliable environments and to reduce business interruptions by offering transparent access to information available in the chain.

How does blockchain work?

The concept of the blockchain (BC) is very simple. It's a distributed ledger of transactions. All participants in the blockchain have a copy of the entire ledger and are informed about every transaction. If one participant is compromised, the other participants note this and exclude that participant until the consistency is restored. A lot of message sequences and transaction protocols support this operation, but the essence is simple: Everyone knows everything. To compromise a BC, an attacker must compromise EVERY device consistently.

Put another way; blockchain is a distributed file system in which participants keep copies of the file and agree to the changes in consensus. The file is composed of blocks, each of which includes a cryptographic signature of the previous block, creating an immutable record.

How is blockchain redefining security?

When we think of blockchain, we see mainly a broader view of information security rather than the traditional endpoint protection tools. This broader view includes the security of the user's identity, transactions, and communication infrastructure through transparent processes. Progressive deployment of blockchain technology helps to improve cybersecurity in healthcare and will help ease the sharing of data among stakeholders.

This vision is increasingly necessary in today's connected world. In a world where companies reinforce their defenses against security breaches, fraud, and hackers, blockchain can be an alternative to digital transactions.

How can artificial intelligence complement blockchain?

It is believed that this combination, when applied in a specific way, could enhance our medical data management systems.

More security: Blockchain aids in safe-keeping data without any manipulation or interference with data security.

More efficiency: Blockchain can assist artificial intelligence by building a database that can be easily expanded or upgraded. With artificial intelligence, it will be possible to have a decentralized and even more efficient system.

Better energy consumption: Some activities in the blockchain require a lot of energy to be completed. AI has already proved to be a great tool to optimize this consumption.

How can blockchain complement artificial intelligence?

Just as AI can complement blockchain, the reverse is also possible and generates very good results for everyone. Here's how it happens:

Improves the explanation: One of the things that bother AI is the difficulty of forming good explanations for the user. Blockchain can establish a clear information chain with a precise route so that it does not get lost.

Increases trust between machines: Another problem found in artificial intelligence is that robots often find it difficult to establish a bond of trust. Therefore, having a chain of blocks helps to track data reliably, in addition to improving communication between machines.

Blockchain offers distribution in interchanging value and energizes parties to participate in such an exchange in a trustless manner, while artificial intelligence requires the extraction of valuable data.

Decentralized planning makes it possible for power and decision to not be focused in the hands of a single individual, an entity, or an object.

More effective: Blockchain can provide more security for learning data, as well as improve actions and standards models, in addition to offering more advantages in terms of results; this will immensely enhance healthcare data storage.

Because AI and blockchain are naturally complementary, they will forever change the healthcare system when applied.

. . . . And at the bleeding edge of technology

G. Brain-Computer Interface (BCI)

For years, science fiction writers have described a future in which the distinction between the fleshy brain and the computer is blurred by a melding of the two.[16] Lately, science fiction has been moving slowly toward science fact.[17] Many researchers have demonstrated how the human brain can be connected directly to a machine to control it with the power of thought. Applications vary; much of the work focuses on the prosthesis demand for amputees.[18]

Research on the Brain-Machine Interface (BMI) aims to establish direct communication between nervous tissue and robotic, electronic, or computational fabrication through the use of neurophysiological signals and cerebral micro-stimulation. Early BCI evolved from the possibilities exposed by R&D efforts on electroencephalogram (EEG), virtual reality, electrocorticography (ECoG), and, latterly, neuro-engineering technologies related to Augmented Reality.

Over the past decade, BMI has quickly become one of the fastest-growing areas of scientific research worldwide. Although BCI research is still in its infancy, emphatic demonstrations of its therapeutic potential for a variety of neurological diseases, such as paralysis, epilepsy, Parkinson's disease, stroke, and depression, have already been carried out. These statements indicate that further research on BMI may soon lead to the arrival of an innovative generation of neuroprosthetic devices capable of restoring a variety of neurological functions in patients severely limited by their disability. The long-term applications of BCI are numerous and go well beyond medicine, as direct brain control of computers, and electronic devices may become possible in the future. For this reason, several developed nations have recently created national BMI programs.

Neuralink is one of the multiple companies developing BCI devices.[19] It aims to build a very powerful device with the ability to handle lots of data that can be inserted in a relatively simple surgery. Neuralink's approach has been to create both a new type of electrode – a neural "lace" or "thread" – and a surgical robot to "sew" the BCI into the brain. Its short-term goal is to build a device that can help people with specific health conditions.

H. Quantum Computing

Thanks to the superposition and entanglement properties of quantum particles, a quantum computer can process a vast number of calculations simultaneously. Whereas a classical computer works with ones and zeros, a quantum computer will have the advantage of using ones, zeros, and "superpositions" of ones and zeros. Quantum computers are expected to be millions of times faster and process a vastly larger amount of data than classical computers. This will revolutionize healthcare practice and research. A particularly important application of quantum computers might be to simulate and analyze molecules for drug development and materials design. A quantum computer is uniquely suited for such tasks because it would operate on the same laws of quantum physics as the molecules it is simulating.

I. Internet of Things (IoT) and Embedded Artificial Intelligence/Internet of Everything

The IoT is described as a network of devices that exchange data using either wired or wireless connectivity.

Medical devices with integrated IoT are already being introduced, but they are expected to proliferate hugely over the next few years. Applications will not be just within hospital and clinical settings, but with patients' homes and as wearables attached to the patient 24 hours a day. These developments will help clinicians identify clinical issues and improve outcomes through early intervention. Assisted living solutions will enable patients to stay in their own homes longer, delaying the transition to care homes and improving the quality of later life.[20] IoT will be useful in monitoring patients remotely and also in remotely observing the treatment progress. AI-augmented IoT is more efficient. It allows medical devices to gather and send essential data to clinicians in real-time.

J. Edge Computing

The importance of edge computing is in its capability to process, analyze, and compute data with the same level of quality as that analyzed in the cloud. It is similar to possessing a peripheral nervous system with localized signal transformation rather than having all the signals proceeding to the central nervous system for scrutiny and processing.

This can improve the patient encounter, enhance efficiency, decrease cost, and bring us a bit closer to autonomous care rather than automated.

Fog and edge computing have advantages compared to cloud computing.

These advantages include lesser dependence on limited bandwidth, greater privacy, and security, greater data transmission speed, greater control over data generated in foreign countries, where laws may hinder or permit the use of governmental access, and lower costs. The reason is that as plenty of sensor-derived data is used locally, less data will be required for it to be transmitted remotely.

Significant benefits can be accrued. First is the ability to stimulate the advancement of medical technology in the world. As we all know, the greater the amount of data, the more opportunity we get. Some edge computing makes it easier for colleagues to share data securely. This will significantly enhance the development of technology by permitting researchers to mine data that was unavailable in the past.

Second, it will lessen the workload of medical practitioners by eliminating less useful tasks such as managing and collecting patient data. The last benefit is that it can make healthcare more accessible and affordable, most importantly in rural areas where medical care is lacking. For instance, a truck outfitted with edge computing devices can visit isolated places and provide them with advanced healthcare by linking residents to telemedicine services.

References/Further Reading

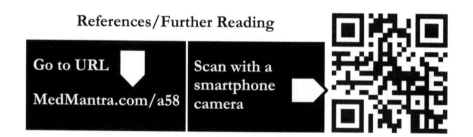

Go to URL
MedMantra.com/a58

Scan with a smartphone camera

"The development of full artificial intelligence could spell the end of the human race ... it would take off on its own, and re-design itself at an ever-increasing rate. Humans, who are limited by slow biological evolution, couldn't compete, and would be superseded."

- Stephen Hawking

SECTION 10

ROLE OF MAJOR CORPORATIONS IN AI IN HEALTHCARE

CHAPTER FIFTY-NINE

IBM WATSON – MAKING INROADS IN THE WORLD OF ARTIFICIAL INTELLIGENCE IN HEALTHCARE

Healthcare is a major area that is targeted by tech firms, as artificial intelligence can play a crucial role in the development of healthcare. Healthcare is understood to be a challenging field, as there are various facets attached to it. The room for personalization is perhaps the biggest challenge in this field. Tech experts believe that healthcare will be revolutionized in the future with the help of AI, as significant inroads have already been made in the field. One of the major obstacles that AI can face in healthcare is the fact that it must understand the challenges that healthcare faces.

When we talk about AI being used to improve the healthcare system, we can't ignore the contribution of IBM Watson. IBM Watson Health's basic purpose is to provide a holistic approach toward solving problems and challenges that are currently faced by healthcare professionals. IBM Watson calls them health heroes and aims to bring about a change in how patients are treated and managed. The 38th J.P. Morgan annual healthcare conference made a lot of headlines, as IBM Watson Health's manager highlighted some of the major areas in which IBM Watson has progressed significantly. This chapter will look at IBM Watson Health's contribution to healthcare and how it plans to completely change the face of the healthcare industry in the future.

Current Achievements and Research

We first need to grasp the reality that many medical professionals are currently using IBM Watson Health. Statistics indicate that nearly 147,000 patients have their healthcare plans managed by IBM Watson.

It is interesting to note that the number of people adopting this technology is increasing by the day. Here are some of the current achievements of IBM Watson Health.[1,2]

- **Faster Access to Knowledge:**

   IBM Watson Health's approach toward diagnosing a disease is quite efficient as it helps a medical doctor identify or diagnose the disease. And we're not talking about a common disease; doctors often get people who have diseases that are not easily identifiable. Diagnosing them can be a tough task requiring a lot of research to reach a conclusion. IBM Watson Health essentially gives your doctor the edge, as he/she will have faster access to knowledge and be able to diagnose a patient in a suitable time frame. Basically, as a doctor, you must vet all the information that gets published in medical forums to look for the right diagnosis. However, with Watson, you won't have to go through the arduous process of reading long research papers, as it conducts all the research.

- **Recommendations for Better Treatments:**

   A doctor's role is to recommend a treatment that would be the best option for the patient. For this, the doctor must spend a significant amount of time and prepare many notes in order to properly look into the patient's health and condition and to provide suitable treatment. **Memorial Sloan Cancer Treatment Center in New York** is currently training IBM Watson to efficiently manage a doctor's time and provide recommendations for a patient's treatment.

   IBM Micromedex Clinical Decision Support Solution (CDSS) can provide efficient delivery of evidence-based specialized care. These CDSS tools can support physicians in making clinical decisions by rapidly mining the major libraries of medical knowledge from around the globe.[1] TidalHealth Peninsula Regional Medical Centre (PRMC), serving nearly 500,000 patients annually, is a great example of using IBM Micromedex Clinical Decision Support Solution. It has decreased clinicians' time spent on clinical searches from 3-4 minutes per clinical search to an average of less than 1 minute per search.

- **IBM Watson Can Help You in Your Home:**

It has never been about the treatment you receive inside a hospital. It's about how a patient acts or follows a doctor's advice after he/she is discharged from the hospital. IBM Watson can help a doctor monitor a patient's progress when the patient has been discharged from the hospital. IBM Watson uses certain wearables that are essentially indicators of whether the patient is on the path of recovery or if potential hurdles are in his way. "HeartBit" is the world's first wearable device aimed for real-time heart monitoring through a wearable ECG device. It immediately alerts customers about warning signs by detecting early signs of atrial fibrillation, arrhythmias, and other potential anomalies.[3,4] HeartBit produces about 10,000 data points per second that are transmitted to the IBM Cloud, processed with IBM Watson's IoT platform, and shared or accessed by customers or their relevant healthcare providers. Through this process, a doctor will get notified if the treatment isn't achieving the desired results. Then the doctor can act accordingly.

- **Use of Health Bots:**

Personal assistants in a healthcare setting are a great achievement for IBM Watson. You can be greeted by a health bot that can answer all sorts of questions for you. A hospital environment is overwhelming for a child, and health bots can make the child feel calm, as they're friendly and can answer whatever question you have in mind.

IBM recently launched "Watson Assistant for Citizens," a new chatbot solution for the healthcare industry, government agencies, and academic organizations to access up-to-date information and guidance recommended by the CDC.[2] Online, by phone, or by text, Watson Assistant for Citizens can answer commonly posed queries such as "What are COVID-19 symptoms?", How should I clean my home properly?" and "How can I protect myself?"

La Trobe University Australia recently deployed Watson Assistant for Citizens to answer commonly asked questions about COVID-19 symptoms, federal and state restrictions, and current university status for all students, faculty, and staff members.[5] At the government level, Andhra Pradesh state in India has deployed the chatbot powered by IBM Watson on the state's health mission portal to answer common queries regarding COVID-19, including central and state government efforts for treatment, prevention, and welfare of the citizens. It is available in the Hindi, Telugu, and English languages.[6]

Currently, IBM Watson Health has a few products that are being offered to healthcare professionals, as IBM Watson certainly believes that these products can make a difference in how patients are treated in a hospital. A patient's overall experience matters for IBM Watson, and the following tools can help a healthcare professional create an optimal environment for patients.

- **IBM Watson Care Manager:**

IBM Watson Care Manager is a tool that can be used to create a personalized plan for optimal treatment. The Care Manager essentially helps one identify the personalized needs of an individual. Then a concise recommendation plan is created that is best suited for the individual. The Care Manager uses multiple care providers and systems to provide a personalized plan—including identifying appropriate treatments and care—for the patient. Watson Care Manager essentially integrates all the facets of a patient's disease while taking into account care management workflows and third-party system integration. Watson Care Manager is helping greatly amid COVID-19. It supports contact tracing with the help of structured interviews to view hotspots, recovery timelines, demographics, and more.[7] Watson Care Manager also provides integrated care management by reviewing an individual's COVID-19 lab results, understanding symptoms, and severity, and supporting clinicians in making clinical decisions about appropriate actions and interventions according to an individual's needs.

Following are the overall features offered in Watson Care Manager:

Health summary

1. Structured programs

2. Third-party system integration

3. Watson Health Cloud

4. Intuitive user interface

5. Summarization of notes

6. Care mentor

7. Interoperability with IBM Watson Health solutions

8. Oversight and management tools

IBM Explorys Platform

The IBM Explorys Platform is a tool that can be used to integrate large amounts of data in a healthcare system. Data sources such as clinical, accounting, billing, communities, and patient-derived are an essential part of an optimal healthcare system. Explorys enables a healthcare system to analyze vital key points such as managing quality of services, risk, cost, and outcomes. Preparing treatment models and obtaining exclusive insights is also a part of Explorys, as it can highlight efficient treatment patterns and how a patient can get a personalized treatment irrespective of the complexity of his condition. As mentioned previously, three major areas that Explorys helps you to analyze are risk, costs, and outcomes, which can help a healthcare system achieve optimal performance. Mercy Healthcare is a premier healthcare service provider in Ohio that uses Explorys to prioritize high-risk and high-cost patients.

During the recent COVID-19 pandemic, the IBM Explorys platform has defined a specific COVID-19 cohort, which includes individuals diagnosed with respiratory problems and other potential COVID-19 symptoms in the past year along with current confirmed COVID-19 diagnosed cases.[8] The database contains real-world, longitudinal EHR data, which is updated every week. These Explorys databases provide a timely analysis to monitor changes or alterations in COVID-19 trends.[9]

Following are some of the related products that Explorys offers:

- **IBM Explorys EPM Inform:** Every time a healthcare professional undertakes an initiative, the EPM monitors the progress and updates regularly if the initiative is on track.

- **IBM Explorys SuperMart:** SuperMart is an ultra-fast search tool that you can use to search billions of patient records and facts. It also supports Business Intelligence tools, which allows a healthcare organization to formulate a cost-efficient strategy. It's a great tool for getting in-depth information.

- **IBM Explorys EPM Registry:** Registry helps to formulate an integrated framework of a healthcare system, as it quickly identifies the target population and views data that can empower decision-making and risk-stratified care management.

- **IBM Explorys EPM Measure:** Measure is an integrated framework for correlating billions of clinical, operational, and financial events into benchmarks and scorecards for comparison. Typically, it can be seen as a tool that compares metrics for providers, groups, and locations.

IBM Watson Care Manager is a tool that can be used to create a personalized plan for optimal treatment. The Care Manager essentially helps one to identify the personalized needs of an individual. Then a concise recommendation plan is given that is best suited for the individual. The ability to carve out personalized routines for patients makes the prospect of IBM Watson a positive one, as it will change the way patients are treated in hospitals.

IBM Explorys Network

Countless strides are being carried out in the world of AI and Healthcare. Explorys gives medical practitioners a chance to help devise new ways of improving healthcare systems. The Explorys Network offers medical experts a place where they can network with each other and strive toward the improvement of healthcare systems. The network actively promotes collaboration between diverse medical fields like biotechnology, pharmaceuticals, and medical device innovators so that extensive research can be accessed and used by people who matter.

The network is essentially a secured one and consists of nearly 100 million patient records that can be accessed for research and plan formulation purposes. Obviously, a healthcare organization might face certain challenges, and this platform provides them with a chance to learn from organizations that have been successful in similar situations. The basic purpose of the Explorys Network is to expand visibility beyond a certain boundary and become limitless. One can do this by gaining access to records of another organization for research purposes, as valuable insights can be deduced from the fact that the other organization is well-versed in its respective field. Collect, link, and combine data to reach an optimal answer that can be implemented.

IBM Explorys EPM: Explore

Explore is a tool offered by IBM Watson that helps a user gain access to billions of data files primarily for treatments, diagnosis, and outcomes. Further, Explore enables a healthcare organization to delve deep into identifying gaps in healthcare management, disease hotspots, and inefficient treatment plans. The tool is used to analyze various facets that can be attached to how a healthcare organization is performing and actively suggests ways to improve.

Future Plans in Healthcare

We have seen that IBM Watson is currently making significant inroads in the world of healthcare by using artificial intelligence, but the company's future plans have the potential to revolutionize the healthcare system. Here are some of those plans for improving healthcare systems:

i. *The Drug Discovery Process:*

Statistics indicate that the pharmaceutical industry, on average, takes ten years to identify a new drug that can treat disease more efficiently. IBM Watson plans to accelerate the process of identifying potential new drugs. Interestingly, IBM Watson has already identified five new proteins that are linked with ALS that haven't been previously linked to ALS. The fact that AI can uncover invisible data gives it the ability to search for new drugs at a much faster rate.

ii. *Care Management:*

Although IBM Watson is already being used in care management in health organizations, the usability will further increase as it provides a great form of assistance to medical staff. It incorporates techniques that assess high-risk patients and can prioritize them. It further improves the care management process by incorporating access to patient records and other organizations.

iii. *Cancer Treatments:*

A medical professional will know that a large amount of time is perhaps wasted on identifying how a cancer patient is to be treated. IBM Watson will be able to identify the treatment plan for doctors in treating cancer. This technology is already in use in nearly 155 hospitals, and IBM plans to expand this to more hospitals in the near future.

iv. *Clinical Trials:*

IBM Watson's AI can be used to identify the right patient for a certain clinical trial. IBM Watson uses CTM (Clinical Trial Matching) to identify patients who are suitable for a clinical trial. The need for manually identifying patients for a trial will be eliminated and, hence, no time will be wasted. Due to the ability of IBM Watson to store billions of patient data, the matchmaking process becomes extremely fast, with chances of a mismatch eliminated.

IBM Watson Health is a leader in, and a testimony to, the significant changes that artificial intelligence is making in the healthcare system. The main aim, however, remains to be accomplished. This primarily involves making the lives of patients and doctors easier and more manageable. Humans obviously have a limit in what they can perform in the medical field, which includes patient management as well as research, but IBM Watson aims to be limitless and to bring in a change to the healthcare system in terms of improving its overall performance.

References/Further Reading

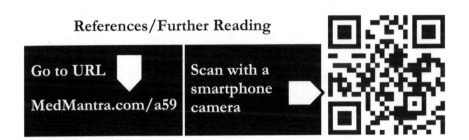

Go to URL

MedMantra.com/a59

Scan with a smartphone camera

CHAPTER SIXTY

ROLE OF GOOGLE & DEEPMIND IN ARTIFICIAL INTELLIGENCE IN HEALTHCARE

Artificial intelligence has the potential to change everything we know about healthcare. Perhaps that is why the number of companies using artificial intelligence and deep learning algorithms is steadily increasing. That is also the reason why tech giants like Google are beginning to explore avenues to dive deeper into the medical industry and see what advancements can be made. Since 2014, Google has been branching into various subsidiaries focused on artificial intelligence and healthcare, making an impact on the present and the future.

Google's Present AI Projects

Google's parent company, Alphabet, currently has three main AI projects related to healthcare:

- *DeepMind* – emphasizes AI research in several medical fields;

- *Verily Life Sciences* – analytical tools, research, and partnerships with current healthcare groups under the umbrella of "life sciences";

- *Calico* – focuses on biotechnology and age-related diseases. Not much is presently known about Calico and its projects.

Interestingly, Verily has grouped with the Nikon subsidiary Optos to begin working on detection methods for diabetic retinopathy using AI. Furthermore, Google and pharmaceutical giant Johnson & Johnson recently partnered to create Verb Surgical. The objective of the company is to build a platform for surgeons and physicians that connects robotics, analytics, medical imaging, and more. Although AI is infused into Verily and Calico, DeepMind is the one that holds the most relevance in present artificial intelligence research and development.

About DeepMind

DeepMind was founded in 2010 as a British AI company and was later acquired by Google in 2014. Aside from creating a neural network that allows machines to play video games the same way people do, DeepMind created the "Neural Turing machine," a neural network that can access external memory, thus granting a computer short-term memory like a human brain.

You may have heard about DeepMind's famous success—the AlphaGo program. In 2016, the company became a sensation when AlphaGo defeated a professional Go player twice, becoming part of a documentary film. Another program, AlphaZero, has also beat players in Go, Chess, and Shogi (Japanese game) with only a couple of hours of reinforcement learning. After AlphaGo, AlphaGo Zero, and AlphaZero, in 2019, DeepMind introduced its newest AI agent, called MuZero. MuZero is a significant step forward, and masters Go, Chess, Shogi, and Atari without even being told the rules. The power of DeepMind's artificial intelligence is worthy of respect, which is certainly a reason why Google has been able to weave its presence into the healthcare industry throughout the world.

DeepMind recently launched AlphaFold, which is an AI program developed to predict protein structures.[10] It was designed by using the deep learning system. AlphaFold is currently helping to understand proteins in the SARS-COV-2 viral genome in order to provide useful insights about virus structure and further mutation capacities.

In the UK, DeepMind also developed a diagnostic app called Streams that partnered with the National Health Service (NHS). Oddly, Streams doesn't use AI. Instead, it uses an algorithm designed solely for the detection of acute kidney injury (AKI). Though the NHS ran into issues when giving Google customer data, the app, which was made to aid doctors and nurses in detecting signs of kidney failure in susceptible patients, was welcomed by healthcare professionals at Royal Free Hospital in London. Soon after, DeepMind decided to turn its attention away from Streams for partnerships like the one with Moorfields Eye Hospital. The goal is to train an algorithm to detect signs of major eye-related diseases like glaucoma, diabetic retinopathy, and macular degeneration.

Thousands of scans have been given to the DeepMind AI, and it is now capable of picking out signs of eye disease more efficiently and swiftly than human optometrists and ophthalmologists. The algorithm is also receiving training to use anonymous 3D retinal scans received from Moorfields Eye Hospital to label images for doctors instead of doctors having to labor on their own

Similar partnerships include the University College London Hospital Foundation Trust (UCLH) to allow machine learning algorithms to study MRI and CT scans of patients with head and neck cancer. Moreover, DeepMind and the Cancer Research UK Imperial Centre embarked on a journey to improve breast cancer detection, diagnosis, and treatment in November 2017.

That is just in the UK alone.

Recent Medical Developments with Google in America

While handling the data controversy in the United Kingdom, Google DeepMind has also been working to bring AI advancements to America. Presently, DeepMind and G Suite are trying to solve the ongoing issue of record complications and data breaches. The idea is to create an accessible yet secure method for patient records that adheres to HIPAA regulations. Using cryptography and blockchain technology, DeepMind can encrypt data while lessening the burden of updating and transferring medical data through a network of healthcare professionals.

The incorporation of blockchain into artificial intelligence will hopefully create a more trustworthy network, seeing as how the main issue of data breaches and ethics has already been touched upon with Streams. However, Google, being the internet powerhouse that it is, should have no issue developing an algorithm that does for the healthcare field what others have done for information on the internet and search engine optimization (SEO).

For example, G Suite will handle patient records, meaning that the storage method will be HIPAA-compliant. Because G Suite is "software-as-a-service (SaaS)," physicians with access to G Suite will have the ability to digitally store many medical files, like x-rays, videos, scans, and records.

Google also has its eye on medical video. The Google Cloud Video API Machine Learning system is being geared to sift through media autonomously. Through application to the healthcare field, the AI will be able to rapidly sort through massive amounts of data, thereby finding and potentially preventing sickness, disease, and untimely death. An example of what could one day be possible would be recognizing signs of cancer through ultrasound scan video.

Google Health and the Mayo Clinic recently announced a partnership to develop an AI algorithm to accelerate the process of planning radiotherapy for cancer care. This collaboration will work to build an algorithm for clinicians in differentiating healthy tissues from tumors and planning precise radiotherapy treatment for metastatic tissues.

Conclusion

Google and its subsidiaries in the healthcare realm—mainly DeepMind—are among the many faces of revolution. Though the developments being made by the data and information technology enterprise rely on sensitive topics like consumer data, there is no doubt that machine learning algorithms like those from Google can change healthcare for the better. Already, advantageous steps have been taken. What Google brings humankind in the future will surely have a positive effect on healthcare and the world.

References/Further Reading

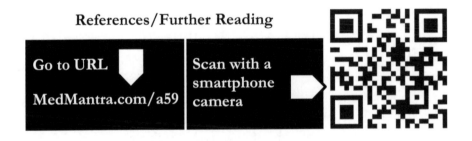

Go to URL

MedMantra.com/a59

Scan with a smartphone camera

CHAPTER SIXTY-ONE

BAIDU: THE FUTURE OF ARTIFICIAL INTELLIGENCE IN HEALTHCARE?

The future is always near and always full of possibilities. Yet, as many invest in technologies like Amazon Alexa and self-driving cars, some brands are using AI for more unique applications. Baidu, the Chinese Google, was once a dark horse in the technology race but has recently come to the forefront of AI research, alongside enterprises like Alibaba and Tencent. With the bounds in AI research that have already been accomplished, it is safe to say that Baidu could be the future of artificial intelligence.

Software Launches

In 2017, the CEO of Baidu, Robin Yanhong Li, decided to invest in restructuring and rebranding the company, thus placing resources into AI, big data, mobile, and cloud research. Since then, Baidu has developed the following software and devices by pairing up with AI-first companies:

- *Baidu Brain* – In December 2017, Baidu and Huawei partnered to blend Huawei's AI projects with a suite of AI services called "Baidu Brain." This gives smartphone developers access to tools that promote AI-powered smartphones, such as an AI-powered voice assistant. At the same time, Baidu paired up with Xiaomi, another smartphone company, to collaborate on voice recognition and computer deep learning. As of September 2020, Baidu Brain had been updated to version 6.0. Baidu Brain 6.0 was developed with about 270 core abilities and more than 310,000 models for developers, making it a major driver of intelligent transformation for a broad range of industries.

- *DuerOS* – Also known as a conversation AI system, this is a Baidu-powered voice-activated assistant designed to provide recommendations. Baidu built its own AI mobile app that can be used by millions of Chinese, just like Siri or Google Now. DuerOS saw a redesign once Baidu teamed up with 130 partners to make an update happen. Thus, DuerOS 2.0 was born. Qualcomm also stepped forward to help integrate DuerOS into smartphones and IoT devices on the Snapdragon Mobile Platform. Baidu recently announced an upgrade of DuerOS to version 6.0. DuerOS 6.0 is the largest system of its kind in China, has more than 40,000 developers, and receives more than 5.8 billion monthly voice queries. DuerOS V6.0 has also been deployed through the Xiadou AI voice assistant.

- *Little Fish VS1* – Once DuerOS 2.0 was unleashed, Baidu had the chance to introduce a DuerOS-integrated smart display, known as Little Fish VS1, at CES 2018. The device can recognize and respond to different faces and comes with media playback and video call capabilities. Little Fish VS1 also has core Baidu services, such as iQiyi streaming, a cloud photo album, and Baidu Search.

- *Self-Driving Cars* – Out of all the technology giants in China, only Baidu has several patents published for space and autonomous vehicles (15 in the U.S. alone), showing that the company is clearly aiming for the stars. In 2018, Baidu's self-driving software, Apollo, took a car for a spin safely. More than 100 companies, including international enterprises like Ford and Nvidia, decided to invest in Apollo software, and it has gotten the green light for road-testing. Recently, Baidu announced major updates regarding its fully autonomous and remotely driven cars by using the Apollo platform. Baidu also noted that its autonomous vehicles have gone through about 6 million kilometers of open-road testing with zero accidents across 27 cities.[11] In addition, Baidu displayed its fully autonomous robotaxi to carry passengers without the need for a backup driver.

- *LinearDesign*

  Baidu launched the LinearDesign web server in collaboration with the University of Rochester and Oregon State University. LinearDesign algorithms can help giant vaccine companies optimize their vaccine designs based on the most stable secondary structure of the viral mRNA sequence.[12]

AI Cameras to Detect Ocular Fundus Diseases

Baidu and Sun yat-sen University co-developed AI-powered cameras that are deployed in the hospitals of Guangdong province. These cameras can detect three types of ocular fundus diseases, i.e., glaucoma, diabetic retinopathy, and macular degeneration. These AI-powered cameras scan the eyes and develop a report in 10 seconds without the need for an ophthalmologist to be present.

Ongoing Research

At Baidu Research, which has three facilities in Beijing, Silicon Valley, and Seattle, incredible minds have come together to research how AI can be merged with natural language and speech, business intelligence, computer vision, and computational biology and bioinformatics. Although Baidu has pulled back from expanding the AI system known as "Medical Brain," which made waves in the healthcare industry, researchers continue to seek new ways to bring AI into healthcare, finance, and education.

Recent research notes hint at a developing software that provides insight into how people learn a language as well as gives machines the ability to learn. The AI starts blank, but soon, by making use of visual and auditory stimuli, it starts to form an understanding of the language. Once the initial stage is over, the AI unit can start recognizing never-before-seen objects. The teaching environment uses Baidu's open-source XWorld and PaddlePaddle, a deep learning platform.

Baidu is in negotiations with giant investors to raise up to $2 billion in the next three years to support a biotech startup. The Baidu-supported biotech startup will use Baidu's powerful AI technology to perform complex computing for drug discovery and the wide diagnosis of diseases.

With such advancements in technology, there is no clear winner in the race just yet. However, Baidu is proving that with a little reshuffling of one's priorities and partnering up with various international teams, AI can be integrated into everything from classrooms to medical exams, cars to assistant robots. Where will Baidu's vision take us next?

References/Further Reading

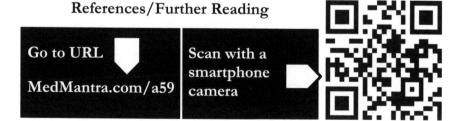

Go to URL
MedMantra.com/a59

Scan with a smartphone camera

CHAPTER SIXTY-TWO

FACEBOOK & ARTIFICIAL INTELLIGENCE IN HEALTHCARE

Facebook has been showing a lot of enthusiasm in redefining the future of healthcare. Through suicide prevention models, Facebook is now showcasing the role of AI in healthcare. It is using AI for the early prediction of suicidal thoughts in users. The main purpose of its AI development program is to learn consumer behavior. The Facebook AI team has conducted several experiments involving hundreds of people. It has advanced its AI activities and is now using AI to prevent suicide. It is making use of various advanced technologies like language processing and speech recognition. It is using user reports as well as human facilitators. When the posts go live, the AI-based software scans them. All signs of distress can be noticed and brought to the attention of the response teams. In this way, Facebook is using AI to rescue humans by combing through video or text data. Facebook has made the reporting options of the site visible to users and can now give information to the concerned authorities faster than in the past.

AI for Fighting the Suicide Epidemic

Every day, no fewer than 20 veterans commit suicide. The same Facebook technology mentioned above is being used to fight this national epidemic in the form of the Durkheim Project. Veterans allow the program to access and analyze their mobile content. If their language indicates a suicidal thought or tendency, the AI software predicts the same. Medical professionals, as well as social workers, are alerted immediately so that they can provide help to the veterans and avert the suicide attempt. The success rate of the initial tests surpassed the rates of the latest methods. Suicidal intent was detected with 65% accuracy, and the software has become a powerful tool for medical professionals to identify people who have potential suicidal tendencies. The government and veterans all over the U.S. strongly supported the project launched by Facebook, whose AI teams are working hard to ensure that all veterans in the U.S. get the benefit of this innovative software.

Saving People from Drug Addiction

Another outcome of this program was the use of AI to detect drug addiction from the data collected using smartphones. Various organizations fighting drug addiction are using AI on mobile platforms. Many new apps are now available to detect drug addiction. These apps collect data regarding screen engagement of the user, phone logs, sleep data, texting habits, and location services. Using the data, the apps help the affected people avoid falling prey to the cravings and triggers that may lead to drug relapse. The information gathered from the person regarding drug preferences, history of drug use, and trigger words is combined with the data collected by the app. AI will provide information about the potential risks and will also send a notification to the person's care team.

Saving Thousands of Lives

Facebook succeeded in showing the world how AI can help people by dealing with serious issues like suicide and drug addiction. AI functions just like vaccines and seatbelts and is saving the lives of many people.

References/Further Reading

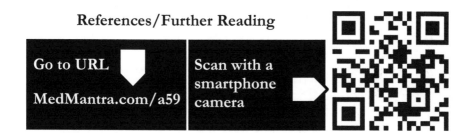

Go to URL
MedMantra.com/a59

Scan with a smartphone camera

CHAPTER SIXTY-THREE

MICROSOFT & ARTIFICIAL INTELLIGENCE IN HEALTHCARE

When it comes to well-known names in innovation, Microsoft is an enterprise that comes to mind. Microsoft has done more than develop computers and software that is widely favored throughout the globe. As one of the major players in technological advancements, Microsoft is now joining in on the emergence of a new trend—the evolution of healthcare as we know it. With artificial intelligence and cloud-based data, Microsoft is seeking to transform the health sector.

According to Microsoft, the medical research being done focuses on creating precision medicine and clinical-grade wearables, crowdsourcing health, and increasing accessibility to medical care through the digital world. Other sections of research include genomics, computational biology, and computational psychology. These are no doubt hot topics when it comes to the blending of AI and healthcare. Having Microsoft targeting the same areas as the competition is bound to accelerate the integration of AI into the public sector, as well as increase the demand for machine learning.

Microsoft stated that the "mission at Microsoft is to empower every person and organization to achieve more, and with that in mind, our ambition is that innovators will be able to use AI and the cloud to unlock biological insight and break data from silos for a truly personal understanding of human health, and in turn, to enable better access to care, lower costs, and improve outcomes".[13]

Judging by the research being done, one can say that Microsoft is staying the course.

Microsoft's AI Initiative

In 2017, Microsoft released Healthcare NexT, a program meant to introduce the world to the benefits of cloud computing and artificial intelligence. Some of the projects that have already started to disseminate into healthcare are the following.

AI Network for Healthcare

What was once known as the Microsoft Intelligent Network for Eyecare has been recently renamed to encompass all facets of healthcare. The main objective is to create an AI-based network for cardiologists. It was founded through a partnership with one of India's largest healthcare systems, Apollo Hospitals.[13]

Project EmpowerMD

True to the mission of Microsoft's AI, Project EmpowerMD was launched to create an AI system that can listen to and learn from human doctors to automate tasks in healthcare. If EmpowerMD is successful, AI will be able to handle simpler tasks while physicians can focus on the primary role of their occupation—caring for others and having more face-to-face time with their patients. The project is based on Microsoft Azure.

Microsoft Healthcare Bot Service

Microsoft Healthcare Bot Service is a solution that uses AI to help the CDC and other organizations respond to common queries, thereby freeing up clinicians, nurses, and other healthcare providers to provide the best care for individuals who need it. Microsoft Healthcare Bot Service is an Azure-based cloud service that helps organizations to develop and deploy an AI-powered bot for their patients or the general public.[14]

One of the largest health systems in the US, "Providence," is using an Azure-powered AI chatbot named "Grace" to answer its patients online. Walgreens, the largest drug store in the U.S., has recently deployed Microsoft's Healthcare Bot to support its customers with common health- and medicine-related queries during the pandemic.

Some interesting features found in the Project EmpowerMD framework include services like Custom Speech Services (CSS) and Language Understanding Intelligent Services (LUIS), which are part of the Intelligent Cloud. The use of such voice recognition and language understanding algorithms will be truly helpful in the future, especially for reaching populations that often forego medical care. Smarter chatbots that can recognize certain vocal cues or receive instructions will allow for quicker online consultations and medical treatment. Plus, CSS and LUIS can both be used for translation services, which is excellent for Doctors Without Borders, for example.[13]

Project InnerEye

Microsoft describes Project InnerEye as a way to develop machine learning for the "automatic delineation of tumors" and other 3D radiological images. The goal of the project is to enable the "extraction of targeted radiomics measurements for quantitative radiology," expedited radiotherapy planning, and "precise surgery planning and navigation".[13]

Project InnerEye uses several algorithms already in operation, such as Deep Decision Forests, seen in Kinect and Hololens technology, and Convolutional Neural Networks (CNN). However, the main point is that InnerEye is meant to aid medical practitioners, helping them adjust their practices to redefine results while increasing the quality of care they can give.

Microsoft Genomics

With the main partner for Microsoft Genomics being St. Jude Children's Research Hospital, the primary goal is to cure various diseases. Made from Microsoft Azure, Genomics research provides medical professionals with a powerful cloud-based genomic processing service. Other projects within Microsoft Genomics include Project Premonition, which involves a partnership with Adaptive Biotechnologies and has the ambitious goal of decrypting the immune system.

HIPAA/HITRUST – Microsoft Azure Security and Compliance Blueprint

With the explosion of electronic data and patient records, it is more important than ever to keep information safe, secure, and accounted for. Furthermore, this vast amount of data contains details about various medical conditions, diseases, and treatments that have gone unnoticed because people simply don't have the time to sift through it all. That is why Microsoft Azure Security and Compliance Blueprint for Health Data & AI is a HIPAA-compliant "end-to-end app" that was made to "help healthcare organizations move to the cloud, with security and compliance at the center." Microsoft Azure Security can be paired with Microsoft 365 Huddle Solution Templates or downloaded separately. Presently, groups like IRIS and KenSci are using the Microsoft Azure Security and Compliance Blueprint.[13]

Microsoft 365 Huddle Solutions

In February 2018, Microsoft released new templates based on the original Office 365 platform that are specific to certain industries. Using Microsoft Teams alongside the templates, healthcare groups can enhance meetings and communication amongst one another by using new SharePoint lists, Power BI tables to create visuals, and a Bot Framework for brainstorming and recording new ideas.

Conclusion

So, what does this mean for healthcare? What does the future, where technology and medical care are interwoven, have in store for Microsoft? Undoubtedly, the advancements that are being made by researchers at Microsoft with mapping DNA, enhancing radiology images, and providing swifter, more accurate care are already influencing healthcare systems throughout the world. With companies like Microsoft combining their efforts to create networks like the earlier version of AI Network for Healthcare, which aids in better eye health screening to combat global blindness, or current projects like InnerEye, healthcare is sure to improve.

Many are saying it, but it is true: The future of healthcare is in the hands of technology companies like Microsoft. Without the innovations that have shaped this world throughout the years, many of the diseases and ailments that are already curable would continue to plague humanity. Therefore, these projects from Microsoft are essential to humankind's future.

References/Further Reading

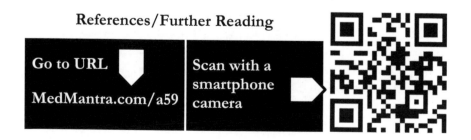

Go to URL
MedMantra.com/a59

Scan with a smartphone camera

CHAPTER SIXTY-FOUR

AMAZON & ARTIFICIAL INTELLIGENCE IN HEALTHCARE

Structured data is indispensable for training machine learning algorithms. Although electronic health records (EHR) have been here for quite a while, they still contain unstructured text that cannot be used satisfactorily. Plus, hand-written notes, admissions forms, prescriptions, and test reports get buried in hordes of hospital charts, which are impossible to process by bots. Manually sorting these medical records and analyzing them is an incredibly difficult and time-consuming job requiring either medical specialists to understand and input data or developers to write custom codes to extract every chunk of information.

Amazon Comprehend Medical (ACM) is Amazon's answer to this perplexing situation. ACM is a fully managed natural language processing service that can analyze and organize data from unstructured medical notes and prescriptions. It can comprehend medical language, anatomic terms, differential diagnoses, medical test reports, treatment options, medication strength, dosage, and frequency from a variety of non-homogenous documents, making it easy to find important stats and correlate information. The software transcribes doctor's handwritten notes, including medical slang and abbreviations, with astonishingly high accuracy. Amazon says that its algorithm is trained to handle the idiosyncrasies of doctors in history-taking and prescribing treatments.

The use of Amazon Comprehend Medical (ACM) doesn't require any machine learning expertise, and the system can be accessed through an API by an end-user without the need to write complicated rules or train models. A user simply enters the unstructured data into the Comprehend Medical interface, which then analyzes the text and extracts relevant medical data and its interlinked relationships into an easy-to-read format. This can be used to build AI-powered applications for prompt diagnosis and better insights to help doctors make more informed medical decisions. When combined with Amazon Alexa, ACM can also help patients proactively manage their health, including reminders for their medications and booking a visit to a physician right from their home.

Amazon HealthLake

Amazon Web Services (AWS) recently launched Amazon HealthLake, a HIPAA-compliant platform that allows healthcare organizations to smoothly store, analyze, and transform data in the cloud. Amazon HealthLake standardizes unstructured clinical data in a way that unlocks meaningful insights.[15] Healthcare IT giant "Cerner" is using Amazon Web Services as its cloud provider. Cerner's cloud-based platform, named "HealtheDataLab" and hosted on AWS, provides medical data to researchers at Children's Hospital of Orange County for their clinical research and data science work.

Amazon Distance Assistant

Amazon recently deployed a new AI-powered technology, "Distance Assistant," for its employees to maintain social distancing. It works through a 50-inch monitor, a local computing device, depth sensors, and an AI-enabled camera to track the real-time movements of the employees. When employees come less than six feet from one another, highlighted red circles around their feet alert them that they should move to a safe distance apart, based on deep algorithm models.[16]

Privacy has always been a big concern when it comes to cloud computing and massive data flow through machine learning systems. Amazon Comprehend Health is a HIPAA-compliant system that can detect protected health information (PHI) present in the medical data, including name, registration numbers, and family history, and anonymize it to maintain the privacy of individuals.

References/Further Reading

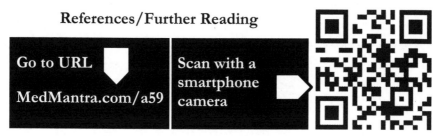

Go to URL	Scan with a smartphone camera
MedMantra.com/a59	

CHAPTER SIXTY-FIVE

APPLE & ARTIFICIAL INTELLIGENCE IN HEALTHCARE

AI in medicine will be a $28 billion industry by 2025, and Apple wants a piece of it. The company already has a handsome reputation across the globe and an immense number of users who can help gather health data. This gives Apple a head start on other startup companies and aggregate leverage when collaborating with existing players.

Apple Watch

Along with recording ECG, the flagship feature of the latest iteration of the Apple Watch is the addition of SPO_2 or a blood oxygen sensor, which was added by Apple due to the need during the COVID-19 pandemic. Blood oxygen has been in the spotlight during this pandemic, which has led to a focus on the Apple Watch.

The latest Apple Watch is very popular due to its fitness tracking element along with an app detailing active calories burned. It has a fitness app that detects and shows steps, standing time, exercise running pace, and walking pace as trends. The sleep tracking app in Apple Watch provides a summary of duration of sleep, consistency of sleep, and time in bed. Overall, it may help you improve your routine and overall health.

Apple Health App

The health app comes pre-installed in all iOS devices and is the building block of Apple's AI strategy. The app keeps step count and tracks wellness metrics, including the amount of physical activity, time spent on the phone, calorie intake, and sleep. Also, there are third-party apps to connect with external sensors and trackers to record vitals and other specific biomarkers. For example, there is continuous glucose monitoring through the Dexcom G5 Mobile CGM System.

Apple is now planning to bring EMR data from hospitals into the phone's health record. HealthKit is a software development kit enabled by FHIR that will allow third-party apps to access a health record application programming interface (API). This will enable users to sync their health data with hundreds of hospitals and clinics. For example, a prescription management app, such as **Medisafe,** can access the Health Records feature using API that will allow consumers to import their prescription lists into the portal without manually entering them and also provide relevant information about the possibility of drug interactions.

Carekit

Carekit is a software development kit (SDK) by Apple that enables developers to create apps that can monitor users in real-time using healthcare sensors and tools in iOS devices. **One Drop** is an app built on this framework that keeps track of food intake, medication reminders, and activity. **Glow nature, Glow baby,** and **Iodine** are some of the most notable health apps made using the Carekit platform, which keeps users better-informed about their pregnancies, provides information about the natural course of a baby's growth, and helps reduce depression, respectively.

References/Further Reading

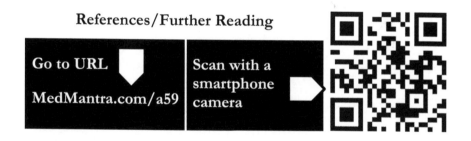

Go to URL
MedMantra.com/a59

Scan with a smartphone camera

CHAPTER SIXTY-SIX

NVIDIA & ARTIFICIAL INTELLIGENCE IN HEALTHCARE

Radiology is one of the first medical fields to feel the seismic activity of powerful AI algorithms. The machine learning algorithms can do a superhuman job in recognizing "patterns" in medical images and providing insights to newer dimensions, thanks to blistering-fast GPU technology available today. GPUs are the nucleus of machines being made to run algorithms for medical image processing, and Nvidia is the uncrowned king of this technology.

Powerful GPU Platforms

A sea of health data is available and is being collected by more powerful and affordable genome sequencing gear and smartwatches, intelligent blood pressure monitors, and glucose monitoring devices. Thus, there is a dire need for advanced computing platforms to harvest all this data for use by deep learning systems. **Nvidia DGX systems** are state-of-the-art technological marvels designed to provide the most powerful computing for AI exploration. They are the world's first purpose-built AI supercomputers made to solve the most intricate machine learning challenges.

BGI Group is a genome sequencing center in China that has more than 1PB of data to be analyzed by its machine learning algorithm, XGBoost. By running its algorithms on the Nvidia DGX-1 system, the team shot the analysis speed by 17x and extended the research to millions of targetable peptides for cancer immunotherapy. **United Imaging Intelligence**, a leading AI company, is partnering with Nvidia to deploy its medical imaging software using DGX systems, enabling it to revolutionize imaging workflows, screening radiographs, and treatment solutions.

Open-Source SDK

NVIDIA Clara enables developers to build GPU-accelerated systems and applications to train AI models with an immense number of medical images and automated healthcare workflows. This opens the door to a universal computing platform for developers to build medical imaging applications in sync with Nvidia GPU hardware and bring about a new wave of AI-powered medical instruments for assisting in the early detection and treatment of many ailments. Nvidia Clara promises to bring to the medical imaging field technological advances that have revolutionized other industries, like gaming, self-driving cars, and cloud computing.

Medical equipment augmented with AI-powered supercomputers and intelligent algorithms will be smaller, cheaper, and more efficient, making them more precise and accessible in revolutionizing the medical field.

Health Data Processing

Recently, Nvidia partnered with Scripps to develop deep learning-based algorithms specifically for the early detection and prediction of grave medical events such as atrial fibrillation, which is the predisposing factor of stroke.

To better train their AI models, Scripps is pulling Fitbit wearable data, which is meant to advance precision in the detection of abnormal heartbeats and arrhythmias. Owing to the immense number of users, this will help build a large-scale dataset from more than a million participants.

To give pace to research, Scripps will also provide metadata and key datasets. One such data set contains heart sensor recordings of more than 1000 continuous normal heart rhythms. Another data set provided by Scripps has the entire genomic sequence of people aged above 80 who have never been sick.

References/Further Reading

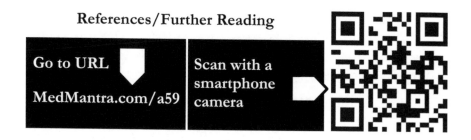

Go to URL
MedMantra.com/a59

Scan with a smartphone camera

CHAPTER SIXTY-SEVEN
ROLE OF GE IN ARTIFICIAL INTELLIGENCE IN HEALTHCARE

Helping Hospitals Run Smoothly

Hospitals are busy places. Thousands of patients come in daily, depending upon the hospital's capacity. These patients come to different departments. Thus, hospitals generate a lot of data daily. Much of that data is not medical-related and is concerned with the management and administrative point of view—for example, insurance information about the patients, biodata, etc. That data is stored daily but never analyzed due to its sheer size. GE Healthcare thought about this problem and created a system using the techniques of artificial intelligence and deep learning to integrate and analyze this data. The system is called **Edison Applications**. By integrating and analyzing these data from different departments in a hospital, the system can help hospitals run more smoothly. Through this system from GE Healthcare, hospitals can improve their patient interaction by better directing the flow of patients. Analyzing the patient demographics and correlating the data with the frequency of various diseases at different times of the year in different patient groups helps hospitals prepare in advance. In the accident and emergency department, just a few seconds can mean the difference between life and death. This system by GE Healthcare can help save valuable minutes, thus saving lives. The interesting thing about this system by GE Healthcare is that it will do all this behind the scenes. It will be an unsung hero. A hospital will use this system to improve its patient care, and its patients will not even know about it.

Analyzing the Medical Data

Now, that was about the administrative data. However, hospitals generate much more medical data than administrative data. This data comes in the form of patient histories, investigations, patient records, and treatment records. Ninety percent of this data is generated by medical imaging, for example, X-rays, MRI, and CT scans. GE Healthcare has also made a system that can analyze this medical data to help improve the healthcare that patients receive.

X-Ray Scan Revolution

X-ray scanning is the most basic and most commonly used investigation tool in hospitals. It composes around two-thirds of the total medical imaging done. However, nearly 25 percent of the scans fall under the category of "quality too bad to be used." This is a huge number considering the total number of X-ray scans being done. GE Healthcare has created this system to help find the causative factors that make an X-ray of bad quality. It will use artificial intelligence, machine learning, and deep learning systems to find out what makes an X-ray a bad one. It can be many factors: operator-dependent, patient-dependent, or machine-dependent. This system will find the causes and offer suggestions on how to minimize the number of these unusable X-rays.

Tackling COVID-19 with GE AI-Powered Technologies

"Critical Care Suite 2.0," with a new AI algorithm, is helping clinicians evaluate the correct placement of the endotracheal tube when ventilating serious COVID-19 patients. "CT in a Box" is another AI-powered solution to enable fast CT scanning with social distancing measures. It is installed in more than 100 locations throughout the world and greatly helps minimize physical contact with COVID-19 patients. The "Thoracic Care Suite" with AI algorithms can analyze the findings of chest X-rays and highlight abnormalities for radiologists' review, including signs of pneumonia, lung nodules, tuberculosis, and other radiological findings that may be indicative of COVID-19.[17]

References/Further Reading

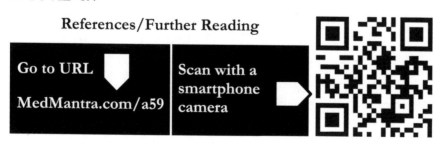

Go to URL

MedMantra.com/a59

Scan with a smartphone camera

CHAPTER SIXTY-EIGHT

ROLE OF SIEMENS IN ARTIFICIAL INTELLIGENCE IN HEALTHCARE

With the amount of development in the world, access to medical help is becoming universal. More people can afford it. Where it is a marker of a country's development and growth, it also puts more stress on healthcare resources. The medical practice these days has also become very dependent on medical imaging, e.g., X-rays, MRIs, and CT scans. This practice has been adopted to make medical practice and diagnoses more accurate. However, it also means that these medical imaging resources have been stretched very thin.

Proper Utilization of Medical Imaging Resources

Siemens Healthcare has developed a system using artificial intelligence and deep learning to address this issue.

It helps doctors throughout the medical imaging process. Not only does it make the test more accurate, but it also helps in analyzing the reports. It has a three-pronged approach for this purpose.

The Three-Pronged Approach

First, by using infrared and other simple cameras and sensors, this Siemens system helps patients to assume the correct posture and position. Correct positioning is very important for a scan. Nearly one-third of the scans must be done again because of the improper position of the patient. Siemens' system prevents this, decreasing the number of unwanted scans and helping to use the limited resources smartly.

Then, the Siemens system tells the doctor about the vulnerable organs of the patients during the scan. The doctor can adjust the strength of radiation accordingly. It also decreases the number of scan slices if an organ is in a vulnerable position.

Finally, and most importantly, this Siemens system, using the techniques of deep learning, machine learning, and artificial intelligence, helps to analyze the scans and produce an accurate diagnosis. It has a vast database. It has collected this database over many decades from many hospitals. It uses this database to help radiologists accurately analyze scans and provide accurate diagnoses.

Thus, this Siemens system helps to reduce stress on medical imaging resources. It reduces the number of bad-quality, unusable scans and also helps doctors analyze and interpret medical images.

References/Further Reading

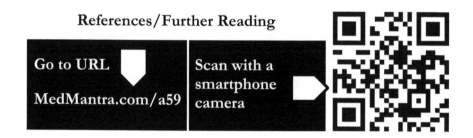

Go to URL

MedMantra.com/a59

Scan with a smartphone camera

CHAPTER SIXTY-NINE
ROLE OF PHILIPS IN ARTIFICIAL INTELLIGENCE IN HEALTHCARE

Philips has many different products that use artificial intelligence systems and deep learning to help the patients as well as the doctors. Let's briefly review the company's products.

Philips Illumeo

This Philips product was developed especially to help radiologists. By using its database and artificial intelligence systems, it helps radiologists better analyze medical images. Using Philips Illumeo for image analysis enables a radiologist to provide better output and feedback reports to physicians whose diagnosis depends upon these reports.

Philips IntelliSpace Portal 12

While Philips Illumeo helps with analyzing images, Philips IntelliSpace Portal 12 has revolutionized the imaging techniques themselves through AVaaS (Advanced Visualization as a Service). Automatic recognition and detection of pulmonary infiltrates in COVID-19 patients is extremely important. The AI-powered quantitative assessment capabilities of IntelliSpace Portal 12 allow radiologists to get useful insights for the identification of COVID-19 pneumonia that is differentiated from other diagnoses.

The latest features in the IntelliSpace Portal 12 include AI algorithms for lung nodule detection, analysis of different cardiac functions, and pulmonary infiltrates associated with COVID-19 patients.

Philips IntelliSpace Portal 12 is changing the imaging techniques in the fields of cardiology, pulmonology, oncology, orthopedics, neurology, and vascular imaging. Their systems are compatible with the machines already being used.

An advanced clinical software package for cardiology is introduced in IntelliSpace Portal 12, which includes MR Cardiac Analysis with CaaS MR

4D flow, to visualize blood flow patterns in the hearts and main arteries of cardiac patients.

Philips Wellcentive

This is an initiative by Philips Healthcare to make quality healthcare available to the masses. Currently, it caters to more than 49 million patients. Patients can get access to healthcare using their phones. It is a health portal. By using the ever-increasing database and sophisticated AI systems, it produces an accurate diagnosis based on the patient's symptoms.

Philips Wellcentive also analyses the population groups for better use of the medical resources in different areas. It also directs its users to the most appropriate healthcare services nearby.

Philips Respironics DreamMapper

Philips Respironics DreamMapper comes with a breathing mask with sensors. This product uses the systems of artificial and deep learning to help patients with sleep apnea get a peaceful night's sleep.

Philips CareSage

Philips CareSage keeps track of the patient's health even after they are discharged from the hospital. Previously, healthcare was limited to the hospital; once the patient left the hospital, no system was in place to continually provide healthcare. Philips CareSage has solved this problem.

References/Further Reading

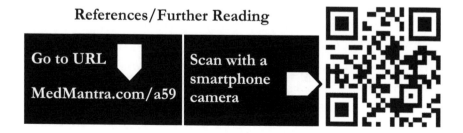

Go to URL

MedMantra.com/a59

Scan with a smartphone camera

"It seems probable that once the machine thinking method had started, it would not take long to outstrip our feeble powers… They would be able to converse with each other to sharpen their wits. At some stage, therefore, we should have to expect the machines to take control."

- Alan Turing

SECTION 11

ROLE OF START-UP COMPANIES IN AI IN HEALTHCARE

CHAPTER SEVENTY
ROLE OF START-UP COMPANIES IN AI IN HEALTHCARE

Start-ups have long been an influence in the economy by introducing new ideas that either explode with popularity or sink beneath the competition. Now, that power has affixed its gaze to healthcare and seeks to recreate the medical system with artificial intelligence. With some countries struggling to keep up with the demand for thorough and affordable care, as well as low doctor-to-patient ratios, the introduction of these start-ups and their artificial intelligence and machine learning systems may have the answer to all healthcare dilemmas.

For a comprehensive list and description of global healthcare AI start-ups, please visit the "Bonus Content" section at MedMantra.com/aih Here are some of the randomly selected start-ups reshaping healthcare with their artificial intelligence and machine learning technology:

1. AtomWise

AtomWise is a company based in the USA. They use their very powerful AI tools to discover and develop new drugs. Their programs screen for potency, selectivity, and polypharmacology and guard against off-target toxicity with unparalleled speed and efficiency.

The epidemics of the Ebola virus have killed thousands of people worldwide. There are thousands of approved medicines for it. Out of these numerous drugs, AtomWise identified a drug that was not even used as an antiviral drug previously. This drug blocked infectivity across multiple strains of the virus.

2. Medopad

Medopad is a UK-based company that aims to play its role as a bridge between the health care providers and the patients. Its wearables can send data to the health providers so that the patients can get optimum health care with minimum visits to the hospitals. Their strong AI systems also help in diagnosing diseases.

3. VoxelCloud

A Chinese company that is revolutionizing the diagnosis and treatment using AI systems. Their powerful analyzers analyze the medical scans and help in reaching a prompt and reliable diagnosis using AI. The company's current products cover lung cancer, retinal diseases, and coronary heart disease. The company has offices both in China and America.

4. Nuritas

Nuritas, an Ireland-based company, believes in the therapeutic potential of naturally occurring bioactive peptides. They do so by utilizing the knowledge of genomics with the help of artificial intelligence. Their aim is to help different pharmaceutical companies in the development of new drugs and other healthcare items.

5. OWKIN

Owkin is a French company. They have a very comprehensive artificial intelligence program that encompasses many a field. They combine and utilize medical data, the knowledge of genomics, biology, and pathology to reach an accurate diagnosis. They have been making ripples since their inception in France.

6. Insilico Medicine

A Russian company that is dedicated to keeping humans young for a longer time. They use AI systems to research and extend healthy longevity. This company is not limited to developing this youth potion only; they also research and help in the development of new effective drugs by partnering with different pharmaceutical companies.

7. Snap40

A Scotland-based company that makes wearables that take your vitals like blood pressure, temperature, heart rate, respiratory rate, blood saturation, etc. These wearables can not only store them in their data but also send them to your healthcare provider so that they can keep an eye on your health 24/7 with a minimum number of visits.

8. Aidoc

Aidoc is a helping tool for radiologists. Aidoc uses a deep learning algorithm to read medical images. It is very helpful in picking up anomalies from the scans. By helping to read the scans and stratifying the vast data, it helps the radiologists to function more efficiently. Aidoc is an Israeli company.

9. Engine biosciences

A Singapore-based company that is helping pharmaceutical companies to develop new drugs by integrating the knowledge of genomics with medical data using AI. They have introduced a way faster method of drug development, combining high-throughput, massively parallel biological experimentation with artificial intelligence to redesign the way drugs are approached.

10. Fronteo Health

Fronteo health is a Japanese company that utilizes AI to facilitate health care in a system. It helps by applying state-of-the-art word and document embedding techniques and rigorous statistical implementations. They deliver objective, transparent, and reproducible analysis to accommodate healthcare professionals' demands. Some of the fields Fronteo health is playing its part in include diagnostics, pharmaceuticals, personalized health care, and data management.

11. Sword Health

This Portugal-based company was the first to develop an AI-based digital physical therapist allowing the patients for the first time to perform their therapy at home, maximizing engagement and clinical outcomes while ensuring full data accountability. They also make wearables that collect and send the data related to the health of an individual, e.g., Vitals, to the healthcare providers.

12. Lunit

A South Korea-based company that uses deep learning AI technology and the vast pool of medical data to discover, design, and develop powerful data-driven imaging biomarkers. They are especially focused on development in the field of pathology and radiology. Lunit has MFDS approval for AI-powered nodule detection in chest X-Ray scan.

13. Life Whisperer

Life whisperer is an Australian company. It utilizes AI systems to detect the healthiest embryo out of those available. This maximizes the chances of pregnancy following IVF. It takes into account different parameters of embryo health and points out the embryo which is most likely to become a fetus in the mother's uterus.

14. Mediktor

A Spanish company that has put up a very reliable symptoms checker. It uses AI and deep learning to provide an accurate diagnosis. This chatbot has made the availability of health care very easy and accessible. It also connects doctors to patients.

15. Kaia health

A German company which allows your phone to take care of your health. Using AI systems, it is making easy health care available to everyone.

16. Top Data Science

A company from Finland aims to use AI to collect medical data, analyze it, and then point out smart patterns which help the doctors in future diagnoses and treatment of different diseases.

17. Geras Solutions

Dementia is a dreadful disease of old age. Geras Solution aims to start AI systems to help old people with dementia lead a relatively normal life of better quality. It is a virtual assistant helping old people. Geras Health is a Sweden-based company.

18. Triage

Triage is a Canadian company. They have developed this smartphone that can help diagnose skin conditions instantaneously. You just have to take a picture and upload it on the app; the AI system will do the rest.

19. Prognica labs

A UAE-based company that aims to revolutionize the field of oncology using AI. They help early detection of cancer patients with the help of a very advanced AI system that scans and analyses the medical images, giving a very reliable diagnosis. They are also playing their role in helping the pathologists by using AI, machine learning, and cloud computing to revolutionize how histological patterns are read on whole slide images.

20. Qure.ai

This Mumbai-based company was established in 2016. They are using artificial intelligence (AI) and deep learning systems to revolutionize the field of medical imaging. They have developed a large database by analyzing thousands of X-rays, CT scans, and MRIs and integrated their data by using AI and deep learning systems. They proudly present their three products:

i) qXR:

qXR uses AI and deep learning to analyze and find anomalies in X-ray films. qXR can identify and localize 15 common abnormalities in chest radiographs. In its database are a huge number of previous X-ray films and records from the X-ray departments worldwide, so it can give accurate diagnosis even with varying X-ray film quality.

ii) qER:

CT scans are the first investigation to be performed in the emergency room in the case of head trauma. qER detects emergencies like hemorrhage in the brain and skull fractures. qER helps in the triaging and evaluation of patients in the ER, especially in crowded and busy emergency rooms.

iii) qQuant:

qQuant boasts of features, including fully automated detection, quantification, and 3D visualization for CT and MRI scans.

Their aim is to assist the doctors so that they are able to give more attention to the patients.

Conclusion

Artificial intelligence is not only a key to unleashing the potential of healthcare technology; it is the doorway through which we see the future. These startups are just a select few that are revamping the entire medical field with their artificial intelligence and machine learning technology. From streamlining the process of creating and archiving medical records to enhancing medical imaging and detecting diseases, these algorithms and AI systems are backing up the capabilities of professionals throughout the world. As the market continues to shift towards AI-based technology, healthcare is bound to improve—and more startups like these are going to appear.

"I think we should be very careful about artificial intelligence. If I had to guess at what our biggest existential threat is, I'd probably say that. So, we need to be very careful."

- Elon Musk

SECTION 12
CONCLUSION

CHAPTER SEVENTY-ONE
CONCLUSION

The emergence of artificial intelligence in society has gained critical acclaim. While some laud it as an advancement in technology, some schools of thought see it as a necessary evil. But one thing is certain, AI has come to stay, and it can only get better. Some people fear that AI may not be a welcome development because of its immense impact on the job market and humans in general. Most of the time, some people do engage in false controversies about what the introduction of AI may mean to the populace, generating open questions and unlimited controversies about this technology.

So, when are these machines expected to overthrow humans or surpass human-level intelligence? Is it even possible? The problem of ultimate certainty plagues the human race. We have often talked about getting superhuman AI in the 21st century. We often over-hype technology, and AI is in the center of it all.

In the healthcare sector, the use of AI presents many organizations with numerous exciting opportunities. Within a short period of time, healthcare can be drastically improved, that too with saving costs. But there is a need to put autonomous systems in order just in case the deployment of AI may affect the workforce. However, the existence of AI is to be a support system to healthcare givers in various institutions as opposed to the general opinion that believes human employment in the healthcare sector may be threatened by this technology.

Few examples of what AI promises to deliver include scan analysis, sample analysis, taking records of vital signs in patients, and all of which that decide their final treatments by the presiding doctor. The development of new drugs follows some sort of guesswork or deployment of instincts by the scientists who select target molecules from a combination of chemicals. Even though AI is termed the 'experimentalist's helper,' it promises to perform this task with more efficiency and effectiveness.

In understanding diseases, healthcare professionals are skilled at this, but the technology serves as a booster in making better and reliable clinical decisions to fast-track innovations. In short, natural intelligence is supposed to be augmented by AI, and this places it second to human intelligence.

Moving forward...

It has been predicted that AI will hit healthcare in the most shocking way. The predicted steps include:

- Care and management of chronic diseases

- Increasing the availability of health data of patients

- Environmental and socio-economic facets of medicine

- Precision medicine and genetic information integrated with care management

Pharmaceutical companies are also joining the bandwagon of the game of technology, and these people are expected to make the best impact. The development of drugs requires efficiency, which AI is capable of to a great extent.

Nevertheless, the worry that AI may replace healthcare providers is just a product of fear and illusion. The technology promises to be a wingman or a research assistant. After all, what better machine is there than the human brain?

In the not-so-distant future, the expenditure on machine intelligence will be very high, contributing immensely to the business of saving lives. More so, when an error can cost the life of a person, one has to be 100% certain about the procedures. Machines should be given a chance to make this difference.

"We have seen AI providing conversation and comfort to the lonely; we have also seen AI engaging in racial discrimination. Yet the biggest harm that AI is likely to do to individuals in the short term is job displacement, as the amount of work we can automate with AI is vastly larger than before. As leaders, it is incumbent on all of us to make sure we are building a world in which every individual has an opportunity to thrive."

- Andrew Ng

SECTION 13
GLOSSARY

Index

Review Request

Reviews are like gold for authors. If you liked this book, please leave me an honest review on any of the following: Amazon, Barnes & Noble, Apple Books, Google Books, Kobo, and Goodreads, or simply send me your personal feedback. I would be so happy.

Review Links

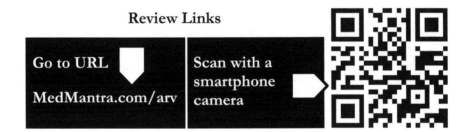

Go to URL
MedMantra.com/arv

Scan with a
smartphone
camera

About the Author – Dr. Parag Mahajan, MD

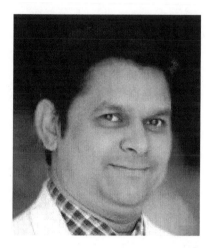

Dr. Parag Mahajan is a radiologist, clinical informatician, teacher, researcher, author, and serial entrepreneur. His current interests include the development of startups in the fields of AI in healthcare, blockchain in healthcare, electronic health records, and medical eLearning systems.

Contact Author

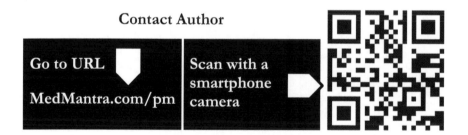

Made in the USA
Middletown, DE
11 March 2022

62466303R00327